Advances in Synaptic Plasticity

Advances in Synaptic Plasticity

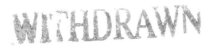

edited by Michel Baudry, Joel L. Davis, and
Richard F. Thompson

A Bradford Book
The MIT Press
Cambridge, Massachusetts
London, England

This book was set in Palatino by Asco Typesetters, Hong Kong and was printed and bound in the United States of America.

Library of Congress Cataloging-in-Publication Data

Advances in synapthic plasticity / edited by Michel Baudry, Joel L. Davis, Richard F. Thompson.
     p.   cm.
Includes bibliographical references and index.
ISBN 0-262-02460-8 (hc. : alk. paper)
  1. Neuroplasticity. I. Baudry, M. II. Davis, Joel L., 1942–   .
III. Thompson, Richard F.
QP363.3.A433   1999
573.8—dc21   98-51887
                                                     CIP

In memory of Helen T. Davis

Contents

Preface

Five years ago, the three of us (M.B., R.F.T., and J.L.D.) edited a book published by The MIT Press, *Synaptic Plasticity: Molecular, Cellular, and Functional Aspects*, which was in part the outcome of an international symposium held at the University of Southern California to celebrate the inauguration of the Hedco Neuroscience Building. This building was and still is the home of many members of the Program in Neural, Informational, and Behavioral Sciences (NIBS), a program that has focused on multidisciplinary studies of synaptic plasticity. The book presented an up-to-date overview of the then status of research in the broad field of synaptic plasticity, including developmental plasticity, responses to neuronal injury, and mechanisms of learning and memory. It was well reviewed and was quite successful among neuroscientists and researchers interested in obtaining an introduction to the field. So much so that The MIT Press asked us to follow up with an update that would represent the current status of the field and that would allow the interested reader to measure the evolution and progress in this field.

We took this opportunity to organize a Second International Symposium on Synaptic Plasticity that included some of the same participants who were present at the first one in order to provide a direct measure of their views of the evolution in the field. Newcomers were also invited to provide a review of new aspects and approaches. We were extraordinarily fortunate that Gilbert Chauvet, one of the participants in both symposia, generously offered his magnificent fifteenth-century castle near Angers in France as the location for the symposium. Whether it was the historical setting and the beauty of the scenery, or the abundance of the delicious local wines and food, the symposium was superb and all the participants certainly used their synaptic plasticity to form long-lasting and rich memories of the event. In addition, some of them agreed to contribute chapters for this update on synaptic plasticity. The book therefore represents only a section of the themes that were discussed during the symposium but we believe that it covers most of the important issues and approaches currently under investigation in many laboratories. As readers will discover, some of the same themes that were discussed five years ago were revisited and the contributions provide a direct measure of the progress made during this period of time. As in the first volume, the approaches range from molecular to cellular and network levels of analysis and the overall unifying theme deals with the relationship between synaptic plasticity and information processing and storage. An edited volume is often a patchwork of chapters that requires the reader to make a considerable effort to fit the pieces of the puzzle together. We believe that this volume provides a clearer picture of current views concerning the mechanisms and functions of synaptic plasticity.

We wish to thank all the persons and organizations who made the symposium and consequently this volume possible. Above all, we wish to thank Gilbert Chauvet and his wife Babette, who spent the last fifteen years working on renovating their castle and who provided not only the conference room but also took care of the local organization, including delicious food and wine, as well as a sophisticated social program. The Office of Naval Research (both the Washington and London offices) was instrumental in providing funding and guidance for the symposium. We wish to thank Dr. Guy Poirier, vice president of the Conseil Regional for his generous financial support, as well as Sanophi, France. The NIBS program from USC as well as MIT Press also contributed to the success of the symposium. Finally, we wish to thank all the participants in the symposium, especially those who contributed a chapter and made this book a reality.

Introduction

Ever since Watson and Crick began the process of showing us how genetic information could be acquired, stored, and transferred from generation to generation, the question of how information could be processed during one lifetime remains one of the great scientific questions of our day. Neuroscientists may differ as to the appropriate level of analysis from which to attack this difficult question, but none would deny the role of neuronal plasticity. Many neurons exhibit plasticity, that is, they can change structurally or functionally, often in a lasting way. Plasticity is evident in such diverse phenomena as drug tolerance, enzyme induction, sprouting of axon terminals after a brain lesion, and strictly synaptic events such as facilitation and depression.

This book represents an attempt to look at a portion of the multitude of mechanisms that provide adaptive properties for a wide variety of phenomena. The editors wanted it to reflect the diversity of phenomena included under the broad concept of synaptic plasticity, and to provide the reader with a glimpse of recent work that currently exemplifies the current approaches to the field.

The first two chapters take a strong gene-oriented approach to plasticity. Although the terminology may be confusing, both chapters describe the activity of a recently discovered gene (*arc*) that helps to regulate the cytoskeleton, or interior structure, of the dendrite. The suggestion is that neural activity changes dendritic structure via the *arc* mechanism. Dietmar Kuhl (chapter 1) suggests that since long-term memory differs from short-term memory in requiring RNA and protein synthesis, retention mechanisms should depend on changes in transcriptional state. A central idea for Kuhl is that plasticity is controlled by activity-dependent changes in gene expression. More specifically, Kuhl's attention is focused on identifying activity-induced genes in cortical and hippocampal neurons, in contrast to the previous non-neuronal "tools" (e.g., proto-oncogenes such as c-*fos* and *zif 268*) used to study the molecular basis of plasticity. Kuhl describes how newly transcribed RNA from gene *arg3.1* is rapidly distributed to dendrites, suggesting that *arg3.1* translation and function may be controlled by the kind of local synaptic events described in long-term potentiation (LTP) studies.

Steward and associates continue the exploration of the relationship between gene expression and synaptic modification. They focus on new findings about the intracellular transport of messenger RNA (mRNA) for an early gene (*arc*) that appears in dendrites after neural excitation due to in vivo manipulations designed to cause enhanced neural activity. Although this *arc* mRNA is only one of many mRNAs changing as a function of neural activity, the sequential coordination of these protein control mechanisms should produce an understanding of how activity-dependent modifications come about.

Chapter 3 (Rivera and Khrestchatisky) is unusual in assigning a role for plasticity to the extracellular matrix (ECM). The ECM is known to play an important role in modulating gene expression, cytoskeletal organization (see the first two chapters), and general survival. A complex family of proteinases keep the ECM in balance. Among these are matrix metalloproteinases (MMPs). The MMPs belong to a group of zinc-dependent endopeptidases. These may provide a link between trace metal metabolism and synaptic function.

LTP was discovered at the end of the 1960s, and now has a long history as a synaptic plasticity model. The review by Muller and colleagues (chapter 4) summarizes some recent results and proposes the idea that LTP could present more than a simple way to modify synaptic strength. Muller's morphological analyses suggest that LTP may produce synaptic changes associated with a wide variety of techniques known to produce plasticity. This chapter also reviews the role of protein phosphorylation in LTP and plasticity. Unfortunately, the question of whether morphological changes and the calcium-calmodulin–dependent protein kinase (CaMKII) are functionally related to LTP manipulation, or are a by-product of this phenomenon, remains unresolved.

The chapter of Muller and associates leads quite nicely to chapter 5, in which the authors present three studies in which mathematical models of a synapse incorporate both known dynamics of synaptic mechanisms and morphological parameters to analyze the impact of alterations in morphology on synaptic transmission and plasticity. This might be a good time to point out to the interested reader that chapters 9, 10, and 12 also involve the use of nonlinear mathematics as a tool for understanding neural function and plasticity. This trend will become stronger as more scientists with training in mathematics and the physical sciences apply their intellectual resources to understanding brain function. The model by Liaw and associates is strongly constrained by neuroscience and predicts some nontrivial factors about 2-amino-3-hydroxy-5-methylisoxazole-propronate acid (AMPA) and N-methyl-D-aspartate (NMDA) postsynaptic receptor distribution in the synapse during LTP.

In a sense, chapter 6 (Linden) continues the approach motivating the work in chapter 3, that is, it would be useful to look outside the neuron itself to find plasticity mechanisms. Although historically glia have been assigned a support function (e.g., transport of nutrients, buffering, neurotransmitter uptake), the development of the patch-clamp technique has demonstrated that glial cells contain voltage-gated ion channels similar to neuron membranes. Linden extends this story to include neurotransmitter and neuromodulator sensitivity. This is work very much in progress because although glial cells would seem to have the potential to signal neurons when activated, there is presently no evidence that this signaling comprises "computation."

The developmental process has long served as a "laboratory" for adult plasticity. In chapter 7, Chesselet and colleagues summarize recent evidence from their laboratory suggesting that robust axonal plasticity and reactive synaptogenesis occur in the striatum, not only during late postnatal development but also in adult rats. The authors extend the locus of axonal plasticity from the hippocampus to the dorsolateral striatum where LTP has been shown to occur. The data present an interesting challenge to the field because many of the molecules that are thought to be associated with anatomical plasticity are absent or expressed at much lower levels in the dorsolateral striatum than in other brain regions believed to be loci of plasticity. This suggests that although axonal plasticity may rely on similar molecular mechanisms in a subset of brain regions, it is likely that regional differences exist in these mechanisms.

The next chapter also extends the plasticity work beyond the traditional anatomical loci. Connors and his group (chapter 8) have studied corticothalamic (CT) slices to study the physiology of CT synapses onto cells of sensory relay nuclei in the somatosensory thalamus. The authors describe synapses in this circuitry that can depress strongly, depress weakly, or facilitate. So far most of these synaptic pathways remain untested, but it is very likely that synapse dynamics is an important variable in analyzing forebrain circuits, and it would be a mistake to assume that any single synapse can serve as a general model for the rest.

As in the previous chapter, the authors of chapter 9 also use frequency-labeled cellular firing to track plasticity in functional nervous circuitry. Laurent and his co-authors have carefully studied a model for insect olfaction in the antennal lobe of the locust and honeybee. Their work suggests that temporal features of spike trains in the highly tuned olfactory apparatus of these animals might play a significant role in information coding. Synchronization and oscillation may be representative of the dynamical systems coding perception. If stimulus representations in the brain rely on spatiotemporal codes, it is likely that the mechanisms for pattern learning and recognition should be reflected in these firing patterns. Unfortunately, the decoding or "readout" mechanism remains unknown.

Chapter 10 also relies on the idea that frequency-dependent synaptic transmission is a "code" or computational element capable of transmitting a limited subset of information contained within the presynaptic action potential train. Markram and associates point out that frequency-dependent synaptic transmission has essentially been ignored in virtually every concept developed for information processing and learning and memory in the mammalian brain—but, see chapters 5 and 12. In a closely reasoned argument, the authors suggest a phenomenological model that represents an integration of previous experiments on synaptic depression. The models and algorithms presented in this chapter are mathematically precise and testable. They represent a new, contrasting approach to the study of neural plasticity at the microcircuit level. Some of their conclusions pose a serious challenge to current views of information transmission by synapses, synaptic plasticity, and information processing in neural networks.

In chapter 11 Roman and colleagues examine the functional interaction between the limbic system and neocortical structures. The authors present data from three experiments that show a temporal sequence or progression of synaptic modification during olfactory conditioning. The authors concentrate on the separate roles of hippocampus and olfactory circuitry in the synaptic plasticity involved in storing associative memories.

Gilbert and Pierre Chauvet, the authors of chapter 12, concentrate on defining circuitry in the cerebellum and how the Purkinje cells in these circuits can be shown to display learning rules of the Hebbian type. One of their contributions is a formalism that simplifies all the coupled motor functions that are being produced by the cerebellum at the same time. The cerebellum is treated as a nonlinear, dynamical system with the Purkinje local circuit as the basic structure. One feature of this chapter is the precisely specified equations and algorithms that can generate testable hypotheses. Whether or not this relatively recent mathematical descriptor approach to plasticity has a permanent influence on the study of plasticity requires a time frame longer than this present volume.

Finally, two of the editors (M.B. and R.F.T.) provide a summary chapter that ties together many of the details alluded to in this introduction. Both bring a unique and extensive background to the study of plasticity.

This book reveals a surprising convergence of experimental and theoretical concepts and suggests that an encompassing theory of neural plasticity may not be far off. Overall, we believe that this book will be extremely useful for scientists and students interested in the mechanisms and functional significance of synaptic plasticity in all its wonderful manifestations.

Advances in Synaptic Plasticity

1　Learning about Activity-Dependent Genes

Dietmar Kuhl

Activity-dependent remodeling of synaptic efficacy and neuronal connectivity is a remarkable property of synaptic transmission and characteristic of plastic events in the nervous system. To understand the brain, both as the organ of mental function and as a target for disease, we need to understand synaptic plasticity at the cellular and molecular levels. A central idea in this entire area of research has been that functional plasticity is subserved by activity-dependent changes in gene expression. A large body of work indicates a broad role for activity-dependent gene products in neuronal plasticity, including cellular processes underlying learning and memory, epileptogenesis, drug abuse, and neurological diseases. In this chapter I will not attempt to review this work but will focus on two specific activity-dependent genes encoding products that might directly modify neuronal function. In the course of this discussion I describe molecular biological approaches developed in our laboratory to identify and study activity-regulated genes specifically involved in synaptic plasticity.

Neuronal plasticity is associated with critical physiological processes in the developing and adult brain. Particularly fascinating examples of naturally occurring neuronal plasticity are seen in studies of learning and memory. Learning is the process by which we acquire knowledge and memory is the process by which we retain that knowledge over time. In both invertebrates and vertebrates, long-term memory differs from short-term memory in that it requires RNA and protein synthesis (Davis and Squire 1984; Castellucci et al. 1989). This suggests that retention mechanisms should depend on changes in transcriptional state (Berridge 1986; Goelet et al. 1986; Curran and Morgan 1987) (figure 1.1). This idea is supported by the demonstration that in invertebrates behavioral training elicits changes in the levels of specific messenger RNAs (mRNAs) in cells involved in learning (Dash et al. 1989; Kennedy et al. 1992; Kuhl et al. 1992; Hu et al. 1993; Alberini et al. 1994; Hegde et al. 1997) and memory critically depends on induced gene expression (Bartsch et al. 1995; Yin et al. 1995; Bailey et al. 1996).

Our attention has been focused on identifying activity-induced genes in the mammalian hippocampus and cortex. Both brain regions are subject to plastic alterations in response to normal levels of neuronal activity as well as

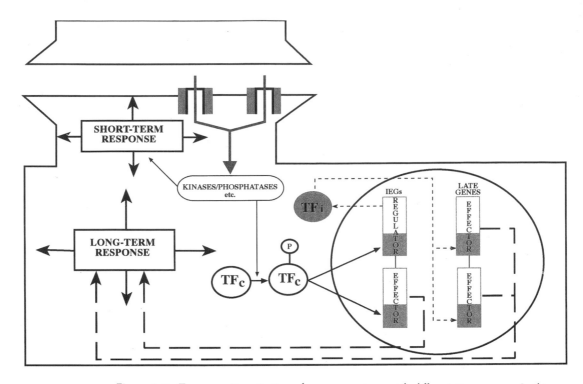

Figure 1.1 Transsynaptic activation of memory systems with different time courses. In this model a synaptic signal acts on the neuron to initiate separate memory processes with various durations. Short-term memory has a time course of minutes to hours and depends on the covalent modification of preexisting proteins. The duration of these covalent modifications determines the retention of short-term memory (short-term response). Unlike these short-term processes, long-term memory requires new RNA and protein synthesis. The same signaling systems activated during the short-term response are used to modify constitutively expressed transcription factors (TF_c). These transcription factors mediate the induced expression of immediate-early genes (IEGs). Some of these IEGs might have effector functions like t-PA or *arg3.1* (see text); others represent regulatory genes encoding inducible transcription factors (TF_i). These inducible transcription factors trigger the expression of late genes. Both early effectors and late genes participate in the maintenance of the long-term response.

in neuropathological states, such as epilepsy. Seizures set in motion a cascade of events that include changes in gene expression, axonal sprouting, and the establishment of new synaptic contacts (Ben-Ari and Represa 1990; Gall 1993; Gall et al. 1997). These long-lasting alterations are remarkably reminiscent of changes that occur during long-term potentiation (LTP) of synaptic transmission in the mammalian brain (Ben-Ari and Represa 1990). LTP is an activity-dependent and persistent enhancement of synaptic efficacy that may underlie certain forms of explicit learning (Bliss and Lomo 1973; Lynch et al. 1991; Staubli 1995; Stevens 1998). Explicit memory requires attention and conscious participation, and involves to an important degree the hippocampus as well as the cerebral cortex (Squire 1992; Eichenbaum 1997). As is the case for memory in the intact animal, LTP is blocked by inhibitors of

RNA and protein synthesis (Krug et al. 1984; Frey et al. 1988; Otani and Abraham 1989; Nguyen et al. 1994; Frey et al. 1996), indicating that neuronal activity resulting in LTP initiates a cascade of changes in gene expression. To understand the underlying genetic program it will be necessary to identify the specific genes that are induced during learning.

HOW CAN WE IDENTIFY ACTIVITY-REGULATED GENES IN THE MAMMALIAN BRAIN?

Until recently, insights into the molecular basis of plasticity in the mammalian brain have been largely dependent on tools originally generated in studies of non-neuronal cells. In this way the proto-oncogenes *c-fos* and *zif268* have been found to be activated by neuronal activity, as have a number of other genes for which probes are available (Morgan and Curran 1986; Greenberg et al. 1986; Dragunow and Robertson 1987; Morgan et al. 1987; Saffen et al. 1988; Gall and Isackson 1989; Cole et al. 1989; Sheng and Greenberg 1990; Gall et al. 1991). To identify novel activity-dependent genes that are induced during plastic events in the brain we and others have made use of differential screens of complementary DNA (cDNA) libraries generated from hippocampi of experimental seizure rats (Yamagata et al. 1993; Nedivi et al. 1993; Qian et al. 1993; Link et al. 1995) (figure 1.2). More recently we developed a subtractive cloning methodology that further improves the sensitivity of these screens (Konietzko and Kuhl 1998). To establish subtractive hybridization and cloning protocols that are well suited for the isolation of functionally important, activity-dependent genes, three main limitations of conventional procedures have to be addressed. First, we and others have shown that even modest changes in gene expression (i.e., three- to five-fold changes in mRNA content) can have consequences for the functional properties of nerve cells (Yamagata et al. 1993; Nedivi et al. 1993; Qian et al. 1993; Link et al. 1995).

These changes are orders of magnitude smaller than those that can be observed in some model systems for gene induction (e.g., see Kuhl et al. 1987; MacDonald et al. 1990). In particular, the commonly used 10- to 100-fold excess of driver sequences derived from the control cell population is therefore prohibitively large to enrich for many genes of interest. Second, problems arise with analysis of brain tissue that are not encountered in studies of cultured cells. An advantage of cloning directly from hippocampus is that it truly reflects brain physiology; that is, genes induced by neuronal activity in vivo are most likely to be physiologically relevant. However, the number of different RNA sequences transcribed in brain tissue is considerably higher than in homogeneous cell cultures. As a result of this complexity, the rate constant of the hybridization reaction will be significantly smaller when working with brain tissue. To drive the hybridization reaction to kinetic termination for low abundance genes, R_{ot} values greater than 1000

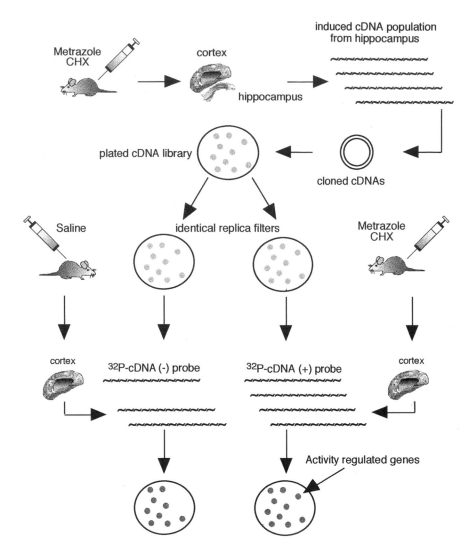

Figure 1.2 Differential screen for activity-regulated immediate-early genes. Immediate-early genes are typically induced only transiently and unlike late genes their transcripts are stabilized and accumulate in the presence of the protein synthesis inhibitor cycloheximide (CHX). We took advantage of this property, known as superinduction, to generate a complementary DNA (cDNA) library enriched for immediate-early genes from hippocampal RNA isolated from rats that had undergone pentylenetetrazole (Metrazole)-induced seizures. Duplicate filters of this library were then screened with two cDNA probes, one derived from seizure-induced animals (+probe), the other from the brain of control animals (−probe). Clones that hybridized preferentially to the + probe represent putative activity-regulated genes and were subjected to further analysis.

have to be achieved (Sargent 1987). This, in turn, requires a driver concentration of at least 3 μg/μL to limit the time of high temperature exposure during hybridization. Since both driver and target sequences have to be isolated from hippocampus, a relatively small area of the brain, the material required in standard subtractive protocols is difficult to obtain. Third, with conventional subtractive hybridization procedures an enrichment of induced sequences is frequently accompanied by an accumulation of sequences unable to form heteroduplexes for purely technical reasons (Li et al. 1994). Consequently the efficacy of the subtractive hybridization is severely limited.

To address these issues we have developed a modified phagemid subtraction protocol (Konietzko and Kuhl 1998) based on previous reports (Duguid et al. 1988; Rubenstein et al. 1990; Gruber et al. 1993; Li et al. 1994). The basic strategy of the method is shown in a flow chart (figure 1.3). As a first step in the subtraction protocol, cDNAs from poly(A)$^+$ RNA of stimulated and control hippocampus were synthesized. These cDNAs were then cloned into phagemid vectors to generate representative control and induced libraries. Analysis of these libraries demonstrated that a vast majority (97%) of clones contained inserts of one to two thousand base pairs on average. The cDNA expression profiles in control and induced libraries were examined in a virtual Northern blot that was probed for constitutively expressed glyceraldehyde-3-phosphate dehydrogenase (GAPDH) transcripts (Fort et al. 1985) and activity-induced tissue plasminogen activator (t-PA) (Qian et al. 1993), nur77 (Dragunow et al. 1996), and c-fos transcripts (Morgan et al. 1987) (figure 1.4A, lane C and C/P; figure 1.4B, lane C and C/P). Virtual Northern blots take advantage of the quantitative representation of cellular RNA populations in cDNA libraries, which therefore may serve as source of population cRNAs. Hybridization signals were comparable to those in standard Northern blots of cellular RNA from hippocampus. The appearance of multiple bands in the virtual Northern blot analysis (figure 1.4 A and B) most likely reflects cDNA clones in the libraries that have different lengths due to incomplete reverse transcription during cDNA synthesis.

Biotinylated driver RNA was then synthesized in vitro from the control cDNA library, and the induced library was used to generate single-stranded phagemid cDNA targets. By this approach, driver and target are renewable and in unlimited supply. Conventional subtraction hybridizations use high driver-to-target ratios; as a consequence they often do not allow the enrichment for moderately induced genes (Fargnoli et al. 1990; Li et al. 1994). This is in agreement with our own results, which have shown that even fivefold excess of driver-to-target sequences leads to a depletion of moderately induced genes in the subtracted library (see figure 1.4B). Hence, we conducted the subtractive hybridization reaction using a low driver-to-target ratio (2 : 1). After hybridization of target and driver, unhybridized single-stranded phagemid target was separated from heteroduplex hybrids using streptavidin-coated magnetic beads. The unhybridized phagemids were rendered double-stranded and transformed into bacteria to produce the first

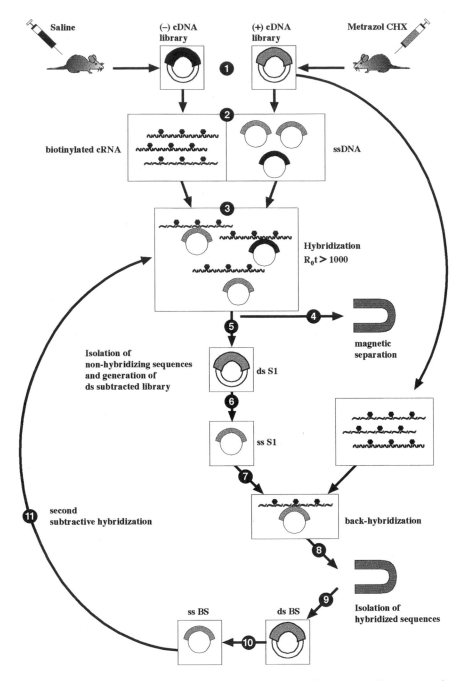

Figure 1.3 Flow chart of the subtractive cloning strategy. A driver cDNA library (−) and a target cDNA (+) from control and stimulated hippocampus, respectively, are generated in phagemid vectors (1). The (+) library is used to produce single-stranded phagemid cDNA target (ssDNA) and the (−) library is in vitro transcribed to synthesize biotinylated cRNA driver (2). Subtractive hybridization is driven to kinetic termination at a low driver-to-target ratio (3). Heteroduplex hybrids are removed in a magnetic separation (4) and unhybridized single-sranded phagemids are rendered double-stranded to generate the first subtracted library (ds S1) (5). This subtracted library was used to produce single-stranded phagemid (ss S1) (6) which served as target in a backhybridization with biotinylated cRNA from the (+) library (7). Heteroduplex hybrids were isolated in a magnetic separation (8) and bound ssDNA was released from the RNA to generate the double-stranded backhybridized library (ds BS) (9). This library was rendered single-stranded (ss BS) and used in a second subtractive hybridization (11).

subtracted library. Notably, the method avoids polymerase chain reaction (PCR) amplification which is less likely to amplify rare mRNAs, presumably owing to competition for amplification with more abundant transcripts (Liang et al. 1993; Bauer et al. 1993; Bertioli et al. 1995).

Virtual Northern blots of the first subtraction library show that low-ratio hybridization effectively depleted the library of GAPDH transcripts while moderately induced transcripts, such as t-PA, *nur77*, and c-*fos*, become highly enriched (figure 1.4A, lane S1; figure 1.4B, lane 2 : 1). The enrichment favored clones with smaller inserts. This result might have been a consequence of heat-mediated degradation processes active during the subtractive hybridization which statistically affect longer sequences more often than shorter sequences. Upon analysis of the subtracted library we observed, in addition to the enrichment of induced sequences, that there was a strong enrichment of phagemids lacking inserts or containing insert sequences of less than fifty base pairs. Whereas the percentage of clones without inserts in the original induced library was very low (3%), this percentage was dramatically increased by the first (52%) and second (85%) subtraction procedure. We assume that the percentage of insertless clones in the target library increased during each subtraction because of the lack of complementary sequences in the driver RNA. This problem has been described for other subtractive hybridization protocols (Herfort and Garber 1991; Li et al. 1994). To remove these clones, we employed a backhybridization procedure wherein the driver RNA was derived from the induced library and the target phagemids were prepared from the subtracted library. After kinetic completion of the hybridization, nonhybridizing sequences were discarded and heteroduplex-forming phagemids were recovered, rendered double-stranded, and transformed into bacteria. The incidence of insertless clones in this purified, subtracted library was reduced to 12%, thereby enabling a further round of subtraction (figure 1.4A, lanes BS and S2). The introduction of the backhybridization step is particularly useful when single-stranded phagemid libraries are used as target. More generally, backhybridization should reduce the incidence of false-positive clones that are not actually enriched in the target tissue but are only enriched by the technique.

Single clones from the backhybridized, once-subtracted library (see figure 1.4A, lane BS) were selected at random and analyzed in a differential Southern blot. Radiolabeled plus and minus, virtual cDNA population probes were prepared by reverse transcription of cRNA that had been in vitro transcribed from the induced and control cDNA libraries, respectively. Figure 1.5 shows an example of a differential Southern blot (i.e., a virtual reverse Northern blot) using induced and control, virtual population probes. In this example two clones exhibited a dramatically increased hybridization signal with the induced probe. However, these clones should only be considered as candidates of interest until the abundance of their corresponding RNA is examined by Northern blots or another quantitative method. Standard Northern blot analysis confirmed that one out of every ten clones in the subtracted

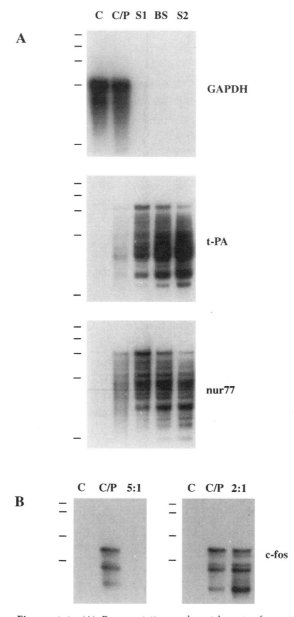

Figure 1.4 (A) Representation and enrichment of constitutive and induced transcripts in cDNA libraries. Autoradiographs of virtual Northern blot analysis of cRNA in vitro transcribed from hippocampal cDNA libraries. A 3-μg sample of cRNA was loaded per lane. The same blot was hybridized to a probe specific for glyceraldehyde-3-phosphate dehydrogenase (GAPDH) (top) and, after stripping of the probe, rehybridized with a probe specific for tissue plasminosen activator (t-PA) (middle). An identical blot was hybridized to a probe specific for *nur77* (bottom). Lane C, cRNA from the control cDNA library prepared from animals four hours after saline injection. Lane C/P, cRNA from the induced library, prepared from animals four hours after the onset of pentylenetetrazole-induced seizures in the presence of cycloheximide. Lane S1, cRNA from a library that was generated after one round of subtraction. Lane BS, cRNA from the back-hybridized, subtracted library. Lane S2, cRNA from a library that was generated after subtrac-

library was induced by stimulation, two of which are shown in figure 1.5 and were identified as t-PA and *nur77*, previously reported to be induced by synaptic activity (Qian et al. 1993; Dragunow et al. 1996). Although the subtractive library includes more than a million independent clones, this does not indicate the number of induced sequences. So far we have repeatedly identified several of the known activity-dependent genes. In addition, we have identified novel sequences, some of which are expressed at an abundance of 1 in 100,000 clones in the induced nonsubtracted library. Based on a nonexhaustive screen of the subtracted library we estimate that there are between 50 and 100 activity-dependent immediate-early genes that are induced at least twofold. This is in good agreement with an estimation based on the reiterative isolation of activity-dependent genes from an independent library (Paul Worley, personal communication, April 2, 1998). Significantly higher numbers of activity-induced immediate-early genes have been reported on the basis of differential display or differential Southern blot (reverse Northern blot) techniques which should be considered semiquantitative at best. Since we feel that even the best quantitative methods such as Northern blots, and S1 or RNase protection assays using an internal standard as control cannot reliably determine small differences in gene expression, we concentrate on genes whose RNA level changes more than twofold with stimulation.

TISSUE PLASMINOGEN ACTIVATOR IS INDUCED AS AN IMMEDIATE-EARLY GENE BY SYNAPTIC ACTIVITY

Differential screening revealed that expression of the gene for t-PA is induced with neuronal activity (Qian et al. 1993). As t-PA is an extracellular protease that is released in association with morphological differentiation (Krystosek and Seeds 1981; Pittman et al. 1989; Neuman et al. 1989), increases in t-PA expression may play a role in the structural changes that are a hallmark of activity-dependent plasticity (Ben-Ari and Represa 1990; Wallace et al. 1991; Cavazos et al. 1991). In quantitative Northern blot and in situ hybridization experiments we found that t-PA expression is induced with different spatial patterns in three activity-generating paradigms: (1) experimentally induced seizures increase t-PA expression throughout the brain; (2) electrical stimulation of the perforant path leading to hippocampal after-

Figure 1.4 (continued)
tion, backhybridization, and a second round of subtraction. Positions of the RNA ladder (GibcoBRL) bands (0.24, 1.35, 2.37, 4.40, and 7.46 kb) are indicated on the left. (B) Driver-to-target ratio is critical for the enrichment of induced sequences. Virtual Northern blots were hybridized to a probe specific for c-*fos*. Lane 5 : 1, cRNA from a library that was generated after one round of subtraction with a driver-to-target ratio of 5 : 1. Lane 2 : 1, cRNA from a library that was generated after one round of subtraction with a driver-to-target ratio of 2 : 1. RNA amounts and abbreviations are as in A. Positions of the RNA ladder (GibcoBRL) bands (1.35, 2.37, 4.40, and 7.46 kb) are indicated on the left. (From (Konietzko and Kuhl 1998.)

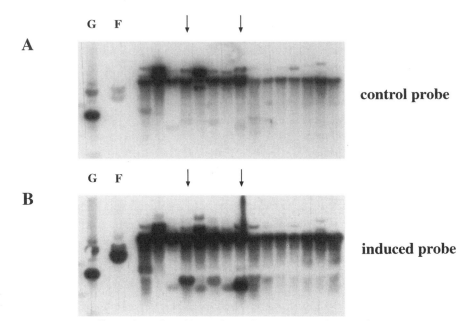

Figure 1.5 Differential Southern blot analysis of cDNA inserts from a subtracted library. (A) Autoradiograph of a Southern blot hybridized to a virtual, control (−) cDNA population probe. (B) Autoradiograph of a duplicate blot hybridized to a virtual, induced (+) cDNA population probe. cDNA inserts were released from fifteen randomly picked clones of the backhybridized, subtracted library. Lane G, cDNA insert released from GAPDH plasmid (Fort et al. 1985) loaded as a control for a constitutively expressed gene. Lane F, cDNA insert released from *c-fos* plasmid (Morgan et al. 1987), loaded as a control for an activity-induced gene. Arrows mark lanes of two clones from the subtracted library with strong differential hybridization signals with the (+) probe that were confirmed in standard Northern blots. For differential screening, single colonies from the backhybridized, subtracted library were picked at random and plasmid DNA was prepared. Exposure time of the autoradiographs was adjusted on the basis of the constitutively expressed GAPDH gene. Clones exhibiting differential hybridization signals were examined in standard Northern blots with cellular hippocampal RNA from control and experimental seizure animals. Sequence analysis of two positive clones shown revealed that they are identical to t-PA and *nur77*. (From Konietzko and Kuhl 1998.)

discharges and kindling increases t-PA mRNA levels throughout the hippocampal neuronal layers bilaterally; and (3) high-frequency, LTP-inducing stimulation of the perforant path in vivo causes an NMDA (N-methyl-D-aspartate) receptor–dependent increase in the t-PA mRNA level which is restricted to the granule cells of the ipsilateral, stimulated dentate gyrus.

In continuation of this work we used t-PA knockout mice to address the question of whether t-PA gene expression was necessary for the establishment and maintenance of LTP (Frey et al. 1996). Specifically, in collaborative studies with Dr. Uwe Frey (IFN, Madgeburg, Germany) we analyzed long-lasting LTP (L-LTP, greater than four hours) in hippocampal slices from mice homozygous for disrupted t-PA genes. The genetically engineered mice develop normally, are fertile, and have a normal life span (Carmeliet et al. 1994). Our histochemical analysis did not reveal any gross anatomical abnormalities in hippocampus or other regions of the brain. Electrical stimulation of the Schaffer collaterals in t-PA-deficient mice elicited LTP in field CA1 that was phenotypically similar to potentiation observed in wild-type mice and was maintained in vitro for at least eight hours (figure 1.6A and B). However, further analysis demonstrated that there were differences in the contribution of GABAergic activities to LTP in wild-type and t-PA knockout animals. In slices of wild-type mice, the γ-aminobutyric acid (GABA$_A$) receptor inhibitor picrotoxin did not disrupt the normal establishment and maintenance of LTP (figure 1.7A and B). By strong contrast, tetanization of slices of t-PA-deficient animals in the presence of picrotoxin failed to induce stable LTP. Mutant mice were completely devoid of late phases of potentiation, showing only a short-lasting potentiation that declined to baseline values within 60 minutes after tetanization (see figure 1.7A and B). These and several other experiments led us to conclude that t-PA-deficient mice exhibit a different form of potentiation that is characterized by NMDA receptor–dependent downregulation of GABAergic transmission in the CA1 region. This form of potentiation provides t-PA-deficient mice with an output of CA1 neurons that is identical to that seen in wild-type mice during conventional L-LTP and may compensate for the absence of L-LTP function. Compensation for deficiencies in conventional LTP by a GABA-dependent potentiation in the hippocampus could explain why spatial memory is not affected in the mutant mice (Huang et al. 1996). However, performance of t-PA-deficient mice was impaired on a two-way active avoidance task which is thought to depend on activities in striatum (Huang et al. 1996). The latter deficit could also reflect impaired motor learning mediated by the cerebellum; in this structure t-PA is induced with complex motor tasks (Seeds et al. 1995) and there may be no compensation for the loss of t-PA expression.

We found that during control stimulation, t-PA-deficient mice are characterized by unusually strong GABAergic transmission in the hippocampal CA1 region. Interestingly, in line with these results, Tsirka, Strickland, and colleagues have reported that t-PA-deficient mice are less susceptible than the control strain to experimentally induced seizures, ischemia, and neuronal degeneration (Tsirka et al. 1995, 1997; Wang et al. 1998). Various human pathologic conditions involve excitotoxic damage to the brain. The contribution of t-PA to the degeneration pathway suggests that inhibitors of t-PA might have therapeutic potential for diseases involving excitotoxic damage. During normal brain function, the action of t-PA might be counterbalanced by naturally expressed serine protease inhibitors of the serpin family (Monard 1988; Krueger et al. 1997; Hastings et al. 1997). Synaptic activity associated with plasticity might lead to the induction and release of t-PA, and other recently described secreted serine proteases (Chen et al. 1995; Okabe et al. 1996; see also chapter 3), thereby shifting the balance between the proteases and their natural inhibitors to favor increased proteolytic activity in the extracellular environment. Such controlled induction and release of t-PA during activity-dependent plasticity could transiently alter adhesive contacts

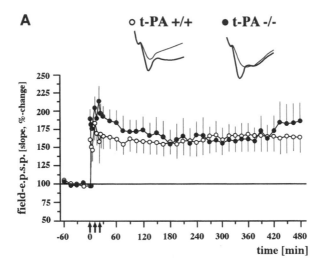

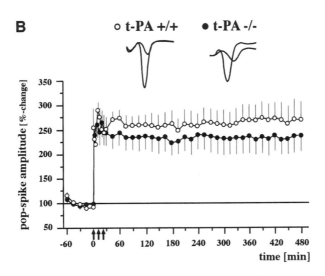

Figure 1.6 Long-term potentiation (LTP) and long-lasting potentiation in hippocampal slices of t-PA$^{+/+}$ and t-PA$^{-/-}$ mice. A, Time course of the percentage change of the slope of field excitatory postsynaptic potentials (EPSPs) and B, of the population spike amplitiude (pop-spike) in t-PA-deficient (filled circles, n = 8) and wild-type mice (open circle, n = 8). Threefold tetanization resulted in stable potentiation in both animal groups for eight hours (each point shown is the mean of averaged potentials ± SEM). Insets show typical examples of superimposed traces of EPSPs (A) and pop-spikes (B) before and eight hours after tetanization for each animal group. Arrows indicate the time point of threefold tetanization. (Adapted from Frey et al. 1996.)

A

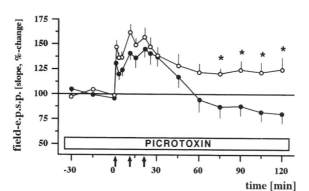

B

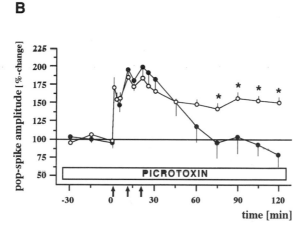

Figure 1.7 Time course of long-lasting potentiation in t-PA$^{+/+}$ and t-PA$^{-/-}$ mice in the presence of picrotoxin. Time course of potentiation of the field EPSP (A) and the pop-spike (B) in wild-type (open circles, n = 10) and t-PA-deficient mice (filled circles, n = 9) after application of picrotoxin. In the latter, only a short-term potentiation could be evoked. Asterisks indicate the statistically significant difference between the mutant and wild-type mice after application of picrotoxin (Mann-Whitney U test, $P < .05$). Arrows indicate the time point of threefold tetanization. (Adapted from Frey et al. 1996.)

between neurons (Pittman et al. 1989). For example, t-PA is capable of converting plasminogen into plasmin which, in turn, can lead to the degradation of laminin in the brain (Chen and Strickland 1997). Limited degradation of the extracellular matrix initiated by the activation of t-PA and other proteases might therefore be a prerequisite for the morphological remodeling of synaptic contacts underlying long-term memory.

Although the above-described experiments establish a link between activity-induced gene expression and physiological and pathological neuronal plasticity, it remains an open question how transcriptional activation taking place in the nucleus can selectively modify stimulated synaptic sites in the distant dendritic compartments of the neuron. Such selective modifications of synapses that have experienced coincident activity are required by the Hebbian rule and might be a prerequisite for the input specificity of LTP (Hebb 1949; Wigstrom and Gustafsson 1986; Frey and Morris 1997). Our analysis of the novel immediate-early gene *arg3.1* might guide our thinking and provide insights into this problem.

SOMATO-DENDRITIC EXPRESSION OF *arg3.1* IS REGULATED BY SYNAPTIC ACTIVITY

We, and independently the laboratory of Paul Worley at Johns Hopkins University, cloned and characterized the novel immediate-early gene *arg3.1/ arc* (activity-regulated gene of 3.1 kb, or, activity-regulated cytoskeleton–associated protein (Link et al. 1995; Lyford et al. 1995). It should be noted that the partial cDNA clone BAD1 (for brain activity-dependent), described by Qian et al. (1993), represents the same mRNA as *arc* and *arg3.1*. The full length cDNA sequence of 3018 nucleotides encodes a predicted open reading frame of 396 amino acids. The putative 5'-noncoding sequence includes two in-frame stop codons. The open reading frame is followed by a termination codon and 1630 nucleotides of 3' sequence with a poly(A) addition signal 12 nucleotides from the 3'-terminal poly(A) tail. The predicted protein is hydrophilic and there are no identifiable signal sequences or hydrophobic stretches of sufficient length for a putative membrane spanning region. The *arg3.1* gene product, and its induction by activity, is particularly interesting for two reasons. First, *arg3.1* shows a modest sequence identity with brain spectrin, a major constituent of the cytoskeletal network (Lazarides and Woods 1989; Wasenius et al. 1989). It has been postulated that calcium-dependent proteolysis of spectrin is critical to local structural and functional changes subserving LTP (Crick 1984; Siman et al. 1985; Lynch and Baudry 1987). Second, as described below, newly transcribed *arg3.1* mRNA is rapidly distributed to dendritic processes, thereby suggesting the possibility that *arg3.1* translation and function may be controlled locally by synaptic events within the dendrites.

Our studies provide evidence of expression and regulation of *arg3.1* mRNA in the brain, where synaptic activity markedly increases mRNA levels in discrete populations of neurons (figure 1.8). Basal expression of *arg3.1* RNA is low in hippocampus, caudate putamen, and some thalamic nuclei (figure 1.8B and C), but is high in cortical areas, particularly in visual cortex. In neocortex NMDA receptors make a major contribution to normal excitatory synaptic transmission (Hagihara et al. 1988; Miller et al. 1989; Fox et al. 1989). We found that blocking the NMDA receptor led to a marked reduction in basal *arg3.1* mRNA levels, thereby suggesting that high constitutive expression in cortex is driven by naturally occurring NMDA receptor activation (e.g., by visual experience). Conversely, synaptic activity induced

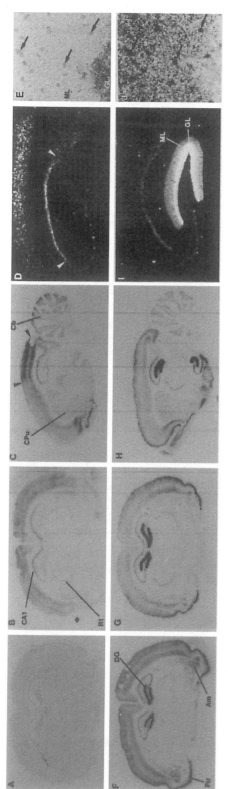

Figure 1.8 Spatiotemporal expression of *arg3.1* messenger RNA (mRNA) in brain after seizure. *arg3.1* mRNA using in situ hybridization with sense (A) and antisense probes (B–J). (B–D) Control animals. F, Animal one hour after seizure. G–J, and E, Animals four hours after seizure. A–C and F–H show film autoradiographs. D, I, and J show dark-field emulsion photomicrographs. E shows bright-field photomicrograph corresponding to J. Hybridization is uniformly distributed and not associated with Nissl-stained somata (arrows). Am, amygdaloid complex; CA1, CA1 field of the hippocampus; Cb, cerebellum; CP$_u$, caudate putamen; DG, dentate gyrus; GL, granular layer; ML, molecular layer; Pir, piriform cortex; Rt, reticular thalamic nucleus; diamond demarcates boundary between temporal and perirhinal cortex; black arrowheads indicate boundaries of occipital cortex; white arrowheads show the borders of the CA1 subfield; arrows point to somata in the molecular layer. (Adapted from Link et al. 1995.)

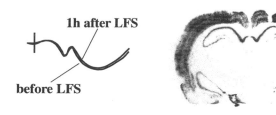

1h after LFS

before LFS

Field Potential ⎤5 mV

2 ms

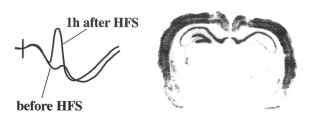

1h after HFS

before HFS

Figure 1.9 Induction of LTP and *arg3.1* mRNA in hippocampal granule cell neurons in freely moving rats. Coronal sections were assayed for *arg3.1* mRNA using in situ hybridization with antisense probe. Representative autoradiographs are shown. (Top) One hour after unilateral application of low-frequency stimulus pulses. (Bottom) One hour after unilateral application of high-frequency stimulus pulses. Field potentials on the left evidence that high-frequency stimulation evokes LTP in freely moving rats, whereas low-frequency stimulation does not. Shown are superimposed field potentials before and one hour after low- or high-frequency stimulation. (Adapted from Link et al. 1995.)

arg.3.1 mRNA expression in hippocampal and cortical neurons. In particular, seizures induced dramatic increases in *arg.3.1* mRNA (figure 1.8F–J); this induction was independent of new protein synthesis, as is typical of immediate-early genes. *Arg3.1* mRNA was also markedly induced by LTP stimulation. To evoke LTP in the granule cells, three bursts of high-frequency stimulation were applied to the perforant path of freely moving rats. This elicited a spatially confined increase in *arg3.1* mRNA levels in the ipsilateral dentate gyrus granule cells. Delivery of the same number of stimulus pulses at low frequency, which did not evoke LTP, also did not alter mRNA levels for *arg3.1* (figure 1.9). Most strikingly, following LTP and seizure activity, the *arg3.1* mRNA was localized to the granule cell dendrites in the stratum moleculare (figure 1.8I and J).

To date only a few mRNAs have been identified to be prominent within dendritic laminae (Steward 1997; Kuhl and Skehel 1998). To my knowledge *arg3.1* represents the first example of a gene that is regulated by neuronal activity and gives rise to dendritic mRNAs. It is known that protein synthesis can take place in dendrites (Torre and Steward 1992; Crino and Eberwine 1996; Tiedge and Brosius 1996; Kang and Schuman 1996) where it can be stimulated by NMDA receptor–dependent afferent synaptic activity (Torre

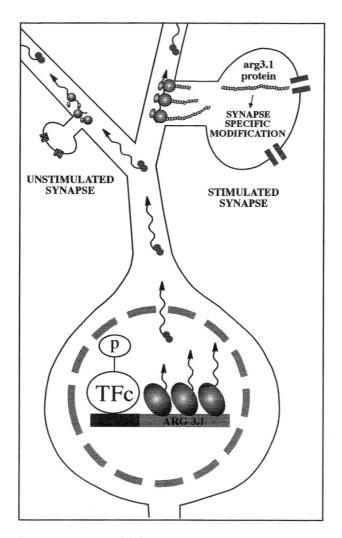

Figure 1.10 A model for synapse-specific modification following activity-induced *arg3.1* expression. Trans-synaptic activation of constitutively expressed transcription factors (TFc) leads to induced transcription of *arg3.1* mRNA. The newly synthesized *arg3.1* transcripts are transported indiscriminately to all dendritic spines, but enhanced translation of *arg3.1* protein takes place only at synaptic sites where the translation apparatus has been trans-synaptically activated.

and Steward 1992; Feig and Lipton 1993). The observations that (1) *arg3.1* protein expression is tightly linked to *arg3.1* mRNA synthesis and (2) accumulations of *arg3.1* protein are apparent at spinelike protrusions suggest the possibility that the translation of *arg3.1* mRNA within dendrites may be locally controlled by synaptic activity. Consequently, regulated *arg3.1* synthesis may play a key role in synapse-specific modifications during plastic events in the brain (figure 1.10).

From this model it becomes clear that RNA transport into the dendrites might be an important mechanism underlying synaptic plasticity. In the next section I describe a new technique that we have developed for the in vivo analysis of RNA-protein interactions and are applying to define the molecular mechanisms of dendritic *arg3.1* mRNA transport. One of the major advantages of the method is that a multiplicity of proteins or RNAs can be tested simultaneously for the interaction with an RNA or protein of interest. The interaction relies solely on the biophysical properties of the recombinant molecules. Consequently, the method is amenable to the analysis of a wide variety of ribonuclear protein complexes.

RNA-PROTEIN INTERACTIONS RECONSTITUTED BY A TRIHYBRID SYSTEM

Interactions between RNAs and proteins are fundamental to many cellular processes. The questions of how a protein recognizes a specific RNA, and which proteins interact with a specific RNA, are thus central to a large number of basic problems in molecular biology. Moreover, a growing body of evidence indicates the importance of RNA binding in a variety of human diseases (Burd and Dreyfuss 1994; Okano and Darnell 1997). Current work on protein-RNA complexes can be roughly divided into two areas: characterization of RNA target sites and identification of proteins and protein structures recognizing RNA.

Traditionally, RNA-protein interactions have been studied using biochemical assays such as RNA bandshifts, footprinting, and RNA-protein cross-linking. One disadvantage of these procedures is that interacting proteins often exist in low abundance and are consequently difficult to detect. In addition, these techniques do not easily allow the identification of target RNAs recognized by a known RNA-binding protein. A further disadvantage is that these techniques do not allow one to identify the genes encoding the proteins or RNAs of interest; instead, they provide reagents for further characterization and cloning of the cognate cDNAs. To obviate some of the difficulties and limitations inherent to the biochemical techniques, investigators have turned to other experimental approaches that permit the analysis of RNA-protein interactions (see, e.g., MacWilliams et al. 1993; Stripecke et al. 1994; Harada et al. 1996; Paraskeva et al. 1998). Recently, two genetic systems capable of rapidly identifying proteins binding to an RNA of interest or finding RNAs binding to a protein of interest have been developed (Putz et al. 1996, 1999; SenGupta et al. 1996).

The yeast two-hybrid system is a widely employed genetic screen for detecting protein-protein interactions (Fields and Song 1989; Allen et al. 1995; Phizicky and Fields 1995). We have developed a modification of this system to detect RNA-protein interactions in order to take advantage of the genetic basis of the system (Putz et al. 1996, 1999). The two-hybrid system utilizes the modular structure of particular transcription activators, allowing the DNA binding and the transcription activation domains to function independently. The DNA binding and transcription activation domains are expressed as two separate polypeptides fused to heterologous sequences. Any interaction between the heterologous polypeptides of the hybrid proteins brings together the two components of the transcription activator leading to the induction of genes under the control of appropriate upstream activating sequences. Select markers such as β-galactosidase or amino acid auxotrophy can then be used to report recombinant protein-protein interactions.

To modify this approach for the detection of RNA-protein interactions, it is necessary to construct a system where the association of the DNA binding and transcription activation domains is dependent on an RNA-protein interaction. The basic strategy of the method is illustrated in figure 1.11. We took advantage of the well-characterized and specific RNA binding activity of the RevM10 mutation of the Rev protein of human immunodeficiency virus type 1 (HIV-1). The wild-type Rev protein enhances the export of viral transcripts out of the nucleus and into the cytoplasm of the host cell. This activity is mediated in part by specific binding of Rev protein to the RRE, a 240-nucleotide-long RNA sequence, located in the viral *env* gene (Zapp and Green 1989; Daly et al. 1989; Battiste et al. 1994). This RNA-protein interaction is initiated with the binding of a Rev monomer to a Rev-binding site in the RRE (Cook et al. 1991). This high-affinity binding site is located to a short stem loop (nucleotide 45 to 75, RRE IIb) (Cook et al. 1991). Both the nucleotide sequence and the secondary structure of the RRE are important for binding (Olsen et al. 1990). Rev is a 116–amino acid protein that contains at least two functional regions. The N-terminal domain confers RNA (RRE) binding, nuclear localization, and also contributes to protein multimerization (Malim et al. 1989; Hope et al. 1990; Zapp et al. 1991). The effector domain contains a signal that promotes export of RNAs from the nucleus to the cytoplasm (Fischer et al. 1995). Consequently, RevM10, which is mutated in the C-terminal region binds with high affinity to the RRE and is localized to the nucleus, but unlike the wild-type protein is unable to promote the export of RNA from the nucleus to the cytoplasm (Malim et al. 1989; Stutz and Rosbash 1994; Fritz et al. 1995).

The three component molecules used in the trihybrid system are the RevM10 protein fused to the DNA-binding domain of GAL4, an RNA-hybrid containing the RRE sequence fused to a target RNA, and a second protein hybrid comprised of the activation domain of GAL4 fused to any protein of interest or to proteins expressed from a library of cDNAs. Each hybrid protein and the hybrid RNA is expressed in yeast cells under the control of independent promoter and termination sequences. Upon productive interaction of the three hybrid molecules a functional GAL4 transcription factor is reconstituted. The activity of this transcription factor is then used to report the RNA-protein interaction.

As an example we expressed both the DNA-binding domain and transcription activation domain of GAL4 as fusion proteins with RevM10. The

A

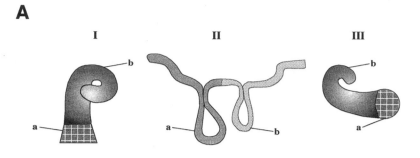

B

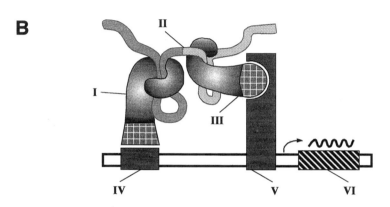

Figure 1.11 The basic strategy of the trihybrid method. (A) Schema of the components. The first hybrid protein (I) contains the DNA-binding domain of GAL4 (Ia) fused to the RRE-RNA-binding protein RevM10 (Ib). A hybrid-RNA (II) containing the RRE sequence (a) and a target RNA sequence X (IIb). The second hybrid protein (III) contains the activation domain of GAL4 (IIIa) fused to a protein Y (IIIb) capable of recognizing the target RNA X on the RNA hybrid. (B) Upon productive interaction of the three hybrids a reconstituted GAL4 transcription factor (I + II + III) bound to a GAL4-responsive promoter (IV) stimulates the basal transcriptional machinery (V) of the *lacZ* gene and the nutritional reporter gene *HIS3* (VI). (Adapted from Putz et al. 1996.)

yeast strain CG-1945 was transformed with plasmids expressing hybrid proteins containing the DNA-binding domain of GAL4 fused to RevM10, the transcription activation domain of GAL4 fused to RevM10, and a recombinant RNA containing two copies of the RRE. The maps and details of construction of the expression plasmids used are given in figure 1.12. Transformants were analyzed for histidine-independent growth and *β*-galactosidase expression. Functional GAL4 activity was detected only when all three recombinant molecules were coexpressed. Results from these experiments are shown in table 1.1. No GAL4 activity was detected in yeast

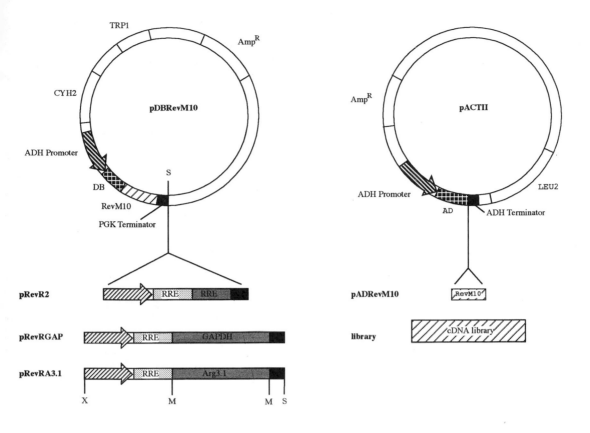

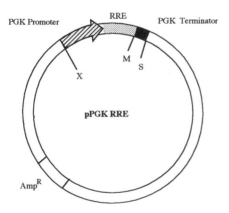

Figure 1.12 The plasmids used in the trihybrid system. The upper plasmids are *Escherichia coli*–yeast shuttle vectors and were used in the transfection and mating experiments of tables 1.1 and 1.2. pPGKRRE was used as an intermediate to clone hybrid RNAs as a transcription unit cassette into pDBRevM10. The transcription units generating the hybrid proteins and the hybrid RNAs are indicated. The respective promoters and terminators are depicted. *E.coli* and yeast replication origins are not shown. *E.coli* selectable marker for ampicillin resistance, Amp^R, and the yeast selectable markers TRP1 and LEU2 are also shown. Cycloheximide sensitivity in yeast is conferred by CYH2. M, *MluI*; S, *SalI*; X, *XhoI*, relevant restriction sites. (Adapted from Putz et al. 1996.)

Table 1.1 Tri-hybrid interaction of RevM10 protein with the RRE RNA sequence

	β-galactosidase activity	
Expressed hybrid-protein	−RRE	+RRE
DB-RevM10 + AD-RevM10	−	+++
DB-RevM10	−	−
AD-RevM10	−	−

Relevant expressed proteins are indicated. +RRE indicates the presence of an RNA containing two copies of the RRE. −RRE indicates the absence of the hybrid RNA. DB, GAL4 DNA binding domain; AD, GAL4 activation domain. Clones that developed visible blue color within four hours were registered as +++. If no color developed after sixteen hours, clones were recorded as −. Transformants were grown on media selective for the given plasmids. When growth was a measure of GAL4 activity the medium lacked histidine and contained 30 mM 3-amino-1,2,4-triazole. (Adapted from Putz et al. 1996.)

expressing these fusion proteins alone or in combination (see table 1.1). However, when a recombinant RNA carrying two copies of the RRE was coexpressed with the two RevM10 fusion proteins, functional GAL4 activity was reconstituted (see table 1.1). Therefore, a trimeric ribonuclear protein complex may be formed in the nucleus, bringing together the GAL4 DNA-binding and transcriptional activation domains and re-creating functional GAL4 activity. These results demonstrate the ability of a recombinant RNA to interact with two fusion proteins in a trihybrid system. The methodology can be extended to detect specific RNA-binding proteins from a library of cDNAs.

SCREENING OF A CDNA LIBRARY FOR SPECIFIC *arg3.1* mRNA-BINDING PROTEINS

The dendritic localization of *arg3.1* mRNA is believed to be achieved by specific RNA-protein interactions, although the identities of the proteins involved are not known. We have used the full-length *arg3.1* transcript fused to an RRE, to screen a library of cDNAs expressed as transcription activation domain fusion proteins. The *arg3.1* mRNA was tethered to the DNA binding domain of GAL4 via the interaction between the RevM10 fusion and the RRE present on the recombinant RNA. Any polypeptide capable of interacting with *arg3.1* mRNA will recruit the transcription activation domain into the ribonuclear protein complex, and reconstitute GAL4 activity.

The yeast strain CG-1945 was cotransfected with pRevRA3.1 (see figure 1.12), expressing both the DNA-binding domain−RevM10 hybrid protein and the RRE-*arg3.1* recombinant RNA, and with a library of pACTII-derived plasmids harboring brain-derived cDNAs expressed as fusions with the GAL4 transcription activation domain. From approximately 10^5 clones analyzed, 110 were initially able to grow on medium lacking histidine and con-

Table 1.2 Detection of polypeptides specifically interacting with the dendritically localized transcript *arg3.1*

	β-galactosidase activity		
Expressed hybrid-protein	RRE	GAPDH	*arg3.1*
DB-RevM10 + AD-protein 1	−	−	+++

Expressed hybrid proteins are indicated. DB, GAL4 DNA.

taining 30 mM 3–amino-1,2,4–triazole. Of these His$^+$ clones, eighty-nine scored positive in a filter assay for β-galactosidase activity. These clones were cured of pRevRA3.1, and reexamined for β-galactosidase activity. Twelve clones were able to activate transcription independently and did not depend on the interaction with the other two hybrids. For twenty-nine clones, β-galactosidase activity could be reconfirmed by mating to a Y187 strain carrying the pRevRA3.1 plasmid. The specificity of the interaction with *arg3.1* mRNA was tested against recombinant RRE RNAs containing an additional RRE (pRevR2), or the GAPDH transcript (pRevRGAP; Fort et al. 1985). In these tests, twenty-one clones interacted with the *arg3.1* transcript but also with control transcripts; these presumably represent general RNA-binding proteins. For the eight remaining clones, β-galactosidase expression was specifically dependent on the presence of *arg3.1* mRNA.

As an example, the data for one clone are shown in Table 1.2. The results demonstrate that the method allows the simultaneous testing of a large number of proteins for specific RNA-binding activity, a feature required for cDNA library screening. The genes encoding the identified proteins are readily available for further analysis. Sequence analyses have revealed that the primary structures of these *arg3.1* RNA-binding proteins have not been previously reported, although several of the encoded polypeptides contain motifs found in other RNA-binding proteins. We are currently using the same genetic system to further analyze the structural requirements and specificity of the identified RNA-protein interactions. For example, to determine the minimal RNA sequence required for binding to the newly identified *arg3.1* RNA-binding proteins, yeast clones expressing these proteins were mated to yeast strains expressing deleted *arg3.1* RNA targets. The identified cDNAs encoding the *arg3.1* mRNA-binding proteins are the subject of continued analysis.

NOVEL EFFECTOR GENES OF SYNAPTIC PLASTICITY, AND FUTURE PERSPECTIVES

Insights into the molecular basis of synaptic plasticity have been largely dependent on studies using tools originally generated in non-neuronal systems. These studies carried with them the concept that biological processes operative in differentiation and development are co-opted by the brain to serve activity-dependent plastic processes. Although it is difficult to exaggerate the profound influence of these studies, much in addition can be learned from differential cloning approaches that do not rely on preconceived concepts. As these techniques allow us to discover genes that so far have been elusive, we begin to understand the neuron-specific genomic response to synaptic activity. While initial studies concentrated on those immediate-early genes that function as transcriptional activators of downstream genes, there is now mounting evidence for a set of activity-regulated immediate-early genes that are more restricted in their expression and that might be capable of directly promoting functional changes in activated neurons (e.g., see Yamagata et al. 1993, 1994; Nedivi et al. 1993; Qian et al. 1993; Link et al. 1995; Andreasson and Worley 1995; Lyford et al. 1995; Tsui et al. 1996; Lauterborn et al. 1996; Kauselmann et al. 1997; Konietzko et al. 1997; Brakeman et al. 1997; Naeve et al. 1997). Inasmuch as these genes bear the potential to act as effectors of neuronal function, they become promising targets for the therapeutic intervention of a variety of diseases that involve disturbances of synaptic plasticity. Moreover, they become amenable to a molecular delineation of their specific function. As exemplified with t-PA and *arg3.1*, we want to move from the identification of activity-regulated genes to the analysis of LTP and to assess the consequences that specific activity-regulated gene products have on behavior and, in particular, on the capability to learn and store memories.

ACKNOWLDGMENTS

I thank Dr. Christine Gall for helpful comments on the manuscript, and Oliver Sperl and Julia Adlivankina-Kuhl for preparation of the figures.

REFERENCES

Alberini, C. M., Ghirardi, M., Metz, R., and Kandel, E. R. (1994). C/EBP is an immediate-early gene required for the consolidation of long-term facilitation in *Aplysia. Cell* 76: 1099–1114.

Allen, J. B., Walberg, M. W., Edwards, M. C., and Elledge, S. J. (1995). Finding prospective partners in the library: the two-hybrid system and phage display find a match. *Trends Biochem. Sci.* 20: 511–516.

Andreasson, K., and Worley, P. F. (1995). Induction of beta-A activin expression by synaptic activity and during neocortical development. *Neuroscience* 69: 781–796.

Bailey, C. H., Bartsch, D., and Kandel, E. R. (1996). Toward a molecular definition of long-term memory storage. *Proc. Natal. Acad. Sci. USA* 93: 13445–13452.

Bartsch, D., Ghirardi, M., Skehel, P. A., Karl, K. A., Herder, S. P., Chen, M., Bailey, C. H., and Kandel, E. R. (1995). *Aplysia* CREB2 represses long-term facilitation: relief of repression converts transient facilitation into long-term functional and structural change. *Cell* 83: 979–992.

Battiste, J. L., Tan, R., Frankel, A. D., and Williamson, J. R. (1994). Binding of an HIV Rev peptide to Rev responsive element RNA induces formation of purine-purine base pairs. *Biochemistry* 33: 2741–2747.

Bauer, D., Muller, H., Reich, J., Riedel, H., Ahrenkiel, V., Warthoe, P., and Strauss, M. (1993). Identification of differentially expressed mRNA species by an improved display technique (DDRT-PCR). *Nucleic Acids Res.* 21: 4272–4280.

Ben-Ari, E., and Represa, A. (1990). Brief seizure episodes induce long-term potentiation and mossy fiber sprouting in the hippocampus. *Trends Neurosci.* 13: 312–318.

Berridge, M. (1986). Second messenger dualism in neuromodulation and memory (news). *Nature* 323: 294–295.

Bertioli, D. J., Schlichter, U. H., Adams, M. J., Burrows, P. R., Steinbiss, H. H., and Antoniw, J. F. (1995). An analysis of differential display shows a strong bias towards high copy number mRNAs. *Nucleic Acids Res.* 23: 4520–4523.

Bliss, T. V., and Lomo, T. (1973). Long-lasting potentiation of synaptic transmission in the dentate area of the anaesthetized rabbit following stimulation of the perforant path. *J. Physiol. (Lond.)* 232: 331–356.

Brakeman, P. R., Lanahan, A. A., O'Brien, R., Roche, K., Barnes, C. A., Huganir, R. L., and Worley, P. F. (1997). Homer: a protein that selectively binds metabotropic glutamate receptors [see comments]. *Nature* 386: 284–288.

Burd, C. G., and Dreyfuss, G. (1994). Conserved structures and diversity of functions of RNA-binding proteins. *Science* 265: 615–621.

Carmeliet, P., Schoonjans, L., Kieckens, L., Ream, B., Degen, J., Bronson, R., De, V. R., van den Oord J. J., Collen, D., and Mulligan, R. C. (1994). Physiological consequences of loss of plasminogen activator gene function in mice. *Nature* 368: 419–424.

Castellucci, V. F., Blumenfeld, H., Goelet, P., and Kandel, E. R. (1989). Inhibitor of protein synthesis blocks long-term behavioral sensitization in the isolated gill-withdrawal reflex of *Aplysia*. *J. Neurobiol.* 20: 1–9.

Cavazos, J. E., Golarai, G., and Sutula, T. P. (1991). Mossy fiber synaptic reorganization induced by kindling: time course of development, progression, and permanence. *J. Neurosci.* 11: 2795–2803.

Chen, Z. L., and Strickland, S. (1997). Neuronal death in the hippocampus is promoted by plasmin-catalyzed degradation of laminin. *Cell* 91: 917–925.

Chen, Z. L., Yoshida, S., Kato, K., Momota, Y., Suzuki, J., Tanaka, T., Ito, J., Nishino, H., Aimoto, S., and Kiyama, H. (1995). Expression and activity-dependent changes of a novel limbic-serine protease gene in the hippocampus. *J. Neurosci.* 15: 5088–5097.

Cole, A. J., Saffen, D. W., Baraban, J. M., and Worley, P. F. (1989). Rapid increase of an immediate early gene messenger RNA in hippocampal neurons by synaptic NMDA receptor activation. *Nature* 340: 474–476.

Cook, K. S., Fisk, G. J., Hauber, J., Usman, N., Daly, T. J., and Rusche, J. R. (1991). Characterization of HIV-1 REV protein: binding stoichiometry and minimal RNA substrate. *Nucleic Acids Res.* 19: 1577–1583.

Crick, F. (1984). Memory and molecular turnover (news). *Nature* 312: 101–114.

Crino, P. B., and Eberwine, J. (1996). Molecular characterization of the dendritic growth cone: regulated mRNA transport and local protein synthesis. *Neuron* 17: 1173–1187.

Curran, T., and Morgan, J. I. (1987). Memories of *fos. Bioessays* 7: 255–258.

Daly, T. J., Cook, K. S., Gray, G. S., Maione, T. E., and Rusche, J. R. (1989). Specific binding of HIV-1 recombinant Rev protein to the Rev-responsive element in vitro. *Nature* 342: 816–819.

Dash, P., Sweatt, J. D., Kennedy, T. E., Barzilai, A., Kuhl, D., and Kandel, E. R. (1989). Molecular mechanisms for long-term memory in *Aplysia*. In *The Biology of Memory*, L. Squire and E. Lindenlaub, eds., pp. 81–88. Stuttgart, F. K. Schattauer Verlag.

Davis, H. P., and Squire, L. R. (1984). Protein synthesis and memory: a review. *Psychol. Bull.* 96: 518–559.

Dragunow, M., and Robertson, H. A. (1987). Kindling stimulation induces c-fos protein(s) in granule cells of the rat dentate gyrus. *Nature* 329: 441–442.

Dragunow, M., Abraham, W., and Hughes, P. (1996). Activation of NMDA and muscarinic receptors induces nur-77 mRNA in hippocampal neurons. *Brain Res. Mol. Brain Res.* 36: 349–356.

Duguid, J. R., Rohwer, R. G., and Seed, B. (1988). Isolation of cDNAs of scrapie-modulated RNAs by subtractive hybridization of a cDNA library. *Proc. Natal. Acad. Sci. USA* 85: 5738–5742.

Eichenbaum, H. (1997). Declarative memory: insights from cognitive neurobiology. *Annu. Rev. Psychol.* 48: 547–572.

Fargnoli, J., Holbrook, N. J., and Fornace, A. J., Jr. (1990). Low-ratio hybridization subtraction. *Anal. Biochem.* 187: 364–373.

Feig, S., and Lipton, P. (1993). Pairing the cholinergic agonist carbachol with patterned Schaffer collateral stimulation initiates protein synthesis in hippocampal CA1 pyramidal cell dendrites via a muscarinic, NMDA-dependent mechanism. *J. Neurosci.* 13: 1010–1021.

Fields, S., and Song, O. (1989). A novel genetic system to detect protein-protein interactions. *Nature* 340: 245–246.

Fischer, U., Huber, J., Boelens, W. C., Mattaj, I. W., and Luhrmann, R. (1995). The HIV-1 Rev activation domain is a nuclear export signal that accesses an export pathway used by specific cellular RNAs. *Cell* 82: 475–483.

Fort, P., Marty, L., Piechaczyk, M., el Sabrouty, S., Dani, C., Jeanteur, P., and Blanchard, J. M. (1985). Various rat adult tissues express only one major mRNA species from the glyceraldehyde-3–phosphate-dehydrogenase multigenic family. *Nucleic Acids Res.* 13: 1431–1442.

Fox, K., Sato, H., and Daw, N. (1989). The location and function of NMDA Receptors in cat and kitten visual cortex. *J. Neurosci.* 9: 2443–2454.

Frey, U., and Morris, R. G. (1997). Synaptic tagging and long-term potentiation [see comments]. *Nature* 385: 533–536.

Frey, U., Krug, M., Reymann, K., and Matthies, H. (1988). Anisomycin, an inhibitor of protein synthesis, blocks late phases of LTP phenomena in the hippocampal CA1 region in vitro. *Brain Res.* 452: 57–65.

Frey, U., Frey, S., Schollmeier, F., and Krug, M. (1996). Influence of actinomycin D, a RNA synthesis inhibitor, on long-term potentiation in rat hippocampal neurons in vivo and in vitro. *J. Physiol. (Lond.)* 490: 703–711.

Frey, U., Mueller, M., and Kuhl, D. (1996). A different form of long-lasting potentiation revealed in tissue plasminogen activator mutant mice. *J. Neurosci.* 16: 2057–2063.

Fritz, C. C., Zapp, M. L., and Green, M. R. (1995). A human nucleoporin-like protein that specifically interacts with HIV Rev. *Nature* 376: 530–533.

Gall, C., Lauterborn, J., Bundman, M., Murray, K., and Isackson, P. (1991). Seizures and the regulation of neurotrophic factor and neuropeptide gene expression in brain. *Epilepsy Res. Suppl.* 4: 225–245.

Gall, C. M. (1993). Seizure-induced changes in neurotrophin expression: implications for epilepsy. *Exp. Neurol.* 124: 150–166.

Gall, C. M., and Isackson, P. J. (1989). Limbic seizures increase neuronal production of messenger RNA for nerve growth factor. *Science* 245: 758–761.

Gall, C. M., Lauterborn, J. C., Guthrie, K. M., and Stinis, C. T. (1997). Seizures and the regulation of neurotrophic factor expression: associations with structural plasticity in epilepsy. *Adv. Neurol.* 72: 9–24.

Goelet, P., Castellucci, V. F., Schacher, S., and Kandel, E. R. (1986). The long and the short of long-term memory—a molecular framework. *Nature* 322: 419–422.

Greenberg, M. E., Ziff, E. B., and Greene, L. A. (1986). Stimulation of neuronal acetylcholine receptors induces rapid gene transcription. *Science* 234: 80–83.

Gruber, C. E., Li, W. B., Lin, J. J., and D'Alessio, J. M. (1993). Subtractive cDNA hybridization using the multifunctional plasmid vector pSPORT 2. *Focus* 15: 59–65.

Hagihara, K., Tsumoto, T., Sato, H., and Hata, Y. (1988). Actions of excitatory amino acid antagonists on geniculo-cortical transmission in the cat's visual cortex. *Exp. Brain Res.* 69: 407–416.

Harada, K., Martin, S. S., and Frankel, A. D. (1996). Selection of RNA-binding peptides in vivo. *Nature* 380: 175–179.

Hastings, G. A., Coleman, T. A., Haudenschild, C. C., Stefansson, S., Smith, E. P., Barthlow, R., Cherry, S., Sandkvist, M., and Lawrence, D. A. (1997). Neuroserpin, a brain-associated inhibitor of tissue plasminogen activator is localized primarily in neurons. Implications for the regulation of motor learning and neuronal survival. *J. Biol. Chem.* 272: 33062–33067.

Hebb, D. O. (1949). *The Organization of Behavior: A Neurophysiological Theory.* New York, John Wiley & Sons.

Hegde, A. N., Inokuchi, K., Pei, W., Casadio, A., Ghirardi, M., Chain, D. G., Martin, K. C., Kandel, E. R., and Schwartz, J. H. (1997). Ubiquitin C-terminal hydrolase is an immediate-early gene essential for long-term facilitation in *Aplysia*. *Cell* 89: 115–126.

Herfort, M. R., and Garber, A. T. (1991). Simple and efficient subtractive hybridization screening. *Biotechniques* 11: 598–604.

Hope, T. J., Huang, X. J., McDonald, D., and Parslow, T. G. (1990). Steroid-receptor fusion of the human immunodeficiency virus type 1 Rev transactivator: mapping cryptic functions of the arginine-rich motif. *Proc. Natal. Acad. Sci. USA* 87: 7787–7791.

Hu, Y., Barzilai, A., Chen, M., Bailey, C. H., and Kandel, E. R. (1993). 5-HT and cAMP induce the formation of coated pits and vesicles and increase the expression of clathrin light chain in sensory neurons of aplysia. *Neuron* 10: 921–929.

Huang, Y. Y., Bach, M. E., Lipp, H. P., Zhuo, M., Wolfer, D. P., Hawkins, R. D., Schoonjans, L., Kandel, E. R., Godfraind, J. M., Mulligan, R., Collen, D., and Carmeliet, P. (1996). Mice lacking the gene encoding tissue-type plasminogen activator show a selective interference with late-phase long-term potentiation in both Schaffer collateral and mossy fiber pathways. *Proc. Natl. Acad. Sci. USA* 93: 8699–8704.

Kang, H., and Schuman, E. M. (1996). A requirement for local protein synthesis in neurotrophin-induced hippocampal synaptic plasticity. *Science* 273: 1402–1406.

Kauselmann, G., Konietzko, U., Wulff, P., Scafidi, J., Stäubli, U., and Kuhl, D. (1997). Induced expression of cell-cycle associated kinases in persistent forms of neuronal plasticity. *Soc. Neurosci. Abstr.* 23 (Part 1): 227.

Kennedy, T. E., Kuhl, D., Barzilai, A., Sweatt, J. D., and Kandel, E. R. (1992). Long-term sensitization training in Aplysia leads to an increase in calreticulin, a major presynaptic calcium-binding protein. *Neuron* 9: 1013–1024.

Konietzko, U., and Kuhl, D. (1998). A subtractive hybridisation method for the enrichment of moderately induced sequences. *Nucleic Acids Res.* 26: 1359–1361.

Konietzko, U., Kauselmann, G., Scafidi, J., Stäubli, U., and Kuhl, D. (1997). Substractive hybridization reveals low abundant genes regulated by synaptic activity. *Soc. Neurosci. Abstr.* 23 (Part 1): 232.

Krueger, S. R., Ghisu, G. P., Cinelli, P., Gschwend, T. P., Osterwalder, T., Wolfer, D. P., and Sonderegger, P. (1997). Expression of neuroserpin, an inhibitor of tissue plasminogen activator, in the developing and adult nervous system of the mouse. *J. Neurosci.* 17: 8984–8996.

Krug, M., Lössner, B., and Ott, T. (1984). Anisomycin blocks the late phase of long-term potentiation in the dentate gyrus of freely moving rats. *Brain Res. Bull.* 13: 39–42.

Krystosek, A., and Seeds, N. W. (1981). Plasminogen activator release at the neuronal growth cone. *Science* 213: 1532–1534.

Kuhl, D., and Skehel, P. (1998). Dendritic localization of mRNAs. *Curr. Opin. Neurobiol.* 8: 600–606.

Kuhl, D., de la Fuente, J., Chaturvedi, M., Parimoo, S., Ryals, J., Meyer, F., and Weissmann, C. (1987). Reversible silencing of enhancers by sequences derived from the human IFN-alpha promoter. *Cell* 50: 1057–1069.

Kuhl, D., Kennedy, T. E., Barzilai, A., and Kandel, E. R. (1992). Long-term sensitization training in *Aplysia* leads to an increase in the expression of BiP, the major protein chaperon of the ER. *J. Cell Biol.* 119: 1069–1076.

Lauterborn, J. C., Rivera, S., Stinis, C. T., Hayes, V. Y., Isackson, P. J., and Gall, C. M. (1996). Differential effects of protein synthesis inhibition on the activity-dependent expression of BDNF transcripts: evidence for immediate-early gene responses from specific promoters. *J. Neurosci.* 16: 7428–7436.

Lazarides, E., and Woods, C. (1989). Biogenesis of the red blood cell membrane-skeleton and the control of erythroid morphogenesis. *Annu. Rev. Cell Biol.* 5: 427–452.

Li, W. B., Gruber, C. E., Lin, J. J., Lim, R., D'Alessio, J. M., and Jessee, J. A. (1994). The isolation of differentially expressed genes in fibroblast growth factor stimulated BC3H1 cells by subtractive hybridization. *Biotechniques* 16: 722–729.

Liang, P., Averboukh, L., and Pardee, A. B. (1993). Distribution and cloning of eukaryotic mRNAs by means of differential display: refinements and optimization. *Nucleic Acids Res.* 21: 3269–3275.

Link, W., Konietzko, U., Kauselmann, G., Krug, M., Schwanke, B., Frey, U., and Kuhl, D. (1995). Somatodendritic expression of an immediate early gene is regulated by synaptic activity. *Proc. Natal. Acad. Sci. USA* 92: 5734–5738.

Lyford, G. L., Yamagata, K., Kaufmann, W. E., Barnes, C. A., Sanders, L. K., Copeland, N. G., Gilbert DJ, Jenkins, N. A., Lanahan, A. A., and Worley, P. F. (1995). Arc, a growth factor and activity-regulated gene, encodes a novel cytoskeleton-associated protein that is enriched in neuronal dendrites. *Neuron* 14: 433–445.

Lynch, G., and Baudry, M. (1987). Brain spectrin, calpain and long-term changes in synaptic efficacy. *Brain Res. Bull.* 18: 809–815.

Lynch, G., Larson, J., Staubli, U., and Granger, R. (1991). Variants of synaptic potentiation and different types of memory operations in hippocampus and related structures. In *Memory: Organization and Locus of Change*, L. R. Squire, N. M. Weinberger, G. Lynch, and J. L. McGaugh, eds, pp. 339–363. New York, Oxford University Press.

MacDonald, N. J., Kuhl, D., Maguire, D., Naf, D., Gallant, P., Goswamy, A., Hug, H., Bueler, H., Chaturvedi, M., de la Fuente, J., Ruffner, H., Meyer, F., and Weissmann, C. (1990). Different pathways mediate virus inducibility of the human IFN-alpha 1 and IFN-beta genes. *Cell* 60: 767–779.

MacWilliams, M. P., Celander, D. W., and Gardner, J. F. (1993). Direct genetic selection for a specific RNA-protein interaction. *Nucleic Acids Res.* 21: 5754–5760.

Malim, M. H., Boehnlein, S., Hauber, J., and Cullen, B. R. (1989). Functional dissection of the HIV-1 Rev trans-activator—derivation of a trans-dominant repressor of Rev function. *Cell* 58: 205–214.

Miller, K. D., Chapman, B., and Stryker, M. P. (1989). Visual responses in adult cat visual cortex depend on N-methyl-D-aspartate receptors. *Proc. Natal. Acad. Sci. USA* 86: 5183–5187.

Monard, D. (1988). Cell-derived proteases and protease inhibitors as regulators of neurite outgrowth. *Trends Neurosci.* 11: 541–544.

Morgan, J. I., and Curran, T. (1986). Role of ion flux in the control of c-fos expression. *Nature* 322: 552–555.

Morgan, J. I., Cohen, D. R., Hempstead, J. L., and Curran, T. (1987). Mapping patterns of c-fos expression in the central nervous system after seizure. *Science* 237: 192–197.

Naeve, G. S., Ramakrishnan, M., Kramer, R., Hevroni, D., Citri, Y., and Theill, L. E. (1997). Neuritin: a gene induced by neural activity and neurotrophins that promotes neuritogenesis. *Proc. Natal. Acad. Sci. USA* 94: 2648–2653.

Nedivi, E., Hevroni, D., Naot, D., Israeli, D., and Citri, Y. (1993). Numerous candidate plasticity-related genes revealed by differential cDNA cloning. *Nature* 363: 718–722.

Neuman, T., Stephens, R. W., Salonen, E. M., Timmusk, T., and Vaheri, A. (1989). Induction of morphological differentiation of human neuroblastoma cells is accompanied by induction of tissue-type plasminogen activator. *J. Neurosci. Res.* 23: 274–281.

Nguyen, P. V., Abel, T., and Kandel, E. R. (1994). Requirement of a critical period of transcription for induction of a late phase of LTP. *Science* 265: 1104–1107.

Okabe, A., Momota, Y., Yoshida, S., Hirata, A., Ito, J., Nishino, H., and Shiosaka, S. (1996). Kindling induces neuropsin mRNA in the mouse brain. *Brain Res.* 728: 116–120.

Okano, H. J., and Darnell, R. B. (1997). A hierarchy of Hu RNA binding proteins in developing and adult neurons. *J. Neurosci.* 17: 3024–3037.

Olsen, H. S., Nelbock, P., Cochrane, A. W., and Rosen, C. A. (1990). Secondary structure is the major determinant for interaction of HIV rev protein with RNA. *Science* 247: 845–848.

Otani, S., and Abraham, W. C. (1989). Inhibition of protein synthesis in the dentate gyrus, but not the entorhinal cortex, blocks maintenance of long-term potentiation in rats. *Neurosci. Lett.* 106: 175–180.

Paraskeva, E., Atzberger, A., and Hentze, M. W. (1998). A translational repression assay procedure (TRAP) for RNA-protein interactions in vivo. *Proc. Natal. Acad. Sci. USA* 95: 951–956.

Phizicky, E. M., and Fields, S. (1995). Protein-protein interactions: methods for detection and analysis. *Microbiol. Rev.* 59: 94–123.

Pittman, R. N., Ivins, J. K., and Buettner, H. M. (1989). Neuronal plasminogen activators: cell surface binding sites and involvement in neurite outgrowth. *J. Neurosci.* 9: 4269–4286.

Putz, U., Skehel, P., and Kuhl, D. (1996). A tri-hybrid system for the analysis and detection of RNA-protein interactions. *Nucleic Acids Res.* 24: 4838–4840.

Putz, U., Kremerskothen, J., Skehel, P., and Kuhl, D. (1999). RNA-protein interactions reconstituted by a tri-hybrid system. In *Yeast Hybrid Methods, in vivo Detection of Interaction Between Protein, DNA, RNA, and Other Molecules*, L. Zhu, ed. Natick, MA, Eaton (in press).

Qian, Z., Gilbert, M. E., Colicos, M. A., Kandel, E. R., and Kuhl, D. (1993). Tissue-plasminogen activator is induced as an immediate-early gene during seizure, kindling and long-term potentiation. *Nature* 361: 453–457.

Rubenstein, J. L., Brice, A. E., Ciaranello, R. D., Denney, D., Porteus, M. H., and Usdin, T. B. (1990). Subtractive hybridization system using single-stranded phagemids with directional inserts. *Nucleic Acids Res.* 18: 4833–4842.

Saffen, D. W., Cole, A. J., Worley, P. F., Christy, B. A., Ryder, K., and Baraban, J. M. (1988). Convulsant-induced increase in transcription factor messenger RNAs in rat brain. *Proc. Natal. Acad. Sci. USA* 85: 7795–7799.

Sargent, T. D. (1987). Isolation of differentially expressed genes. *Methods Enzymol.* 152: 423–432.

Seeds, N. W., Williams, B. L., and Bickford, P. C. (1995). Tissue plasminogen activator induction in Purkinje neurons after cerebellar motor learning. *Science* 270: 1992–1994.

SenGupta, D. J., Zhang, B., Kraemer, B., Pochart, P., Fields, S., and Wickens, M. (1996). A three-hybrid system to detect RNA-protein interactions in vivo. *Proc. Natal. Acad. Sci. USA* 93: 8496–8501.

Sheng, M., and Greenberg, M. E. (1990). The regulation and function of c-fos and other immediate early genes in the nervous system. *Neuron* 4: 477–485.

Siman, R., Baudry, M., and Lynch, G. (1985). Regulation of glutamate receptor binding by the cytoskeletal protein fodrin. *Nature* 313: 225–228.

Squire, L. R. (1992). Memory and the hippocampus: a synthesis from findings with rats, monkeys, and humans [published erratum appears in *Psychol. Rev.* (1992) 99: 582]. *Psychol. Rev.* 99: 195–231.

Staubli, U. (1995). Parallel properties of long-term potentiation and memory. In *Brain and Memory: Modulation and Mediation of Neuroplasticity*, J. L. McGaugh, N. M. Weinberger, and G. Lynch, eds, pp. 303–318. New York, Oxford University Press.

Stevens, C. F. (1998). A million dollar question: does LTP = memory? *Neuron* 20: 1–2.

Steward, O. (1997). mRNA localization in neurons: a multipurpose mechanism? *Neuron* 18: 9–12.

Stripecke, R., Oliveira, C. C., McCarthy, J. E., and Hentze, M. W. (1994). Proteins binding to 5′ untranslated region sites: a general mechanism for translational regulation of mRNAs in human and yeast cells. *Mol. Cell Biol.* 14: 5898–5909.

Stutz, F., and Rosbash, M. (1994). A functional interaction between Rev and yeast pre-mRNA is related to splicing complex formation. *EMBO J.* 13: 4096–4104.

Tiedge, H., and Brosius, J. (1996). Translational machinery in dendrites of hippocampal neurons in culture. *J. Neurosci.* 16: 7171–7181.

Torre, E. R., and Steward, O. (1992). Demonstration of local protein synthesis within dendrites using a new cell culture system that permits the isolation of living axons and dendrites from their cell bodies. *J. Neurosci.* 12: 762–772.

Tsirka, S. E., Gualandris, A., Amaral, D. G., and Strickland, S. (1995). Excitotoxin-induced neuronal degeneration and seizure are mediated by tissue plasminogen activator. *Nature* 377: 340–344.

Tsirka, S. E., Rogove, A. D., Bugge, T. H., Degen, J. L., and Strickland, S. (1997). An extracellular proteolytic cascade promotes neuronal degeneration in the mouse hippocampus. *J. Neurosci.* 17: 543–552.

Tsui, C. C., Copeland, N. G., Gilbert, D. J., Jenkins, N. A., Barnes, C., and Worley, P. F. (1996). Narp, a novel member of the pentraxin family, promotes neurite outgrowth and is dynamically regulated by neuronal activity. *J. Neurosci.* 16: 2463–2478.

Wallace, C. S., Hawrylak, N., and Greenough, W. T. (1991). In *Long-Term Potentiation*, M. Baudry and J. L. Davis, eds, pp. 189–122. Cambridge, MA, MIT Press.

Wang, Y. F., Tsirka, S. E., Strickland, S., Stieg, P. E., Soriano, S. G., and Lipton, S. A. (1998). Tissue plasminogen activator (tPA) increases neuronal damage after focal cerebral ischemia in wild-type and tPA-deficient mice [see comments]. *Nat. Med.* 4: 228–231.

Wasenius, V. M., Saraste, M., Salven, P., Eraemaa, M., Holm, L., and Lehto, V. P. (1989). Primary structure of the brain alpha-spectrin [published erratum appears in *J. Cell Biol.* (1989) 108: following 1175]. *J. Cell Biol.* 108: 79–93.

Wigstrom, H., and Gustafsson, B. (1986). Postsynaptic control of hippocampal long-term potentiation. *J. Physiol. Paris* 81: 228–236.

Yamagata, K., Andreasson, K. I., Kaufmann, W. E., Barnes, C. A., and Worley, P. F. (1993). Expression of a mitogen-inducible cyclooxygenase in brain neurons: regulation by synaptic activity and glucocorticoids. *Neuron* 11: 371–386.

Yamagata, K., Sanders, L. K., Kaufmann, W. E., Yee, W., Barnes, C. A., Nathans, D., and Worley, P. F. (1994). rheb, a growth factor- and synaptic activity-regulated gene, encodes a novel Ras-related protein. *J. Biol. Chem.* 269: 16333–16339.

Yin, J. C., Del, V. M., Zhou, H., and Tully, T. (1995). CREB as a memory modulator: induced expression of a dCREB2 activator isoform enhances long-term memory in *Drosophila*. *Cell* 81: 107–115.

Zapp, M. L., and Green, M. R. (1989). Sequence-specific RNA binding by the HIV-1 Rev protein. *Nature* 342: 714–716.

Zapp, M. L., Hope, T. J., Parslow, T. G., and Green, M. R. (1991). Oligomerization and RNA binding domains of the type 1 human immunodeficiency virus Rev protein: a dual function for an arginine-rich binding motif. *Proc. Natal. Acad. Sci. USA* 88: 7734–7738.

2 Synaptic Regulation of Messenger RNA Trafficking within Neurons

Oswald Steward, Christopher S. Wallace, and
Paul F. Worley

There is increasing evidence that enduring forms of activity-induced synaptic plasticity require protein synthesis during a critical time window (for recent reviews, see Bailey et al. 1996; Mayford et al. 1996; Nguyen and Kandel 1996). This conclusion is based on the fact that the establishment of enduring synaptic modifications (the cellular homolog of memory consolidation) can be interrupted by inhibiting protein synthesis. Although there are numerous possible interpretations of this general finding, probably the most widely accepted view is that appropriate patterns of activity at individual synapses induce the synthesis of particular proteins which then are critical for establishing enduring modifications. These modifications involve select populations (synapse-specificity) and occur during a critical time window. Hence, in molecular terms, the epoch of consolidation involves stepwise molecular modifications that are precisely timed and that occur selectively in certain populations of synapses. The steps in the process are not known, and there are several possible mechanisms. In considering the possibilities, it is useful to consider some of the steps that might be involved.

A dependence on protein synthesis could indicate that the required proteins are made from messenger RNAs (mRNAs) that are present constituitively or mRNAs that are synthesized as a consequence of transcriptional activation. If the required proteins are made using existing mRNAs, one would expect there to be some mechanism for regulating translation via synaptic activity. If new gene expression is required to bring about activity-dependent synaptic modifications, there must be some mechanism that would allow signaling from the synapse to the transcriptional machinery of the neuron. This could be directly mediated by signal transduction events triggered specifically by the synapses to be modified, or could be a general signal related to postsynaptic activity. In addition, there must be some means to assure synapse-specificity, because known forms of activity-induced synaptic plasticity apparently occur selectively as a function of the history of activity at individual synapses. Hence, newly synthesized proteins critical for modification could be delivered selectively to the synapses that are to be modified, or could be widely distributed, with synapse-specificity being conferred by some interaction between the newly synthesized proteins and other molecules at synapses that had been modified by synaptic activity.

Are there molecular mechanisms available to neurons that could mediate these functions? The answer is a definite yes. A number of signal transduction pathways have been identified that could regulate translation or mediate signaling from the synapse to the transcriptional machinery of the neuron. Many of these signal transduction pathways have been shown to be activated in situations that lead to enduring synaptic modification.

Also, there are clearly a number of ways that newly synthesized gene products can be delivered to particular synapses in a way that would assure synapse-specificity. For example, neurons could take advantage of known protein transport and targeting mechanisms coupled with some enduring "synaptic tag" brought about as a result of synaptic activity (Frey and Morris 1997). But for maximal economy, it is reasonable to pay special attention to mechanisms that can mediate several of the required functions simultaneously. It is in this regard that evidence demonstrating a mechanism for "synapse-specific gene expression" is of particular interest.

Synapse-specific gene expression refers to the capability that neurons have for transporting particular mRNAs to synaptic sites on dendrites where the mRNAs can be locally translated. This idea had its roots in the discovery of 'synapse-asssociated polyribosome complexes' (SPRCs)—polyribosomes and associated membranous cisterns that are selectively localized beneath postsynaptic sites on the dendrites of central nervous system (CNS) neurons (Steward 1983; Steward and Fass 1983; Steward and Levy 1982). Based on the assumption that form implies function, the highly selective localization of SPRCs beneath synapses suggested the following working hypotheses: (1) that the machinery might synthesize key molecular constituents of the synapse, and (2), that translation might be regulated by activity at the individual postsynaptic site. As discussed below, these working hypotheses have been confirmed, and the idea that these elements may be involved in synaptic plasticity has been reinforced and refined. Moreover, many of the mRNAs that are present in dendrites have been identified, and there is now considerable evidence that these mRNAs do enable a local synthesis of the encoded proteins (Steward et al. 1996; Steward and Singer 1997).

What has been missing until recently is evidence of a linkage between synaptic activation and either the transport of mRNAs into dendrites or the local translation of these mRNAs on site. In this chapter, we summarize some of the recent data that establish that a linkage does exist, and that begin to define the nature of the underlying mechanisms (figure 2.1).

We begin with a brief update regarding mRNAs that are localized in dendrites (and thus potentially present at SPRCs). We summarize recent evidence that local translation of mRNA at the synapse may be regulated by synaptic actvity, and then summarize new information regarding how afferent activity regulates the expression and trafficking of the mRNA for an unusual immediate-early gene (IEG, the mRNA for *arc*, also known as *arg3.1*).

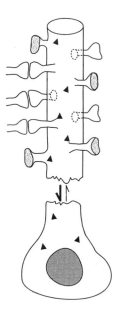
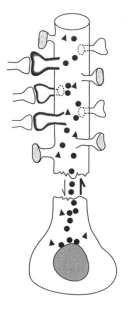
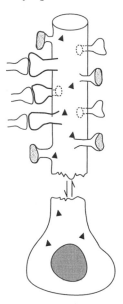

A) Synaptic Activation   **B) Induction and Delivery of *Arc***   **C) Enduring Functional Synaptic Modification?**

Figure 2.1 This schematic diagram illustrates how mRNA trafficking within dendrites (as exemplified by *arc* mRNA) might play a key role in the consolidation of synaptic modifications induced by activity. Hypotheses about the role that a dendritic mRNA might play are based on the fact that synaptic modifications (1) occur at selected synapses on an individual neuron; (2) are triggered by certain patterns of synaptic activity; and (3) require protein synthesis to consolidate a short-term change into an enduring one. The mRNA for *Arc* is induced and regulated in a way that would be consistent with what might be expected for a molecule that is involved in activity-dependent synaptic modifications. The schematic illustrates a potential scheme linking neuronal activation, induction of nuclear gene expression, dendritic transport of mRNA, and translation of the mRNA at synaptic sites that are to be modified. Other mRNAs that are present constitutively in dendrites provide a substrate whereby synaptic activation can also activate translation, thus mediating a local synthesis of other molecules at or near the synaptic sites that are to be modified.

The patterns of expression of the *arc* gene, and the characteristics of the gene product implicate *arc/arg3.1* in activity-dependent synaptic plasticity. We briefly consider very recent evidence indicating that the delivery of other mRNAs into dendrites is also regulated by activity. Finally, we consider how these pieces might fit together to suggest a mechanism through which gene expression at the synapse mediates long-term synaptic modifications induced by activity.

MESSENGER RNAS THAT ARE LOCALIZED IN DENDRITES

It seems a reasonable assumption that important clues about the significance of protein synthesis at the synapse will come from the identification of the proteins that are synthesized at SPRCs. In this regard, important information can be obtained by identifying the mRNAs that are present in dendrites. It is important to recall, however, that the localization of a particular mRNA in dendrites is not ironclad evidence that the mRNA is translated by SPRCs; there are polyribosomes in dendrites which are not localized beneath synapses, and these polyribosomes could be associated with a different set of mRNAs than are translated in the postsynaptic cytoplasm (see Steward and Reeves 1988). Nevertheless, identification of mRNAs that are present in dendrites provides candidates for synapse-associated mRNAs that can be further evaluated in other ways.

As discussed in more detail in previous reviews (Steward et al. 1996; Steward and Singer 1997), most dendritic mRNAs have been identified as such through incidental findings made in the course of in situ hybridization analyses of the cellular distribution of the transcripts of newly cloned genes. Dendritic localization has been inferred by the pattern of labeling in brain regions where neurons are collected in discrete layers, and where there are distinct neuropil layers that contain dendrites and axons but few neuronal cell bodies (cortical regions including the hippocampus and the cerebellar cortex). The presence of labeling in neuropil layers suggests that the mRNA under investigation is localized in dendrites. It is important, however, to exlude the possibility that the labeling reflects the expression of the relevant mRNA by glia, and in this regard, the dendritic localization of many of the mRNAs have been confirmed by studies of neurons in culture.

Table 2.1 lists the mRNAs for which the evidence for dendritic localization in vivo is strong. All of the RNAs listed extend for several hundred micrometers from the cell body. Certain other mRNAs that are localized primarily in cell bodies may extend slightly into proximal dendrites. For example, it has been reported that the mRNA for two protein kinase C substrates (F1, or growth-associated protein-43[GAP-43], and RC3) extend somewhat further into the proximal dendrites of many forebrain than other "cell body" mRNAs. (Laudry et al. 1993). It must be said, however, that the differences in the distribution of mRNAs encoding F1/GAP-43 and RC3 vs. other cell body mRNAs are slight, and indeed were not evident in recent studies using nonisotopic in situ hybridization techniques that produced heavy labeling over cell bodies (Paradies and Steward 1997).

There are several other mRNAs that are detectable by in situ hybridization in the dendrites of young neurons developing in vitro that are not evident in the dendrites of mature neurons in vivo (e.g., the mRNAs for brain-derived neurotrophic factor (BDNF) and trkB receptors; see below). Finally, there are also other "possible" dendritic mRNAs for which the evidence regarding dendritic localization is incomplete or controversial (e.g., the mRNA for a "fragile X"—related protein; see below). Even though there are a number of unresolved issues, the evidence allows several generalizations.

1. There are actually a number of different patterns of mRNA distribution. Some mRNAs are present at relatively high levels throughout dendrites,

Table 2.1 Messenger RNAs that have been shown to be localized within dendrites of neurons in vivo by in situ hybridization. Not shown are mRNAs that are localized only in the most proximal segments

mRNA	Cell type	Localization in dendrites	Class of protein	Protein function
MAP-2 (1)	Cortex, hippocampus dentate gyrus	Proximal 1/3–1/2	Cytoskeletal	Microtubule-associated
CAMII kinase (2) alpha subunit	Cortex, hippocampus dentate gyrus	Throughout	Membrane-associated post-synaptic density	Multifunctional kinase Ca^{2+} signaling
arc/arg 3.1 (3)	Cortex, hippocampus, dentate gyrus, depending on inducing stimulus	Throughout (when induced)	Cytoskeleton-associated	Actin-binding, ?
Dendrin (4)	Hippocampus, dentate gyrus, cerebral cortex	Throughout	Putative membrane	Unknown
G protein (5) gamma subunit	Cortex, hippocampus, dentate gyrus, striatum	Throughout	Membrane-associated	Metabotrophic receptor signaling
Calmodulin (6)	Cortex, hippocampus, Purkinje cells	Proximal-middle (during synaptogenesis)	Cytoplasm and membrane-associated	Ca^{2+} signaling in conjunction with CAMII kinase
NMDAR1 (7)	Dentate gyrus	Proximal-middle?	Integral membrane	Receptor
Glycine receptor (8) alpha subunit	Motoneurons	Proximal	Integral membrane	Receptor
Vasopressin (9)	Hypothalamo-hypophyseal	Proximal-middle	Soluble	Neuropeptide
Neurofilament protein 68 (10)	Vestibular neurons	Proximal-middle	Cytoskeletal	Neurofilament
InsP$_3$ receptor (11)	Purkinje cells	Throughout (concentrated proximally)	Integral membrane (endoplasmic reticulum)	Ca^{2+} signaling
L7 (12)	Purkinje cells	Throughout	Cytoplasmic?	Homology to *c-sis* PDGF oncogene Signaling?
PEP19 (11)	Purkinje cells	Proximal 1/3	Cytoplasmic	Ca^{2+} binding

MAP, microtube-associated protein; CAM, cell adhesion molecule; NMDAR, N-methyl-D-aspartate receptor; InsP$_3$, inosital 1,4,5-triphosphate.
(1) Garner et al., 1988; (2) Burgin et al., 1990; (3) Lyford et al., 1995; (4) Herb et al., 1997; (5) Watson et al., 1994; (6) Berry et al., 1996; (7) Benson et al., 1997; (8) Racca et al., 1997; (9) Prakash et al., 1997; (10) Paradies et al., 1997; (11) Furuichi et al., 1993; (12) Bian et al., 1996.

whereas other mRNAs are concentrated in particular dendritic domains (Paradies and Steward 1997). Also, the degree to which certain mRNAs are localized in dendrites varies across neuron types (Paradies and Steward 1997). We list in table 2.1 only those mRNAs that have a distinctly dendritic distribution in most of the neuron types that express the genes in question. Not included are mRNAs that seem to extend somewhat into proximal dendrites, but which are localized primarily in neuronal cell bodies (the mRNAs for GAP-43 and RC3, for example).

2. All of the dendritic mRNAs that have been identified so far are expressed differentially by different types of neurons. This is especially evident when considering the mRNAs that are present in the dendrites of forebrain neurons vs. cerebellar Purkinje cells.

3. The proteins encoded by the dendritically localized mRNAs include different classes of protein (cytoplasmic, cytoskeletal, integral membrane, and membrane-associated). These proteins have very different functions. This means that it is unlikely that there will be a single purpose for mRNA localization in dendrites (for additional discussion of this point, see Steward 1997).

To elaborate briefly on the implications of these generalizations, the fact that a different mixture of mRNAs is present in the dendrites of different cell types and even different dendritic regions of individual neurons has important implications for understanding the significance of local protein synthesis. For example, although a number of mRNAs are present in the dendrites of cortical neurons, hippocampal pyramidal cells, and dentate granule cells, the patterns of expression and subcellular distributions of the mRNAs are different. The mRNAs for (calcium-calmodulin protein kinase II) (CaMKII), dendrin, and *arc* (when induced) are localized throughout the neuropil layers. In contrast, microtubule-associated protein 2 (MAP-2) mRNA is concentrated in proximal dendrites, and is not detectable in distal dendrites. The mRNAs that are present in the dendrites of Purkinje cells also exhibit different localization patterns; the mRNA for the inosol 1,4,5-triphosphate (InsP$_3$) receptor is present throughout dendrites but is concentrated in the proximal third of the dendrite, whereas L7 mRNA appears to be more uniformly distributed in Purkinje cell dendrites (Bian et al. 1996). These findings indicate that the capability exists for a different mixture of proteins to be synthesized locally in different neuron types and different dendritic domains.

A MUCH LARGER NUMBER OF DIFFERENT mRNAs MAY BE PRESENT IN DENDRITES BUT IN LOW ABUNDANCE

The mRNAs considered above are present in dendrites at levels that are easily detectable by in situ hybridization. Indeed, the localization of these mRNAs in dendrites was established on the basis of in situ hybridization analyses. It is likely that there are more dendritic mRNAs yet to be found. For example, biochemical studies of proteins synthesized within "synaptodendrosomes" (preparations of pinched-off terminals with attached dendritic fragments) suggest that several of the protein constituents of synaptic junctions are locally synthesized within dendrites (Rao and Steward 1991; Steward et al. 1991). The most prominent of these are not in a molecular-weight range that would be consistent with their being the translation products of known dendritic mRNAs.

Systematic searches for new members of the family of dendritic mRNAs must deal with the problem of how to obtain sufficient quantities of mRNA from dendrites that are not contaminated by mRNA from neuronal cell bodies or supporting cells. One approach has been to use patch pipettes to aspirate the cytoplasmic contents of individual dendrites of neurons grown in culture and then use RNA amplification techniques to clone the mRNAs (Miyashiro et al. 1994). This study provided intriguing evidence that there may be a substantial number of mRNAs in dendrites, many of which remain to be characterized. However, certain of the findings are problematic. In particular, the mRNAs for GluR1 receptors were detected, although the mRNAs for these receptors have not been detected in dendrites of neurons in vivo or in vitro. The reason for the disparity of results is not clear. One possibility is that Miyashiro et al. analyzed cytoplasm from dendrites of young neurons developing in culture. These might contain a different complement of mRNAs than the dendrites of mature neurons. Another possibility is that the amplification techniques detect mRNAs which are present in such low abundance that they are not easily detected using routine in situ hybridization techniques. It is also conceivable that some of the mRNAs in dendrites are in a form that somehow interferes with hybridization by complementary probes.

SYNAPTIC REGULATION OF mRNA TRANSLATION AT THE SYNAPSE

As noted above, the selective localization of SPRCs at synapses provides a potential mechanism for locally regulating the production of key proteins that are necessary for synaptic modification. Presumably, these proteins would be synthesized during the period that the synaptic modification was being "consolidated" into a durable form. This local synthesis could either involve mRNAs already in place, or mRNAs that are induced by synaptic activity and delivered into dendrites (like the mRNA for *arc*; see below).

In the case of mRNAs already in place, modulation of the production of proteins during a particular time window would require translational regulation. Is there evidence for such translational regulation of mRNAs at synapses? The answer is a provisional yes. For example, studies involving hippocampal slices have provided evidence that afferent stimulation (activation of the Schaffer collateral system), in conjunction with neurotransmitter application, leads to increases in protein synthesis in the activated dendritic laminae (stratum radiatum). This study evaluated the distribution of newly synthesized protein using autoradiographic techniques after pulse labeling of hippocampal slices with a ^{3}H-labeled protein precursor. Although the results suggest local synthesis within dendrites, the possibility of rapid transport of the newly synthesized proteins from the cell body in these intact neurons cannot be excluded in these experiments.

Other evidence suggesting synaptic regulation of translation within dendrites comes from studies that use synaptoneurosome preparations (a subcellular fraction containing terminals and dendrites isolated by filtration techniques). Both depolarization and neurotransmitter activation lead to an increase in the proportion of mRNA associated with polysomes, and in the levels of protein synthesis within cell fragments in the preparation (Weiler and Greenough 1991, 1993). One important caveat is that it has not yet been established that increases in translational activity reflects events within dendritic fragments rather than events within other cellular elements in the fractions.

In terms of regulating translation in synaptodendrosomes, an especially interesting line of evidence has come from the study of fragile X mental retardation protein (FMRP) and its homologs. FMRP is encoded by a gene called *FMR1* which is affected in human fragile X syndrome. Recent evidence suggests that the protein plays some role in the mechanism through which certain mRNAs are translated at synaptic sites on the dendrites of CNS neurons (Feng et al. 1997; Weiler et al. 1997). This evidence has led to the idea that the neuronal dysfunction that is part of fragile X syndrome may result from a disruption of local synthesis of protein at synapses, which in turn would disrupt synaptic function, especially the capability to undergo long-lasting forms of synaptic plasticity (Comery et al. 1997; Weiler et al. 1997).

The evidence that *FMR1* mRNA itself or its homologs are among the mRNAs that are localized in dendrites and translated at synapses is of two sorts. First, a clone obtained by amplifying mRNAs from cytoplasm that had been aspirated from the dendrites of hippocampal neurons in culture was found to have sequence homology with *FMR1* and a fragile X–related protein termed FRX1 (Weiler et al. 1997). Second, using "synaptoneurosome" preparations and oligonucleotides derived from the *FMR1* sequence, it was shown that activation of metabotropic glutamate receptors increased the proportion of *FMR1* mRNA that was associated with polysomes, implying neurotransmitter-mediated activation of FMRP translation (Weiler et al. 1997). Neurotransmitter activation also increased the total amount of FMR protein in the fractions, implying an increased synthesis of the protein. Also, immunocytochemical studies of brain tissue using antibodies to FMRP revealed immunostaining localized in or very near postsynaptic membrane specializations. Based on this evidence, it was suggested that the *FMR1* mRNA was translated at synapses, and that the newly synthesized protein was then delivered to the synaptic junctional region where it played a key role in synapse maturation or plasticity.

There are some important unresolved issues regarding the hypothesis that FMRP is synthesized at synapses. One key piece of information that is problematic is that *FMR1* mRNA has not been detected in dendrites in vivo by in situ hybridization, despite the fact that the mRNA can be easily detected in neuronal cell bodies (Hinds et al. 1993). It should be emphasized, however, that the study by Hinds et al. did not explicitly set out to assess whether *FMR1* mRNA might be present in dendrites, and so did not undertake an exhaustive analysis. In their study, light labeling can be seen in laminae that contain dendrites (e.g., superficial layers of the cortex). This labeling could be tissue background or might reflect the presence of *FMR1* mRNA in dendrites at relatively low levels with respect to its concentration in cell bodies. In any case, the issue of the presence and especially the distribution of *FMR1* mRNA in dendrites remains to be resolved.

AFFERENT REGULATION OF mRNA TRAFFICKING IN DENDRITES: LESSONS FROM THE STUDY OF *arc*

Of the mRNAs that are present in dendrites, *arc* is of particular interest in terms of a possible involvement in activity-dependent synaptic plasticity. *Arc* was initially discovered in screens for novel *immediate-early genes*, defined in this case as genes that are induced by activity in a protein syn-thesis—independent fashion (Link et al. 1995; Lyford et al. 1995). Like other IEGs, *arc* expression is strongly induced by neuronal activity. However, in dramatic contrast to the mRNAs of other IEGs, *arc* mRNA is rapidly deliv-ered into dendrites. Analysis of a synthetic peptide (based on the sequence deduced from the mRNA) suggests that the protein associates with the cytoskeleton, and that this association is regulated by Ca^{2+} (Lyford et al. 1995). Immunocytochemistry using antibodies against the synthetic peptide indicates that the newly synthesized protein is localized dendrites (Lyford et al. 1995). The other reason that *arc* is of particular interest, considered in more de-tail below, is that *arc* expression is strongly regulated by behavioral experience.

The fact that *arc* mRNA is rapidly delivered into dendrites, whereas the mRNAs for other IEGs remain tightly localized within the cell body, indi-cates that sorting of newly synthesized mRNAs is a highly regulated process (Wallace et al. 1998). Moreover, the fact that *arc* is normally expressed at low levels and is strongly induced by synaptic activity provides an opportu-nity to evaluate the kinetics of the transport and localization processes. Indeed, *arc* has a number of features that would be consistent with it playing a key role in the enduring forms of synaptic modification that require new gene expression (see figure 2.1).

KINETICS OF DELIVERY OF *arc* mRNA INTO DENDRITES

Arc was discovered because it was induced after a single electroconvulsive seizure (ECS). ECS was used because it induces a period of very intense neu-ronal activity within a defined time window. In this way, the pattern of gene induction after a discrete episode of activity can be evaluated.

The time course of *arc* mRNA induction in the hippocampal formation following a single ECS is shown in figure 2.2. Note that basal expression of *arc* mRNA is undetectable in most dentate granule cells in nonstimulated rats, but one hour after ECS, *arc* mRNA levels are massively elevated in most (perhaps all) dentate granule cells. Analysis of the kinetics of *arc* mRNA induction yielded the first estimate of transport rate for an individual dendritic mRNA (approximately 300 μm/hour (see Wallace et al. 1998)). It is noteworthy that this estimate is more than an order of magnitude faster than the rates that had been estimated previously based on the transport of metabolically labeled RNA, most of which is probably ribosomal RNA (Davis et al. 1990). These data also define the interval between the onset of synaptic activation and the arrival of newly synthesized mRNA in dendrites.

Also noteworthy is the fact that *arc* mRNA is present in dendrites transiently after neuronal activation. Peak levels are seen one to two hours after a single ECS; thereafter, the levels of *arc* mRNA rapidly decline. To a first approximation, this time interval corresponds to the period during which synaptic mofifications are sensitive to inhibition of protein synthesis. Hence, the timing of *arc* delivery is synchronous with the protein synthesis—dependent phase of synaptic modification.

Arc mRNA is also induced in dentate granule cells following the induction of LTP in the perforant path (Link et al. 1995; Lyford et al. 1995). Although not evaluated in detail, the kinetics of induction and dendritic delivery appear to be comparable following ECS and the induction of long-term potentiation (LTP). It remains to be seen whether there is any selective targeting of either newly synthesized *arc* mRNA or protein to the synapses that were activated. Selective targeting would be predicted if this general mechanism underlies synapse-specific modifications.

Arc mRNA IS STRONGLY INDUCED BY A NOVEL BEHAVIORAL EXPERIENCE

Obviously, an important motivation for studying molecular processes that are triggered by neuronal activity is to define mechanisms that might be important for the sorts of functional plasticity that are important for behavior. If *arc* mRNA is involved in functional plasticity, the threshold for its induction must extend to behavioral stimuli. As an initial approach to determining whether behavioral experience can regulate the expression and dendritic transport of *arc* mRNA, we employed the environmental complexity paradigm (Wallace et al. submitted). Originally devised by Hebb (Hebb 1949), this manipulation has demonstrated the capacity of experience to significantly alter the postsynaptic structure of a variety of neurons in the CNS (Black et al. 1990; Chang and Greenough 1984; Comery et al. 1995; Greenough and Volkmar 1973; Sirevaag and Greenough 1985). If expression of *arc* mRNA is involved in experience-dependent synaptic modification, more of it should be present in dendrites of rats exploring a complex environment as a

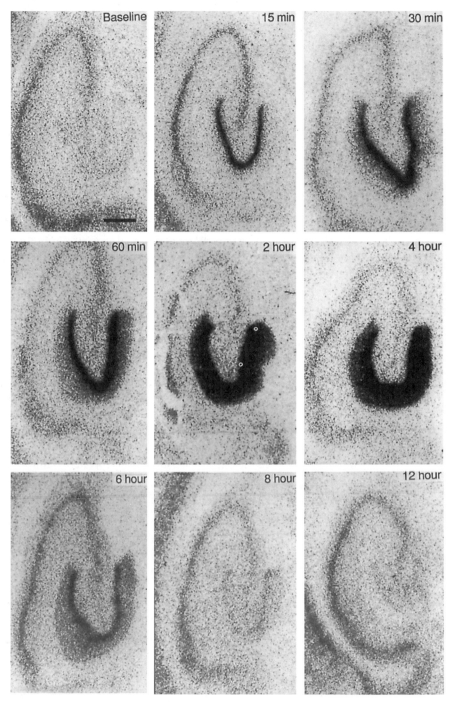

Figure 2.2 Kinetics of *arc* mRNA induction in dentate granule cells following a single electro-convulsive seizure (ECS). Sheet film autoradiograms show labeling of an ^{35}S-labeled cRNA probe for *arc* mRNA in the dentate gyrus at a series of time points after a single ECS. Widespread expression of *arc* mRNA in the somata of a large population of dentate granule cells could be seen within fifteen minutes of ECS. By 30 minutes the labeling extended into the dentate molecule layer, indicating transport of *arc* mRNA into dendrites. Within an hour, labeling was elevated to the distal extent of granule cell dendrites, a distance of up to approximately 300 μm. Levels of *arc* mRNA continued to increase, reaching a peak at two to four hours. By six hours, the amount of *arc* mRNA over the molecular layer was in decline and fell to basal levels by twelve hours. Scale bar: 500 μm. (From Wallace et al. 1998.)

group (EXP) than in cohorts housed undisturbed in standard laboratory cages.

In light of the kinetics of *arc* induction, the expression of *arc* mRNA was examined immediately after brief exposure (fifteen minutes to two hours) to a novel complex environment (EXP) and compared with homecage controls (HC) using nonradioactive in situ hybridization. The experiment was carried out using young rats (twenty-five to forty days old) because of the considerable database available on the long-term consequences of exposure to a complex environment at this age.

As shown in figure 2.3, exposure to a novel complex environment strongly induced *arc* expression in neurons throughout the forebrain. Focusing first on the hippocampal formation, levels of expression were dramatically higher in pyramidal neurons in all CA subfields. While the same exposure also induces mRNAs encoding IEG transcription factors such as *c-fos*, the mRNAs for the other IEGs remain in the cell bodies of hippocampal pyramidal cells at the same time that *arc* mRNA migrates into dendritic laminae (Wallace et al. 1998). Thus, the rapid differential sorting of *arc* mRNA to dendrites represents a new aspect of the primary genomic response to behavioral novelty. Within the context of what is known about trafficking of dendritic mRNA, however, this behavioral induction was surprising both in its magnitude and pattern.

Levels of *arc* mRNA were also dramatically increased in an array of forebrain regions. The pattern of induction (in terms of the neurons exhibiting increased expression) appeared qualitatively similar to that reported previously for the mRNA encoding the IEG transcription factor NGFI-A (i.e., neocortex, striatum, and hippocampal formation; Wallace et al. 1995). Although the general pattern of induction appeared similar, it remains to be determined whether individual neurons upregulate their expression of a number of IEGs or whether different IEGs are induced in different neuron types.

Arc mRNA IS INDUCED IN DIFFERENT POPULATIONS OF NEURONS UNDER DIFFERENT CONDITIONS

The pattern of induction of *arc* expression within the hippocampal formation was especially noteworthy because labeling was most prominent in CA1 pyramidal cells and not dentate granule cells as observed after ECS. This distinct difference is illustrated in figure 2.4, which presents a side-by-side time course of *arc* mRNA induction by behavioral exploration and ECS. Transcriptional activation and dendritic transport appear to occur with similar kinetics, but the induction occurs most prominently in dentate granule cells after ECS, and in hippocampal neurons after exploration. This result suggests that multiple types of neurons have the capacity to deliver newly synthesized *arc* mRNA to their dendrites rapidly, but that this translocation is invoked in different activational contexts depending upon the neuron type.

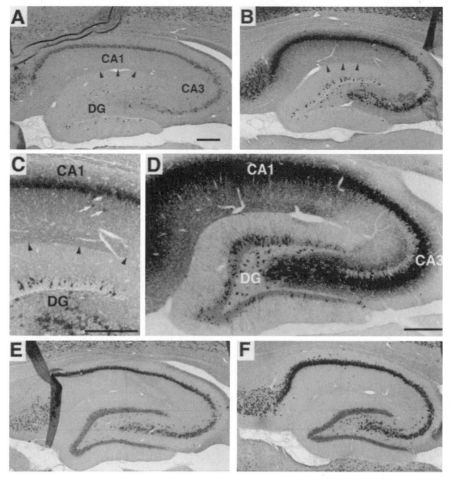

Figure 2.3 Brief exposure to a novel environment induces the expression and dendritic transport of *arc* mRNA. The induction of and intracellular localization of *arc* mRNA was evaluated in the dorsal hippocampal formation of one-hour EXP and HC rats by nonisotopic in situ hybridization using digoxygenin-labeled antisense cRNA probes. Exposure to behavioral novelty resulted in an increase of *arc* mRNA expression by the vast majority of CA1 pyramidal cells (A vs. B) accompanied by an increase in labeling throughout the CA1 molecular layer reflecting dendritic transport of the newly synthesized mRNA. Although *arc* mRNA labeling was detected in the somata of interneurons (C), these cells cannot account for the extent and pattern of labeling within the CA1 molecular layer because of their scarcity and anatomical distribution. Within the dentate gyrus, *arc* expression was restricted to a small subset of granule cells, but the number present in the dorsal blade of the dentate gyrus was increased significantly after exposure to EXP (cf. A and B). D shows a one-hour EXP case hybridized with twice the usual amount of probe to illustrate the heterogeneity of patterns of *arc* expression among principal neurons of the hippocampal formation. Expression and dendritic delivery of *arc* mRNA appeared to occur in nearly every CA1 pyramidal cell, but only a few dentate granule cells. *Arc* mRNA was widely expressed by CA3 pyramidal cells, but dendritic levels were distinctly lower than CA1. *NGFI-A* mRNA (also known as *zif/268*, *egr-1*, and *Krox 24*) is induced by exploration with similar kinetics to *arc* (E vs. F), but remained restricted to the cell body layer, demonstrating that *arc* mRNA is sorted differentially to dendrites. CA1, CA3, hippocampal subfields; DG, dentate gyrus. Black arrowheads mark the hippocampal fissure separating the DG and CA1 dendritic laminae. White arrowheads indicate interneurons in the CA1 molecular layer. DB, VB, dorsal and ventral blades of the dentate gyrus. Scale bar = 300 μm. (From Wallace et al. submitted).

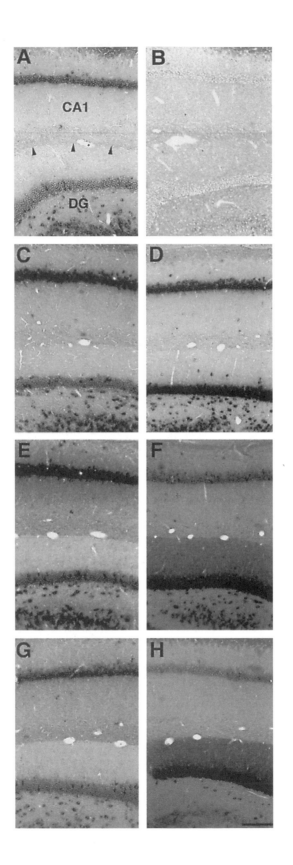

Steward, Wallace, and Worley

IMPLICATIONS OF TRANSIENT VS. CONTINUOUS SUPPLY OF DENDRITIC mRNA TO SYNAPSE FUNCTION

The transient induction of *arc* represents a distinctly different mode of dendritic mRNA supply than is the case for the dendritic mRNAs that are expressed constitutively. After an inducing stimulus, levels of *arc* mRNA rise dramaticaly within dendrites (probably by several orders of magnitude) but then return to control levels within a few hours. Hence, between episodes of massive delivery of *arc* mRNA to dendrites are intervals where the mRNA is quite scarce. In contrast, the mRNAs stationed in dendrites constitutively provide a substrate for synthesizing new proteins, but any regulation would have to be at the level of translation of the mRNA. For these mRNAs, the potential exists for an uncoupling of nuclear transcription and local synaptic translation. In this way, the mixture of proteins that can be synthesized within dendrites varies as a function of the mRNAs that are present.

The transient presence of a dendritic mRNA might allow a protein involved in a specialized physiological adaptation to be present selectively at a critical period during its production-degradation cycle. This would be consistent with a special role for this protein during a particular phase of synaptic modification. In this regard, it is intriguing that the time window when *arc* mRNA is present in dendrites is quite similar to the period during which protein synthesis must occur for synaptic modifications to be consolidated (Frey et al. 1988; Krug et al. 1984; Otani and Abraham 1989; Otani et al. 1989). Additional clues about what the actual role of the protein may be will likely come from studies of the protein itself, and its interactions with other functional molecules of the synaptic junctional region.

ACTIVITY-DEPENDENT TARGETING OF OTHER mRNAs TO THE DENDRITES OF NEURONS DEVELOPING IN VITRO

Recent findings resulting from studies of neurons in culture suggest that there are other mRNAs that are delivered into dendrites in an activity-

Figure 2.4 Exploration and ECS induce *arc* mRNA maximally in separate regions of the hippocampal formation. Detail of the hippocampal formation showing the kinetics of expression and pattern of induction of *arc* mRNA following exposure to a novel complex environment (EXP) and ECS. (A) *arc* mRNA expression in a rat housed undisturbed in a familiar homecage (HC) shown by in situ hybridization using digoxygenin-labeled antisense cRNA probes. (B) Control section showing background labeling observed with sense probe. *Arc* mRNA induction by exposure to a novel environment (EXP) at fifteen minutes (C), one hour (E), and two hours (G). EXP induces *arc* mRNA. Induction by ECS at fifteen minutes (D), one hour (F), and two hours (H). Using the hippocampal fissure (marked in A) as a landmark, it is obvious that these two treatments induce striking different regional patterns of *arc* mRNA expression and dendritic delivery. EXP triggers induction most prominently in pyramidal cells of CA1, whereas after ECS induction is most pronounced in granule cells of the dentate gyrus. Scale bar = 300 μm. (From Wallace et al. submitted.)

dependent fashion. For example, in hippocampal neurons growing in culture, the mRNAs for *BDNF* and *Trkb* are localized primarily in the cell body when the neurons are maintained in standard medium. If, however, neuronal activity is transiently induced by transferring neurons to a medium containing high K^+ (10 or 20 mM) for several hours, the mRNAs for *BDNF* and *TrkB* migrate for considerable distances into dendrites (Tongiorgi et al. 1997).

It is noteworthy that intense neuronal activity also upregulates *BDNF* expression by neurons in vivo (Hughes et al. 1993). Indeed, the pattern of induction following ECS is similar to that seen for *arc*, in that dentate granule cells exhibit especially high levels of induction. Nevertheless, despite the similar patterns of induction, *BDNF* mRNA remains tightly localized in the region of the neuronal cell body during the same time periods and in the same neuronal types in which *arc* mRNA is delivered into dendrites. It may be that the activity-dependent dendritic localization in neurons in vitro is unique to the in vitro setting or to neurons at a particular developmental age. Alternatively, the manipulations that cause dendritic localization in vitro were of long duration (several hours of exposure to high K^+), whereas the ECSs that induce *BDNF* expression in vivo produce only brief periods of increased activity. Hence, it is possible that dendritic transport of *BDNF* would be seen if neuronal activity was maintained at a high level after inducing *BDNF* expression. These and other questions remain to be addressed.

BRINGING IT BACK TO THE SYNAPSE: ARE NEWLY SYNTHESIZED mRNAs OR PROTEINS TARGETED SELECTIVELY TO SYNAPSES UNDERGOING MODIFICATION?

Studies of the induction and dendritic transport of *arc* mRNA have so far revealed that neurons possess mechanisms that would be quite useful for mediating activity-induced protein synthesis—dependent synaptic modifications. To briefly summarize the key findings regarding *arc*: (1) *arc* mRNA is induced in cells known to be undergoing enduring synaptic modification in response to patterned afferent activation and behavioral experience; (2) *arc* mRNA is present in dendrites during the period in which synaptic modifications are sensitive to protein synthesis inhibition; (3) *arc* protein has features that would be consistent with its involvement in synaptic modification; and (4) *arc* expression is induced by the sorts of behavioral experience that lead to long-lasting synaptic modifications. These features of *arc* certainly motivate continued interest.

There are a number of pieces of the puzzle that are still missing, however. First, it remains to be seen whether *arc* mRNA or protein can be selectively targeted to the synapses that are to be modified. Such evidence would close the signaling loop by providing the first example of activity-regulated synapse-specific gene expression. Second, it remains to be established whether *arc* in fact plays a role in activity-induced synaptic modification. But even if *arc* does turn out to be a "red herring," the way that *arc* is handled by neurons reveals the presence of RNA trafficking mechanisms that could be used for sorting other mRNAs that *do* play a key role in bringing about activity-dependent modifications.

At the same time, it is important not to lose sight of the fact that other mRNAs are present in dendrites constitutively, including the mRNAs for molecules that have already been strongly implicated in activity-dependent synaptic modification (the mRNA for the alpha subunit of CaMII kinase, for example). These mRNAs that are present constitutively provide an opportunity for local regulation of the synthesis of key signaling molecules (via translational regulation). Hence, gene expression at individual synapses may be regulated in a complex fashion, first through the regulation of the mRNAs available for translation (i.e., *arc*) and then by regulation of the translation of the mix of mRNAs that are in place, including those present constitutively (a model of which might be the translational regulation of fragile X; see Weiler et al. 1997). How this is coordinated, and how all of these molecules actually fit into the molecular consolidation process remains to be established.

ACKNOWLEDGMENTS

Thanks to Christine Duncan, Paula Falk, Debbie Keelean, and Leanna Whitmore for technical assistance. Supported by NIH NS12333 (O.S.), NSF IBN92–22120 (O.S.), NIH MH 53603 (P.F.W.), NIH/NINDS Individual NRSA NS0973 (C.S.W.).

REFERENCES

Bailey, C. H., Bartsch, D., and Kandel, E. R. (1996). Toward a molecular definition of long-term memory storage. *Proc. Natl. Acad. Sci. USA* 93: 13445–13452.

Benson, D. L. (1997). Dendritic compartmentation of NMDA receptor mRNA in cultured hippocampal neurons. *Neuroreport* 8: 823–828.

Berry, F. B., and Brown, I. R. (1996). CaM I mRNA is localized to apical dendrites during post-natal development of neurons in the rat brain. *J. Neurosci. Res.* 43: 565–575.

Bian, F., Chu, T., Schilling, K., and Oberdick, J. (1996). Differential mRNA transport and the regulation of protein synthesis: Selective sensitivity of purkinje cell dendritic mRNAs to translational inhibition. *Mol. Cell. Neurosci.* 7: 116–133.

Black, J. E., Isaacs, K. R., Anderson, B. J., Alcantara, A. A., and Greenough, W. T. (1990). Learning causes synaptogenesis, whereas motor activity causes angiogenesis, in cerebellar cortex of adult rats. *Proc. Natl. Acad. Sci. USA* 87: 5568–5572.

Burgin, K. E., Washam, M. N., Rickling, S., Westgate, S. A., Mobley, W. C., and Kelly, P. T. (1990). *In situ* hybridization histochemistry of CA^{++}/calmodulin-dependent protein kinase in developing rat brain. *J. Neurosci.* 10: 1788–1798.

Chang, F.-L. F., and Greenough, W. T. (1984). Transient and enduring morphological correlates of synaptic activity and efficacy change in the rat hippocampal slice. *Brain Res.* 309: 35–46.

Comery, T. A., Shah, R., and Greenough, W. T. (1995). Differential rearing alters spine density on medim-sized spiny neurons in the rat corpus striatum: evidence for association of morphological plasxticity with early response gene expression. *Neurobiol. Learn. Mem.* 63: 217–219.

Comery, T. A., Harris, J. B., Willems, P. J., Oostra, B. A., Irwin, S. A., Weiler, I. J., and Greenough, W. T. (1997). Abnormal dendritic spines in fragile X knockout mice: maturation and pruning deficits. *Procl. Natl. Acad. Sci. USA* 94: 5401–5404.

Davis, L., Burger, B., Banker, G., and Steward, O. (1990). Dendritic transport: quantitative analysis of the time course of somatodendritic transport of recently synthesized RNA. *J. Neurosci.* 10: 3056–3058.

Feng, Y., Gutekunst, C.-A., Eberhart, D. E., Yi, H., Warren, S. T., and Hersch, S. M. (1997). Fragile X mental retardation protein: nucleocytoplasmic shuttling and association with somatodendritic ribosomes. *J. Neurosci.* 17: 1539–1547.

Frey, U., and Morris, R. G. M. (1997). Synaptic tagging and long-term potentiation. *Nature* 385: 533–536.

Frey, U., Krug, M., Reymann, K. G., and Matthies, H. (1988). Anisomycin, an inhibitor of protein synthesis, blocks late phases of LTP phenomena in the hippocampal CA1 region in vitro. *Brain Res.* 452: 57–65.

Furuichi, T., Simon-Chazottes, D., Fujino, I., Yamada, N., Hasegawa, M., Miyawaki, A., Yoshikawa, S., Guenet, J.-L., and Mikoshiba, K. (1993). Widespread expression of inositol 1,4,5–trisphosphate receptor type 1 gene (Insp3r1) in the mouse central nervous system. *Receptors Channels* 1: 11–24.

Garner, C. C., Tucker, R. P., and Matus, A. (1988). Selective localization of messenger RNA for cytoskeletal protein MAP2 in dendrites. *Nature* 336: 674–677.

Greenough, W. T., and Volkmar, F. R. (1973). Pattern of dendritic branching in occipital cortex of rats reared in complex environments. *Exp. Neurol.* 40: 491–504.

Hebb, D. O. (1949). *The Organization of Behavior*. New York, John Wiley & Sons.

Herb, A., Wisden, W., Catania, d. M. V., Marechal, D., Dresse, A., and Seeberg, P. H. (1997). Prominent dendritic localization in forebrain neurons of a novel mRNA and its product, dendrin. *Mol. Cell. Neurosci.* 8: 367–374.

Hinds, H. L., Ashley, C. T., Sutcliffe, J. S., Nelson, D. L., Warren, S. T., Housman, D. E., and Schalling, M. (1993). Tissue specific expression of FMR-1 provides evidence for a functional role in fragile X syndrome. *Nat. Genet.* 3: 36–43.

Hughes, P., Beilharz, E., Gluckman, P., and Dragunow, M. (1993). Brain-derived neurotrophic factor is induced as an immediate early gene following N-methyl-D-aspartate receptor activation. *Neuroscience* 57: 319–328.

Krug, M., Lossner, B., and Ott, T. (1984). Anisomycin blocks the late phase of long-term potentiation in the dentate gyrus of freely moving rats. *Brain Res. Bull.* 13: 39–42.

Laudry, C. F., Watson, J. B., Handley, V. W., and Campagnoni, A. T. (1993). Distribution of neuronal and glial mRNAs within neuronal cell bodies and processes. *Soc. Neurosci. Abstr.* 19: 1745.

Link, W., Konietzko, G., Kauselmann, G., Krug, M., Schwanke, B., Frey, U., and Kuhl, K. (1995). Somatodendritic expression of an immediate early gene is regulated by synaptic activity. *Proc. Natl. Acad. Sci. USA* 92: 5734–5738.

Lyford, G., Yamagota, K., Kaufmann, W., Barnes, C., Savokrs, L., Capelard, N., Gilbert, D., Jenkins, N., Lanohar, A., Warley, P. (1995). Arc, a growth factor and activity-regulated gene, encodes a novel cytoskeleton-associated protein that is enriched in neuronal dendrites. *Neuron* 14: 433–445.

Mayford, M., Bach, M. E., Huang, Y.-Y., Wang, L., Hawkins, R. D., and Kandel, E. R. (1996). Control of memory formation through regulated expression of a CaMKII transgene. *Science* 274: 1678–1683.

Miyashiro, K., Dichter, M., and Eberwine, J. (1994). On the nature and differential distribution of mRNAs in hippocampal neurites: implications for neuronal functioning. *Proc. Natl. Acad. Sci. USA* 91: 10800–10804.

Nguyen, P. V., and Kandel, E. R. (1996). A macromoleular synthesis-dependent late phase of long-term potentiation requiring cAMP in the medial perforant pathway of rat hippocampal slices. *J. Neurosci.* 16: 3189–3198.

Otani, S., and Abraham, W. C. (1989). Inhibition of protein synthesis in the dentate gyrus, but not the entorhinal cortex, blocks maintenance of long-term potentiation in rats. *Neurosci. Lett.* 106: 175–180.

Otani, S., Marshall, C. J., Tate, W. P., Goddard, G. V., and Abraham, W. C. (1989). Maintenance of long-term potentiation in rat dentate gyrus requires protein synthesis but not messenger RNA synthesis immediate post-tetanization. *Neuroscience* 28: 519–526.

Paradies, M. A., and Steward, O. (1997). Multiple subcellular mRNA distribution patterns in neurons: a nonisotopic in situ hybridization analysis. *J. Neurobiol.* 33: 473–493.

Prakash, N., Fehr, S., Mohr, E., and Richter, D. (1997). Dendritic localization of rat vasopressin mRNA: ultrastructural analysis and mapping of targeting elements. *Eur. J. Neurosci.* 9: 523–532.

Racca, C., Gardiol, A., and Triller, A. (1997). Dendritic and postsynaptic localizations of glycine receptor alpha subunit mRNAs. *J. Neurosci.* 17: 1691–1700.

Rao, A., and Steward, O. (1991). Evidence that protein constituents of postsynaptic membrane specializations are locally synthesized: analysis of proteins synthesized within synaptosomes. *J. Neurosci.* 11: 2881–2895.

Sirevaag, A. M., and Greenough, W. T. (1985). Differential rearing effects on rat visual cortex synapses. II. Synaptic morphometry. *Dev. Brain Res.* 19: 215–226.

Steward, O. (1983). Polyribosomes at the base of dendritic spines of CNS neurons: Their possible role in synapse construction and modification. *Cold Spring Harbor Symp. Quant. Biol.* 48: 745–759.

Steward, O. (1997). mRNA localization in neurons: a multipurpose mechanism. *Neuron* 18: 9–12.

Steward, O., and Fass, B. (1983). Polyribosomes associated with dendritic spines in the denervated dentate gyrus: evidence for local regulation of protein synthesis during reinnervation. *Prog. Brain Res.* 58: 131–136.

Steward, O., and Levy, W. B. (1982). Preferential localization of polyribosomes under the base of dendritic spines in granule cells of the dentate gyrus. *J. Neurosci.* 2: 284–291.

Steward, O., and Reeves, T. M. (1988). Protein synthetic machinery beneath postsynaptic sites on CNS neurons: association between polyribosomes and other organelles at the synaptic site. *J. Neurosci.* 8: 176–184.

Steward, O., and Singer, R. H. (1997). The intracellular mRNA sorting system: Postal zones, zip codes, mail bags and mail boxes. In *mRNA Metabolism and Post-Transcriptional Gene Regulation*, J. B. Hartford and D. R. Morris, eds., pp. 127–146. New York, Wiley-Liss.

Steward, O., Pollack, A., and Rao, A. (1991). Evidence that protein constituents of postsynaptic membrane specializations are locally synthesized: time course of appearance of recently synthesized proteins in synaptic junctions. *J. Neurosci. Res.* 30: 649–660.

Steward, O., Falk, P. M., and Torre, E. R. (1996). Ultrastructural basis for gene expression at the synapse: synapse-associated polyribosome complexes. *J. Neurocytol.* 25: 717–734.

Steward, O., Kleiman, R., and Banker, G. (1996). Subcellular localization of mRNA in neurons. In *Localized RNAs Molecular Biology Intelligence Unit Series*, H. D. Lipshitz, ed, pp. 235–255. Boca Raton, FL, CRC Press.

Tongiorgi, E., Righi, M., and Cattaneo, A. (1997). Activity-dependent dendritic targeting of BDNF and TrkB mRNAs in hippocampal neurons. *J. Neurosci.* 17: 9492–9505.

Wallace, C. S., Lyford, G. L., Worley, P. F., and Steward, O. (1998). Differential intracellular sorting of immediate early gene mRNAs depends on signals in the mRNA sequence. *J. Neurosci.* 18: 26–35.

Wallace, C. S., Withers, G. S., Ivan, J. W., George, J. M., Clayton, D. F., and Grenough, W. T. (1995). Correspondence between sites of NGFI-A induction and sites of morphological plasticity following exposure to environmental complexity. *Mol. Brain Res.* 32: 211–220.

Wallace, C. S., Mehra, A., Lyford, G. L., Worley, P. F., and Steward, O. (submitted). Brief exposure to a novel environment induces the expression and differential dendritic transport of *arc* mRNA.

Watson, J. B., Coulter, P. M., Margulies, J. E., de Lecea, L., Danielson, P. E., Erlander, M. G., and Sutcliffe, J. G. (1994). G-protein γ_7 subunit is selectively expressed in medium-sized neurons and dendrites of the rat neostriatum. *J. Neurosci. Res.* 39: 108–116.

Weiler, I. J., and Greenough, W. T. (1991). Potassium ion stimulation triggers protein translation in synaptoneuronsomal polyribosomes. *Mol. Cell. Neurosci.* 2: 305–314.

Weiler, I. J., and Greenough, W. T. (1993). Metabotropic glutamate receptors trigger postsynaptic protein synthesis. *Proc. Natl. Acad. Sci. USA* 90: 7168–7171.

Weiler, I. J., Irwin, S. A., Klintsova, A. Y., Spencer, C. M., Brazeltan, A. D., Miyashivo, K., Comery, T. A., Patel, B., Eberwine, I., Greenough, W. T. (1997). Fragile X mental retardation protein is translated near synapses in response to neurotransmitter activation. *Proc. Natl. Acad. Sci. USA* 94: 5395–5400.

3 Matrix Metalloproteinases and Tissue Inhibitors of Metalloproteinases in Neuronal Plasticity and Pathology

Santiago Rivera and Michel Khrestchatisky

The term *plasticity* carries the notion of irreversibility. Neuronal plasticity involves, in part, changes in cell morphology and environment. By virtue of their irreversible nature, proteolytic modifications of proteins are ideally suited to promote plasticity. An important component of the cellular environment is the extracellular matrix (ECM), which is composed of glycoproteins, proteoglycans, and glycosaminoglycans that are secreted and assembled locally into an organized network to which cells adhere (see Adams and Watt 1993 for review). The ECM plays an important role in modulating gene expression, cytoskeletal organization, cell differentiation, and migration, and there is now convincing evidence that the ECM also functions as a survival factor for many cell types (Meredith et al. 1993). ECM integrity in normal physiological conditions depends on a refined balance between the activity and inhibition of ECM proteinases. When this balance is altered, limited proteolysis necessary for physiological remodeling of tissue is no longer under control and pathologic changes may ensue. Among the different families of ECM proteinases, the family of matrix metalloproteinases (MMPs) have been in the scope of intensive research in peripheral tissues. The MMPs belong to a rapidly growing family—to date at least 19 members have been identified—of Zn^{2+}-dependent endopeptidases, including gelatinases, collagenases, stromelysins, the membrane-type MMPs (MT-MMPs) (reviewed in Borden and Heller 1997), and other MMPs that do not belong to these subfamilies (table 3.1). The MMPs are expressed as zymogens that are activated upon proteolytic cleavage of the propeptide region. They are able to cleave protein components of the ECM and to process a number of cell surface receptors, cytokines, and other soluble proteins. Their proteolytic activity is controlled by the tissue inhibitors of metalloproteinases (TIMPs), a family of secreted glycoproteins that comprises at least four members (TIMP-1 through 4), with 30% to 40% sequence similarity (Edwards et al. 1996; Greene et al. 1996). All TIMPs are able to inhibit the active forms of all MMPs by forming tight noncovalent 1 : 1 complexes with them; TIMP binding to latent forms of MMPs has also been demonstrated (reviewed in Kleiner and Stetler-Stevenson 1993). There is evidence that in addition to

Table 3.1

Group	Members	Nomenclature	kDa	Known substrates
Collagenases	Interstitial collagenase	*MMP-1	54	Collagen type I, II, III, VII, X, gelatins, entactin, link protein, aggrecan, α_2-macroglobulin.
	Neutrophil collagenase	MMP-8	53	L-selectin, IGF-binding protein, pro-MMPs (2, 9), α_2-macroglobulin.
	Collagenase-3	MMP-13	54	α_1-proteinase inhibitor, tenascin, pro-TNF-α
	Collagenase-4	xCol4	57	Collagens
Gelatinases	Gelatinase-A	*MMP-2	72	Gelatins, collagen type I, IV, V, VII, X, XI, elastin, fibronectin, laminin, link protein, aggrecan, galectin-3, IGF-binding protein, vitronectin.
	Gelatinase-B	*MMP-9	92	FGF receptor-1, pro-MMPs (2, 9, 13), thrombospondin, substance P, amyloid precursor protein, amyloid-β peptide, myelin basic protein, TNF-α, interleukin-1β
Stromelysins	Stromelysin-1	*MMP-3	54	Proteoglycans, laminin, aggrecan, fibronectin, gelatins, collagen type III, IV, V IX, X, XI, link protein, fibrin/fibrinogen, entactin, tenascin, vitronectin.
	Stromelysin-2	MMP-10	54	L-selectin, pro-MMPs (1, 2, 7, 8, 9, 13), α_1-proteinase inhibitor, α_2-macroglobulin, pro-TNF-α
	Matrilysin	*MMP-7	30	
	Stromelysin-3	MMP-11	55	Laminin, fibronectin, aggrecan, α_1-proteinase inhibitor, α_2-macroglobulin
MT-MMPs	MT1-MMP	*MMP-14	63	Collagen type I, II, III, fibronectin, laminin, vitronectin, proteoglycans
	MT2-MMP	*MMP-15	64	gelatins, pro-MMPs (2, 13), α_1-proteinase inhibitor, α_2-macroglobulin.
	MT3-MMP	*MMP-16	64	pro-MMP-2, collagens, gelatins
	MT4-MMP	*MMP-17	72	
Others	Macrophage metalloelastase	MMP-12	54	Elastin, fibrin/fibrinogen, fibronectin, laminin, proteoglycans, plasminogen, myelin basic protein, α_1-proteinase inhibitor
	Enamelysin	MMP-20	54	Amelogenin
	Xenopus MMP	XMMP		Not known
		MMP-18		Not known
		MMP-19		Aggrecan

TIMPs			
*TIMP-1	28	Pro-MMP-9, all MMPs except MT1-MMP
*TIMP-2	21	Pro-MMP-2, all MMPs
*TIMP-3	24	MMPs
*TIMP-4	22	MMPs

MMP, matrix metalloproteinases; I6F, insulin-like growth factor; TNF-α, tumor necrosis factor-α; F6F, fibroblast growth factor; TIMP, tissue inhibitors of metalloproteinases; MT-MMPs, membrane-type matrix metalloproteinases.

their antiproteolytic activity, TIMPs possess growth-promoting properties and mitogenic activity in a variety of cultured cells (reviewed in Edwards et al. 1996).

The knowledge of the biology of TIMPs and MMPs has blossomed over the past few years, and there is increasing evidence to suggest that they may be instrumental in a large spectrum of physiological and pathological processes, including those associated with the degeneration of connective tissue such as rheumatoid arthritis and osteoarthritis, cancer progression, and the formation of metastasis, arteriosclerosis, inflammatory processes, and autoimmune diseases (Werb 1997). Metalloproteinases have thus become pharmacological targets of primary importance in peripheral tissues. In comparison, little attention has been paid to the role of MMPs and TIMPs in the physiopathology of the central nervous system (CNS) while it is established that MMPs and TIMPs are expressed in the CNS (see table 3.1). This chapter summarizes recent findings concerning the modulation of MMPs and TIMPs in the nervous system and discusses their potential roles as modulators of neuronal plasticity and pathologic processes via their interactions with matrix and nonmatrix substrates (figure 3.1).

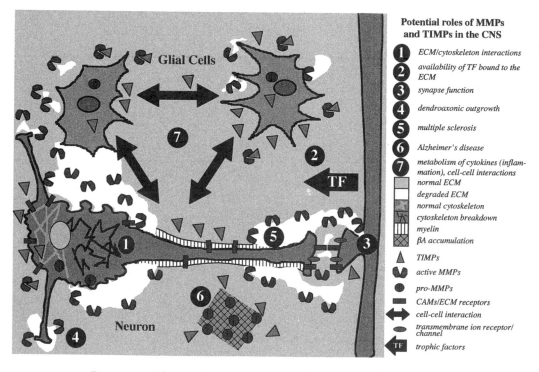

Figure 3.1 Schematic drawing representing the potential roles of matrix metalloproteinases (MMPs) and tissue inhibitors of metalloproteinases (TIMPs) in CNS plasticity and pathologic conditions.

Rivera and Khrestchatisky

THE EXTRACELLULAR MATRIX IN THE CENTRAL NERVOUS SYSTEM

This section is dedicated to a brief overview of some families of ECM components and cell adhesion molecules (CAMs) that are relevant to cell-cell and cell-ECM interactions in the CNS and that are known to interact with the MMPs (see table 3.1). More exhaustive reviews on the ECM in the CNS have been published elsewhere (Letourneau et al. 1994; Perris 1997).

Camillo Golgi described many years ago (Golgi 1889) perineuronal nets enveloping the cell bodies and proximal dendrites of certain neurons in the adult mammalian CNS, suggestive of a supportive and protective scaffolding. The netlike appearance is due to the perisynaptic arrangement of the astrocytic processes and extracellular components that are confined to the space interposed between glial processes and the nerve cells they outline (Koppe et al. 1997). A better understanding of the composition and role of the extra- and pericellular molecules in the CNS is necessary for an insight into the involvement of MMPs in neural plasticity and pathological conditions. Indeed, a large body of evidence implies a role for the ECM in neural cell motility, in neurite outgrowth, growth cone targeting, synapse-specificity and stabilization, in plasticity, and in tissue remodeling during or following lesions. ECM constituents may arbitrarily be subdivided into permissive, nonpermissive, and inhibitory molecules with respect to their action on cell motility and neurite outgrowth. Many ECM molecules have all three properties, depending on the cell types, stages of development, and extensive structural variability (alternative splicing, post-translational modifications). The ECM also promotes development, differentiation, and plasticity by regulating signal transduction, local concentrations of growth factors, and relationships (trophic, inflammatory) between glia and neurons. Until substrate-specificity is determined for each proteinase, all extracellular molecules of the CNS are potential substrates for extracellular proteinases in general and for MMPs in particular.

ECM Diversity and Involvement in Development and in Tissue Remodeling in Pathological Conditions

In the following paragraphs we first describe the expression and suggested functions of glycoproteins and of proteoglycans, a diverse class of glycoproteins, present both as ECM components and as cell surface molecules. Second, we address cell surface molecules and receptors that mediate neural interactions with the ECM and their environment.

Glycoproteins and Proteoglycans *Glycoproteins* are involved in a large diversity of interactions since several of them bind in both a homophilic and heterophilic manner to components of the ECM and of the cell surface. *Fibronectin* and *laminin* participate in differentiation, neuronal migration, and neurite outgrowth during ontogenesis and they have high neurite-promoting activity on primary cultured neurons from the embryonic brain (reviewed in Frisen 1997). Fibronectin expression is increased during neurite regeneration in situations of lesion, and by reactive astrocytes following seizure-induced hippocampal lesions (Niquet et al. 1994). The proteolytic digestion of fibronectin by both MMP-3 and plasmin, a secreted serine proteinase that activates MMPs (Werb et al. 1977), releases a fibronectin fragment that inhibits Schwann cell proliferation (Muir and Manthorpe 1992). Laminin, which is also a substrate of MMPs, preserves neuron-ECM interactions in the adult brain. Laminin immunoreactivity is increased in areas of axonal sprouting after seizures (Represa et al. 1994) and its proteolytic degradation by a plasmin-activated pathway contributes to neuronal death in the hippocampus (Chen and Strickland 1997).

Vitronectin is an ECM glycoprotein involved in axonal growth. Following seizures, reactive glial cells express a vitronectin-like protein which may contribute to the sprouting of mossy fibers in the hippocampus (Niquet et al. 1996). *Thrombospondin (TSP)* is a secreted, trimeric glycoprotein associated with neurons in the brains of adult mice (Hoffman et al. 1994; Iruela-Arispe et al. 1993) that mediates cell-ECM interactions and that modulates neurite outgrowth, migration, and proliferation. TSP is also expressed by brain microglia and by reactive astrocytes, which may contribute actively to neurite growth or regeneration during development or in pathological contexts (Chamak et al. 1995; Eddleston and Mucke 1993). *Tenascin-cytotactin (tenascin-C)* regulates cell migration and neurite outgrowth in the developing CNS. In vitro studies show that tenascin can both promote and inhibit neuronal migration and neurite elongation (Lochter et al. 1991). In developing tissues, tenascin expression correlates with the maintenance of synaptic malleability, while in the adult it is restricted to brain areas known for their plasticity. We and others have shown a correlation between tenascin-C expression and remodeling in animal models of epilepsy and synaptic activation (Ferhat et al. 1996; reviewed in Schachner 1997). *Tenascin-R* and *janusin* are structural homologs of tenascin-C. The first inhibits fibronectin-dependent cell adhesion and neurite outgrowth (Pesheva et al. 1997), and the second promotes axonal but not dendritic growth (Lochter et al. 1994).

Proteoglycans (PGs) are a class of glycoproteins involved in cell-cell and cell-ECM interactions; in growth factor binding, sequestration, and presentation; and in signal transduction. They are expressed in developing and mature brains not only as ECM components but also in cell surface, membrane spanning, and soluble forms. Proteoglycans have a high content of *glycosaminoglycan* sugar moieties that include dermatan sulfate, keratan sulfate, chondroitin sulfate (CS), hyaluronic acid (HA), and heparan sulfate (HS) (reviewed in Letourneau et al. 1994).

Chondroitin sulfate proteoglycans (CSPGs) and chondroitin unsulfated proteoglycans are detected in perineuronal nets that ensheath subsets of neurons in the adult mammalian brain (Bertolotto et al. 1996). CSs are mostly implicated as active components of barriers that cause the repulsion of advancing axons in vivo and in vitro (Snow et al. 1990; Brittis et al. 1992). It has also been shown that CSPGs have a protective action against cell death induced by glutamate (Okamoto et al. 1994). The *aggrecan* family, *or lecticans*, are a family of CSPGs characterized by the presence of a C-terminal lectin-like domain (that binds the ECM protein tenascin-R) and an N-terminal HA-binding domain that confers cell- and tissue-specific functions via HA-binding proteins.

Five lectican family proteoglycans have been characterized by molecular cloning, namely brevican, neurocan, phosphacan, aggrecan, and versican. *Brevican*, which is produced by astrocytes (Yamada et al. 1997), is one of the most abundant CSPGs in the adult brain and its expression increases in the course of ontogeny (reviewed in Yamaguchi 1996). *Neurocan* is synthesized by neurons and undergoes extensive proteolytic processing during the course of brain development (Friedlander et al. 1994). *Phosphacan* is an astroglial proteoglycan. Both neurocan and phosphacan can bind with high affinity to neural cell adhesion molecules (Ng-CAMs/L1/NILE, NCAM, TAG-1/anoxin-1) (Milev et al. 1997), thus inhibiting neuronal and glial cell adhesion and neurite outgrowth. *Aggrecan* is a CSPG expressed in the developing brain and participates in the migration and establishment of neuronal nuclei (Schwartz et al. 1996). *Versican* is an HA-binding proteoglycan that is mainly expressed postnatally in the rat brain. Versican is present in gray matter (Bignami et al. 1993) and in white matter with a distribution identical to that previously reported for brain-specific *glial hyaluronate-binding protein (GHAP)*, probably a proteolytic product of versican, corresponding to its HA-binding N-terminal domain. There is evidence that MMPs are involved in this proteolytic cleavage (Perides et al. 1995). *Appicans* are secreted or cell-associated CSPG forms of amyloid precursor protein (APP) (Pangalos et al. 1996). Appicans are produced by glial cells, and when expressed in C6 glioma cells, promote adhesion of neural cells to the ECM (Wu et al. 1997). It has been suggested that proteolytic cleavage and release of the membrane-anchored APP by MMP-2 could prevent the formation of the amyloid-β peptide (Miyazaki et al. 1993).

Heparan sulfate proteoglycans (HSPGs) are also found on the surface of all adherent cells where they participate in the binding of growth factors, ECM glycoproteins, CAMs, proteinases, and antiproteinases. Among them, *glypican* is a cell-surface glycophosphatidylinositol (GPI)-anchored HSPG expressed in the developing and adult rat nervous system, including hippocampus, amygdala, and cerebral and piriform cortex. *Cerebroglycan* is a nervous system–specific GPI-anchored HSPG expressed during neuronal differentiation (Stipp et al. 1994). N-*Syndecan (syndecan 3)* is an ECM-associated protein that belongs to a family of differentiation and growth factors and that contains mainly HS glycosaminoglycan chains (Raulo et al. 1994). Since basic fibroblast growth factor (bFGF) exhibits significant N-syndecan binding and both are abundant in the neonatal brain, it is possible that N-syndecan functions as a coreceptor for bFGF during nerve tissue development (Chernousov and Carey 1993). *Agrin*, an ECM HSPG (Tsen et al. 1995) important in the formation of the neuromuscular junction, is widely expressed during mammalian embryogenesis, including brain development. Agrin is a potent inhibitor of the proteinases trypsin, chymotrypsin, and plasmin, but not thrombin or the plasminogen activators. Hence, agrin may regulate proteolysis in the ECM (Biroc et al. 1993).

Cell Adhesion Molecules   CAMs are cell surface macromolecules involved in the maintenance of neuronal networks, in processes of network reorganization in situations of plasticity and pathological conditions, and, importantly, in signal transduction and interaction with cytoskeletal components (reviewed in Schachner 1997). Their extracellular domains are potential targets for extracellular proteinases. With the exception of integrins discussed below which interact with the ECM, CAMs bind essentially through homophilic or heterophilic interaction with molecules on adjacent membranes (*cis*- or *trans*-). On the basis of molecular structures and cell-binding properties, cell-cell adhesion molecules in nervous tissues are categorized in distinct groups.

Plexin (Ohta et al. 1995) and the Ca^{2+}-*dependent cadherin* family (reviewed in Barth et al. 1997) mediate cell-cell interactions by means of Ca^{2+}-dependent homophilic protein-protein interactions. Cadherins are expressed during ontogeny and in the adult. They are likely to be involved in synapse formation and in synapse modifications and they convey signals from the cell surface to the cytoplasm via *catenins*, which are cytoskeletal linker proteins.

Members of the *immunoglobulin/fibronectin III* (Ig/FnIII) family belong to a large class of Ca^{2+}-independent CAMs. Some members of the Ig superfamily such as neural CAM (NCAM) and F3/F11 are expressed either bound to cell surfaces by transmembrane domains or by a GPI membrane anchor, or they can be released or secreted into the ECM (Sonderegger and Rathjen 1992). Molecular complexity stems from post-translational glycosylation of CAMs: NCAMs carry *polysialic acid* (PSA), a homopolymer whose expression is highly regulated and that serves as a modulator of cell interactions, and whose levels can be altered by synaptic plasticity (reviewed in Rutishauser and Landmesser 1996). MMPs are involved in the shedding of CAMs. For example, this is the case with the astrocytic intercellular CAM-1 (ICAM-1), a member of the Ig superfamily (Lyons and Benveniste 1998).

Neuroligins and β-neurexins are distinct neuronal cell surface proteins localized on separate cells, which bind to each other forming a heterotypic intercellular junction (Ichtchenko et al. 1995, 1996; Ushkaryov et al. 1992). Interestingly, neuroligins bind to PSD-95 (Irie et al. 1997), an intracellular protein enriched in postsynaptic densities (Kennedy 1997). This protein binds the intracellular C-terminal tails of a variety of receptors and channels, including the Shaker-type K^+ channels and the N-methyl-D-aspartate (NMDA) receptors (Sheng and Wyszynski 1997; Kornau et al. 1995), which contribute to synaptic plasticity and neuropathology.

ECM Receptors   Cell adhesion to the ECM is mediated by cell surface receptors. The activity of these transmembrane protein complexes may be affected by ECM metabolism and they are potential targets for extracellular proteinases.

Nonintegrin ECM receptors are cell surface proteoglycans such as syndecan, thrombospondin-binding glycoprotein, and certain laminin-binding proteins (Adams and Watt 1993). Among the nonintegrin receptors, the cell surface $\beta 1$, 4-galactosyltransferase is a laminin receptor that mediates cell attachment and migration by binding to terminal N-acetylglucosamine residues of laminin (Begovac and Shur 1990).

Integrin ECM receptors make up a large family of proteins that are the primary receptors for ECM components such as tenascin (Varnum-Finney et al. 1995), fibronectin, laminin, and vitronectin (Akiyama 1996; Perris 1997), and that are also involved in cell-cell interactions (Hynes 1992). Integrin subunits are expressed in the developing and adult mammalian brain where they may participate in neuronal migration and in the formation, maintenance, or plasticity of synapses (Bronner-Fraser 1994; Einheber et al. 1996). Integrins, via their intracellular domains, also establish a mechanical link between the ECM and the actin cytoskeleton through several intermediate proteins such as talin, α-actinin, tensin, and vinculin. Integrins trigger a number of intracellular signaling pathways that control cell shape, gene regulation, growth, and survival. Moreover, the loss of integrin-mediated cell matrix contact induces apoptosis ("anoikis") in certain cell types (reviewed in Frisch and Ruoslahti 1997). Cells engaged in cell-cell interactions (as is the case with the majority of cells in the nonpathological brain) are sensitive to anoikis. Thus, in pathological situations, the breakdown of these interactions by overactivated extracellular proteinases might contribute to some extent to neuronal apoptosis. It is known that the expression of MMPs can be regulated by modifying the integrin-ligand interactions in a variety of cells (Romanic and Madri 1994), and evidence has been provided that a proteolytically active MMP-2 binds directly $\alpha v \beta 3$ integrin in invasive cells; thus, by promoting MMP binding or expression, cell surface receptors may regulate both matrix degradation and cell motility (Brooks et al. 1996).

In conclusion, in nervous system tissues, a number of ECM molecules and CAMs that interact with MMPs play a critical role in promoting cell survival, cell adhesion, neurite outgrowth, and synaptic plasticity by modulating cell or synapse adhesion or by modulating signal transduction cascades.

REGULATORY INTERACTIONS OF MMPs AND TIMPS WITH OTHER FACTORS

MMP and TIMP expression and activity are under the control of a variety of transcription factors, oncogenes, growth factors, cytokines, hormones, and proteinases. Many of these regulatory factors are involved to some degree in brain plasticity or pathological conditions.

Transcriptional Regulation of MMPs and TIMPs

The transcriptional control of TIMPs and MMPs has been central to cancer research; it is becoming apparent that oncogenes control the expression of proteins that modulate ECM metabolism. Many MMPs and TIMPs are highly inducible through a variety of stimuli, whereas others are expressed constitutively. Their inducibility is generally associated with the presence in their promoter regions of regulatory sequences, including binding sites for AP-1, Ets, and STAT (signal transducer and activator of transcription) proteins. These regulatory sequences may operate synergistically, for instance, through composite Ets/AP-1 in tumor cells (Gum et al. 1996; Logan et al. 1996) or through STAT/AP-1 in astrocytes and fibroblasts (Korzus et al. 1997). Protein kinase C seems to be an important second messenger in the signal transduction pathway (McDonnell et al. 1990; Takahashi et al. 1993). The connection between MMP and TIMP expression and AP-1 binding proteins is particularly relevant in light of evidence that links AP-1 binding proteins of the Fos and Jun families with neuronal plasticity (Dragunow 1996) and with neuronal death (Smeyne et al. 1993; Ham et al. 1995). MMP-3, which like MMP-1 and other collagenases, possesses an AP-1 binding site in the promoter region, requires the induction of *c-fos* and *c-jun* for its transcriptional activation (McDonnell et al. 1990). Early work by Estus et al. (1994) showing that, in sympathetic neurons deprived of nerve growth factor (NGF), the induction of *c-fos* and *c-jun* is followed by a peak in MMP-1 and MMP-3 messenser RNA (mRNA) expression, provided the evidence for a transcriptional cascade involving AP-1 proteins and MMPs in neurons. More recently, Estus et al. (1997) reported a similar transcriptional cascade in cultured hippocampal neurons treated with amyloid-β protein. In vivo, in animal models of cerebral ischemia and epilepsy, there is indirect spatiotemporal evidence that inducible transcription factors may influence the expression of MMPs and TIMPs.

The relatively rapid activation of MMP-9 after focal cerebral ischemia (Rosenberg et al. 1996) also correlates with the earlier induction of Fos and Jun in this experimental paradigm (Uemura et al. 1991; An et al. 1993). In contrast, MMP-2, which unlike MMP-9 is not responsive to AP-1-binding proteins, is activated only much later (Rosenberg et al. 1996). The finding that TIMP-1 mRNA levels peak in the stratum granulosum of the dentate gyrus approximately four hours after global cerebral ischemia (Rivera et al. 1996) is also in spatiotemporal agreement with the induction of AP-1 proteins (Wessel et al. 1991). Taken together, these data suggest that the induction of certain MMPs and TIMPs might be coordinated in the nervous system through transcriptional mechanisms likely to require AP-1 protein synthesis. However, the fact that the activity-dependent induction of TIMP-1 mRNA after seizures is not blocked by the inhibition of protein synthesis provides ground for an alternative control of TIMP-1 expression by constitutively expressed transcription factors (Rivera et al. 1997).

We suggest that STAT-3 is a putative candidate. This protein is constitutively expressed in the brain (Planas et al. 1996) and is identified in rat hepatocytes as a major regulator of rat TIMP-1 expression through its interaction with the interleukin-6—oncostatin M (OSM) site at the TIMP-1 promoter (Bugno et al. 1995). Similarly, analysis of the signal transduction pathways leading to the MMP-1 gene induction in astrocytes revealed in the promoter the presence of an OSM-responsive element (OMRE) encompassing the AP-1 binding site and a STAT-binding element (Korzus et al. 1997). These findings support the contention that in brain cells, STATs could modulate expression of the MMP-TIMP system. STAT-3, as is the case with other members of the STAT family, is activated upon phosphorylation and translocates to the nucleus where it modulates the expression of specific sets of genes (Schindler and Darnell 1995). The expression of STAT-3 and STAT-1 has been recently reported to be induced in the brain after cerebral ischemia (Planas et al. 1996, 1997), and the activation of STAT proteins has been reported after axotomy of the superior cervical ganglia (Rajan et al. 1995), linking their expression to situations of neuronal injury. Whether STATs are phosphorylated in the nervous system after seizures or glutamate-driven responses remains to be determined.

Regulation of MMPs and TIMPs by Trophic Factors

It has been extensively documented that brain expression of genes encoding trophic factors, that is, neurotrophins, bFGF, interleukin-1 (IL-1), tumor necrosis factor-α (TNF-α), transforming growth factor-β (TGF-β), is modulated in various physiological and pathological situations (Isackson et al. 1991; Lindvall et al. 1992; Castrén et al. 1992; Tchelingerian et al. 1993; Dragunow et al. 1993; Logan and Berry 1993; Bugra et al. 1994; Feuerstein et al. 1994; Khrestchatisky et al. 1995; Rothwell and Hopkins 1995; Lauterborn et al. 1996). Neurotrophic factors are thought to play an important role in synaptogenesis, dendroaxonic outgrowth, neuronal survival, and tissue remodeling in the developing and the injured brain (see Lu and Figurov 1997 for review). How they contribute to the structural changes underlying these processes is largely unknown. One possibility is that their actions are mediated by proteins that have the catalytic capacity to remodel the neural environment. Indeed, it is well-known that the expression and activity of MMPs and TIMPs in non—nervous system tissues are modulated by growth factors and inflammatory cytokines (see Borden and Heller 1997 for review). Several lines of evidence indicate that trophic factors may also regulate the expression of MMPs and TIMPs in the nervous system. In the peripheral nervous system (PNS), NGF-mediated induction of MMP-2 is required for neurite outgrowth of dorsal root ganglia (DRG) neurons (Muir 1994), whereas the induction of MMP-3 expression by NGF, and also by aFGF and bFGF, is associated with the differentiation of PC12 cells (Machida et al. 1989; Fillmore et al. 1992).

Recent work demonstrated that TNF-α, TGF-β, and IL-1α regulate TIMP-1 expression during sciatic nerve repair (La Fleur et al. 1996). In the CNS, NGF suppresses the expression of MMP-9 and activates MMP-2 in brain-metastatic melanoma cells (Herrmann et al. 1993). It has been reported that the activity of MMP-9 and MMP-2 increases in cultured rat astrocytes in the presence of IL-1 (α or -β) (Gottschall and Yu 1995) and in activated microglia (Gottschall et al. 1995). Giraudon et al. (1995) have also documented an increase in MMP-9 activity in neuroectodermal cells treated with TNF-α and increased expression of MMP-9, MMP-3, and TIMP-3 in human and rat astrocytes after TNF-α or IL-1 treatment (Giraudon et al. 1997). It is thus plausible that TIMP-1 and MMP-9 induction observed in reactive astrocytes after brain seizures (Rivera et al. 1997) or after global forebrain ischemia (Rivera et al., unpublished results), is regulated by some of these trophic factors whose expression is known to be induced by seizures and ischemia (Gall and Isackson 1989; Minami et al. 1990, 1992; Feuerstein et al. 1994; Bugra et al. 1994; Wang et al. 1995). In turn, MMPs may regulate the bioavailability and limit the diffusion of matrix-bound trophic factors that are released upon proteolysis of ECM components (Adams and Watt 1993).

It is hypothesized that HSPGs in the ECM serve as storage sites for bFGF and assist in the bFGF-induced activation of the high-affinity FGF receptors linked to astroglia and neurons in areas where they codistribute (Fuxe et al. 1994). TGF-β, another important MMP and TIMP modulator, binds to ECM glycoproteins such as fibronectin, thrombospondin, and proteoglycans (Adams and Watt 1993), all of them substrates for MMPs. These modulatory interactions and the increasing evidence that MMPs and TIMPs are expressed not only by brain glial cells but also by neurons (Backstrom et al. 1996; Lim et al. 1996; Rivera et al. 1997), supports the contention that regulatory loops between trophic substances and the MMPs and TIMPs are implicated in the organization of the pericellular environment and in the crosstalk between neurons and glia (figure 3.2). In this regard, it is interesting to note that the neuronal induction of TIMP-1 mRNA after seizures (Rivera et al. 1997) occurs earlier or at least in tandem with the activation of trophic factors in similar experimental conditions (Dugich-Djordjevic et al. 1992; Gall et al. 1994). This raises the possibility, at least shortly after seizure onset, that TIMP-1 expression does not depend on the trophic reaction triggered by hyperactivity, and experimental evidence suggests that in some situations, TIMP-1 is expressed in the CNS as an immediate early gene (Rivera et al. 1997).

Interactions of the MMPs with Other Proteinases

The MMPs are expressed as latent forms that become active by proteolytic cleavage of the N-terminal propeptide domain within the highly conserved amino acid sequence PRCGXPDV. The activation may occur by autocleavage,

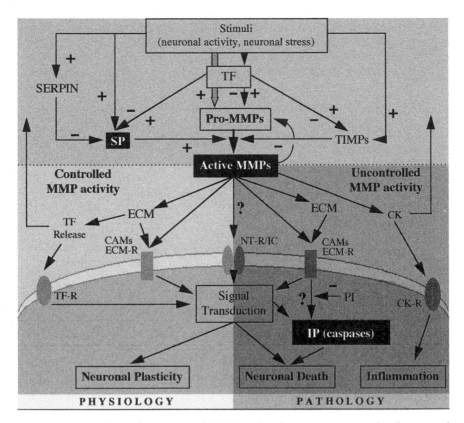

Figure 3.2 Regulatory interactions of MMPs with other proteinases, trophic factors, and matrix and nonmatrix substrates in physiological and pathological situations. MMPs, matrix metalloproteinases; TIMPs, tissue inhibitors of MMPs; SP, serine proteinases; SERPIN, serine proteinase inhibitor; IP, intracellular proteinases; PI, proteinase inhibitors; TF, trophic factors: growth factors and cytokines; CK, cytokines; NT-R/IC, neurotransmitter receptor/ion channel; ECM, extracellular matrix; CAMs, cell adhesion molecules; R, receptor.

but also by the proteolytic action of other family members or members of other proteinase families (see figure 3.2). Among the pro-MMP convertases of the MMP family, the stromelysins appear to be particularly active; MMP-3 cleaves the nonactive forms of MMP-1, MMP-8, MMP-7, and MMP-9 (Murphy et al. 1987; Knauper et al. 1993; Ogata et al. 1992; Imai et al. 1995), whereas MMP-7 can cleave the MMP-1, MMP-2, and MMP-9 (Imai et al. 1995; Sang et al. 1996). This indicates that stromelysins may function upstream of other MMPs in the proteolytic cascade. Pro-MMP-2 and pro-MMP-13 can be cleaved in the proximity of the cell membrane by the MT1-MMP in a complex with TIMP-2, which acts as a receptor for MMP-2 (Sato et al. 1994). Most interestingly, MT2-MMP, whose expression in the brain is highest among other tissues, can process pro-MMP2 into its active form (Takino et al. 1995). This finding suggests that in vivo the tandem MT2-MMP and MMP-2 may play a role in the processing and activation of membrane-bound proteins in neural cells.

When considering the interactions with other proteinase families, the serine proteinases are of particular interest for the nervous system. Urokinase plasminogen activator (u-PA) and tissue plasminogen activator (t-PA) have attracted much attention over the last years because of their possible role in adult brain plasticity and pathologic changes (see below). Plasminogen activators (PAs) can cleave plasminogen into active plasmin, which in turn catalyzes the conversion of pro-MMPs into active MMPs (Werb et al. 1977). Thrombin, a multifunctional serine proteinase involved in CNS development, plasticity, and disease (Turgeon and Houenou 1997), includes pro-MMP-2 among its substrates (Zucker et al. 1995). The transmembrane serine proteinases furins can activate MMP-11 (Pei and Weiss 1995) and MT-MMPs (Sato et al. 1996). It appears that the proteolytic capacities of MMPs depend, at least in part, on serine proteinases. Conversely, it is possible that serine proteinase activity is modulated by MMPs via their interaction with serine proteinase inhibitors (serpins) such as the α_1-proteinase inhibitor (Ohuchi et al. 1977). In vivo, the existence of these cascades, which combine rapid amplification of the proteolytic signal with tight control through multiple inhibitory relays, would fit the requirements for a finely tuned proteolysis linking environmental stimuli to plastic changes (see figure 3.2).

Nonmatrix Components as Potential Targets for MMPs

The ECM per se and latent forms of various secreted proteinases are not the only targets of pericellular proteolysis. During cellular responses to developmental, physiological, and pathological cues, cell surface proteins, neuropeptides, cytokines, receptors, and transmembrane ECM proteins are altered by proteolysis. For instance, MMP-9 cleaves neuroactive peptides such as substance P with a $k$cat per Km thirtyfold higher than that of the collagen-based peptide. The Km for other tachykinin peptides, such as neurokinin A and B, is much lower, suggesting that MMP-9 may regulate the bioavailability of specific neuroactive peptides (Backstom and Tökes 1995). A recent report (Ito et al. 1996) documents that MMP-1, MMP-2, and MMP-9 can specifically degrade IL-1β but not IL-1α. MMPs might also mediate the shedding of IL-6 receptor, since this is abolished by a synthetic metalloproteinase inhibitor (Mullberg et al. 1995). In accordance with this possible regulation of cytokines by MMPs, it has been reported that MMPs (MMP-1, MMP-2, MMP-3, MMP-7, and MMP-9) can proteolytically process the inactive pro-TNF-α into biologically active TNF-α (Gearing et al. 1994, 1995). Nevertheless, the recently cloned TNF-α-converting enzyme (TACE) (Black et al. 1997; Moss et al. 1997), a Zn^{2+}-dependent disintegrin metalloproteinase of the adamalysins family, is most efficient in processing the immature TNF-α, suggesting that it could be the physiologically relevant enzyme in vivo. To date, little is known about the precise tissue distribution or the mechanisms of action of these TNF-α convertase candidates. Therefore, the question remains open as to what enzyme(s) releases TNF-α in the brain.

Shedding of TNF receptors 1 and 2 is blocked by inhibitors of metalloproteinases (Crowe et al. 1995; Mullberg et al. 1995; Williams et al. 1996), although the proteinase(s) involved remains to be determined. MMP-2 can cleave and release an active soluble ectodomain of the FGF receptor-1 (FGF-R1) (Levi et al. 1996). The data mentioned above, linked to the fact that interleukins, TNF-α, and FGFs are among the most important regulators of pro-MMP synthesis and secretion, indicate that MMP and trophic factor bioavailability are interdependent (see figure 3.2). Furthermore, MMPs may regulate the bioavailability of IGF by degradation of the IGF-binding protein-3 (IGFBP-3), which is thought to modulate the binding of the IGF to its receptor (Fowlkes et al. 1994). MMPs have also been associated with the cleavage of myelin basic protein and of the amyloid-β peptide with logical implications for neuropathology, as discussed below. The diversity of known nonmatrix substrates for MMPs suggests that the functions of these enzymes go far beyond the regulation of the ECM metabolism. In this regard, Arribas et al. (1996) have suggested the existence of a general system for the shedding of membrane protein ectodomains involving metalloproteinases. Considering the above, it is conceivable that extracellular proteinases also target the extracellular domains of neurotransmitter and neuropeptide receptors, or of channels, thus modulating their functions.

ECM PROTEINASES AND INHIBITORS IN NEUROPLASTICITY

There is a large body of evidence indicating that during development proteinases and their inhibitors control cell migration and neuritic growth via the regulation of the ECM, CAMs, and receptors (Monard 1988). Controlled local proteolytic activities may be necessary for assembly and disassembly of ECM components allowing cell motility and axonal pathfinding. Experimental evidence supporting this hypothesis comes from early work demonstrating that cultured peripheral neurons spontaneously release PAs and metalloproteinases from their distal processes or growth cones (Krystosek and Seeds 1984; Pittman 1985), and that Ca^{2+}-dependent metalloproteinase activities are necessary for neurite penetration into collagen matrices (Pittman and Williams 1988). More recently Muir (1994) has reported that the expression and activation of MMP-2 is increased by NGF, which enhances MMP-dependent neuritic outgrowth of DRG neurons within a reconstituted extracellular matrix. Similarly, neurite outgrowth from pheochromocytoma cells (PC12) through the ECM was found to be dependent on growth factor–induced MMP production (Machida et al. 1989).

Remodeling of the ECM or the modulation of associated extracellular molecules (i.e., glycoproteins, integrins, and CAMs) has been suggested in models of synaptic plasticity (Rauvala and Peng 1997; Rutishauser and Landmesser 1996; Schachner 1997). Although to date there is no direct evidence for MMP contribution to synaptic plasticity, a number of MMP substrates have been implicated in this process. A correlation has been established between the expression of tenascin-C (a substrate for MMPs), and the induction of changes in synaptic efficiency and remodeling in animal models of epilepsy (Ferhat et al. 1996; Nakic et al. 1996). In addition, mutant mice expressing decreased levels and abnormal forms of tenascin-C show alterations in neurotransmitter systems and behavioral deficits (Fukamauchi et al. 1996). As mentioned above, an interaction between integrins and MMPs has recently been demonstrated (Brooks et al. 1996). Interestingly, Bahr et al. (1997) have shown that an integrin-like matrix receptor is implicated in the stabilization of potentiated synapses following induction of long-term potentiation (LTP), a cellular substrate for learning processes. Furthermore, studies in *Drosophila* reveal that a member of the integrin family is crucial in olfactory learning (Grotewiel et al. 1998). Metabolism of the ECM by MMP activities could induce signal transduction pathways via integrins that may contribute to plasticity. APP, another cell surface substrate of MMPs, is involved in LTP and in learning and memory in mice (Fazeli et al. 1994; U. Muller et al. 1994).

Serine proteinases of the ECM, which modulate MMP activity, have recently been associated with plasticity. t-PA is induced in adult rats during kindling and by stimuli leading to LTP, two forms of synaptic potentiation (Qian et al. 1993). t-PA-deficient mice have a different form of LTP, characterized by an NMDA receptor–dependent modification of γ-aminobutyric acid transmission in the hippocampal CA1 region (Frey et al. 1996). Seeds et al. (1995) have shown that t-PA is specifically induced in the cerebellum during learning tasks controlled by this brain region. Meiri et al. (1994) have reported that mice overexpressing u-PA have impaired learning while preserving normal sensory and motor functions. Protease nexin I, a serine proteinase inhibitor known to promote neurite outgrowth, modulates epileptic activity and hippocampal LTP (Lüthi et al. 1997). The close functional interactions between serine proteinases and MMPs and TIMPs (see above) allows one to speculate that the latter may also participate in neuronal plasticity associated with learning processes. Consistent with this idea, Nedivi et al. (1993) reported that TIMP-1, which was isolated in a subtractive library from the dentate gyrus of kainate-injected rats, is induced in vivo after LTP and suggested that this MMP inhibitor is a candidate plasticity gene. The spatiotemporal correlation found between the activity-dependent induction of TIMP-1 and the maturation of the limbic connectivity (Rivera et al. 1997) provides further evidence for a possible contribution of TIMP-1 in plasticity.

MMP activities may contribute to plasticity, not only through the processing of cytokine receptors (see above) but also by the regulation of neurotransmitter receptors or ion channels. It is already becoming evident that the intracellular domains of receptors or channels are cleaved by intracellular proteinases: Bi et al. (1996, 1997) demonstrated that calpain activation produces a partial proteolysis in the intracellular C-terminal domain of the

GluR1 subunits of the α-amino-3-hydroxy-5-methylisoxazole-4-propionic acid (AMPA) receptors. Calpain also cleaves an L-type Ca^{2+} channel in hippocampal neurons, leading to a truncated channel with increased activity (Hell et al. 1996). Interestingly, a secreted serine proteinase regulates the activity of a *Xenopus* epithelial amiloride-sensitive sodium channel (Vallet et al. 1997). Members of this channel family are known to be expressed in the brain, suggesting that similar mechanisms of ion channel regulation may occur in the CNS. From these observations, it is conceivable that the extracellular domains of receptors or channels may also be targets for secreted proteinases providing additional mechanisms for regulating neuronal plasticity.

ECM PROTEINASE INHIBITORS AND NEUROPATHOLOGY

There is convincing evidence that physiological and pathological processes in the brain share common cellular mechanisms (reviewed in Lynch et al. 1986). It is widely assumed that stimulation of glutamate receptors induces LTP (Collingridge et al. 1983) and excitotoxicity associated with seizures and cerebral ischemia (Ben-Ari 1985; Rothman and Olney 1986). In the rat hippocampus, brief seizure episodes (Ben-Ari and Represa 1990) and in vitro anoxia (Hammond et al. 1994), induce LTP. In our laboratory and elsewhere, it has been found that excitotoxicity may involve an exacerbated cascade of molecular and cellular events that contribute to neuronal apoptosis (Charriaut-Marlangue et al. 1996; Khrestchatisky et al. 1996), and to tissue remodeling and formation of aberrant synapses (Ben-Ari and Represa 1990; Represa et al. 1995). As discussed above, it is likely that in physiological conditions, matrix proteinases modulate neuronal plasticity. When the equilibrium between proteolytic and inhibitory activities is altered, pathological changes may occur (see figure 3.2).

The expression of several MMP substrates such as fibronectin, vitronectin, and tenascin is upregulated by reactive glial cells in areas of mossy fiber sprouting after kainate (Niquet et al. 1994, 1996; Ferhat et al. 1996). In this context, ECM proteinases and their inhibitors are perfectly suited as modulators of cell death and tissue reorganization. In agreement with this idea, we and others (Nedivi et al. 1993; Rivera et al. 1997) have shown that seizures induced by kainate lead to TIMP-1 induction in the rat brain. More precisely, we have shown that this upregulation occurs first in neurons and then in astrocytes in vulnerable regions of the limbic system. Moreover, the inducibility of TIMP-1 during development correlates well with the ontogeny of neuronal vulnerability to seizures (Tremblay et al. 1984; Nitecka et al. 1984). We and others have also observed TIMP-1 induction in lesioned areas after ischemia (Rivera et al. 1996; Wang et al. 1998). Therefore, we hypothesize that TIMP-1 could participate in tissue remodeling in lesioned areas after excitotoxicity. Additionally, TIMP-1 upregulation in the resistant hippocampal neurons is consistent with the trophic activities attributed to TIMPs (Edwards et al. 1996). The idea that TIMPs and MMPs are mobilized in excitotoxicity is reinforced by work in cerebral ischemia. Focal ischemia in rats induces an early activation of MMP-9 and delayed activation of MMP-2 (Rosenberg et al. 1996), suggesting that MMP-9 could contribute to tissue damage while MMP-2 is involved in tissue repair. In the same experimental paradigm, specific inhibition of MMP-9 with neutralizing antibodies reduces infarct size (Romanic et al. 1998). Consistent with this hypothesis, we have found that following global ischemia in rats, MMP-9 is induced in astrocytes in areas of neuronal death (Rivera et al., unpublished results). A series of recent reports further emphasizes the implication of the MMPs and TIMPs system in excitotoxicity. Indeed, seizures triggered by kainate induce MMP-3 mRNA expression (Reeben et al. 1996), and MMP-9 and MMP-2 activity (Zhang et al. 1998; A. W. Szklarczyk and L. Kaczmarek, personal communication 1998) in areas of the rat limbic system, whereas the stimulation of the NMDA receptors induces MMP-3 mRNA in cortical neuronal cultures (Bazan et al. 1997).

MMPs could participate in brain disorders as part of a proteolytic cascade in cooperation with serine proteinases (see figure 3.2). The hypothesis is based on (1) the fact that plasmin has the capacity to activate latent forms of MMPs, and (2) on the important role that the activation of the t-PA-plasmin axis seems to play in excitotoxic damage. Qian et al. (1993) showed that the expression of t-PA was activity-dependent during LTP and seizures. Research from the same laboratory supports the implication of the t-PA-plasmin axis in neuronal degeneration accompanying seizures (Tsirka et al. 1995, 1997; Chen and Strickland 1997). These authors found that t-PA and plasminogen-deficient mice are resistant to kainate-mediated hippocampal neuronal degeneration, and that inhibition of plasmin confers neuroprotection to kainate-treated wild-type mice. Furthermore, the rapid cleavage of laminin and the subsequent destabilization of the neuron-ECM interaction appears to be a key step in the development of disease. As mentioned previously, laminin is a substrate of plasmin, but also of MMPs. An emerging question is whether MMPs can be activated in vivo by plasmin or by other serine proteinases in situations of excitotoxicity and reactive plasticity.

Although it is widely assumed that excessive MMP activation may be toxic to different organs and tissues, the opposite could also be true, and insufficient MMP activity could contribute to fibrotic states with aberrant accumulation of ECM components. In accordance with this hypothesis it is interesting to note that the latent form of MMP-9 is increased in the hippocampus of Alzheimer's disease (AD) patients (Backstrom et al. 1996) and in aged dogs exhibiting AD-like features (Lim et al. 1997). In addition, TIMP-1 has been localized to the senile plaques of brains from AD patients (Peress et al. 1995). When considered together, these results suggest that reduced MMP activity contributes to the accumulation of amyloid-β peptide in amyloid plaques. In vitro assays show that MMP-9 (Backstrom et al. 1996) and MMP-2 (Roher et al. 1994) cleave the amyloid-β peptide at several sites, thus providing a possible mechanism whereby reduced MMP activity could promote amyloid-β peptide deposition. Moreover, it has been suggested that proteolytic cleavage and release of nonamyloidogenic forms of APP by MMP-2 could prevent the formation of toxic amyloid-β peptide (Miyazaki et al. 1993). However, controversy is raised by data showing that mice lacking MMP-2 exhibit a normal secretion of APP, indicating that MMP-2 may not be the unique secretase to generate soluble forms of APP (Itoh et al. 1997).

Further insights into the molecular interactions between amyloid-β peptide and MMPs have been obtained by exposing amyloid-β peptide to either mixed glial-neuronal cultures (Deb and Gottschall 1996) or to neuronal cortical cultures (Estus et al. 1997). MMP expression was increased in both cases and in the cortical cultures was associated with apoptosis. Estus et al. (1994) had already documented the induction of MMP-1 and MMP-3 in sympathetic neurons undergoing apoptosis upon NGF withdrawal. Alexander et al. (1996) have shown that in transgenic mice, mammary epithelial cells overexpressing MMP-3 undergo unscheduled apoptosis, which can be abrogated when these transgenic mice are crossed with mice overexpressing TIMP-1. These results strongly suggest that MMPs and TIMPs may participate in apoptotic processes. A plausible molecular mechanism for such contingency has been advanced by Boudreau et al. (1995). These authors suggest that apoptosis induced by MMP-3 overexpression in mammary epithelial cells is mediated by cysteine proteinase caspases. It is tempting to speculate that similar extracellular-intracellular proteolytic cascades are activated in the CNS and that they contribute to neuronal death, a process in which caspases have already been largely implicated (reviewed in Pettmann and Henderson 1998).

Other neurodegenerative diseases in which the MMPs and TIMPs system has been implicated include senile dementia (Bigmami et al. 1994), in which partial degradation of brain proteoglycans found in the brain of patients is associated with MMP-3 activity. Two forms of retinal degeneration may also be included as MMP-TIMP–associated diseases: simplex retinitis pigmentosa (Jones et al. 1994; Jomary et al. 1995) and Sorby's fundus dystrophy that is linked to mutations in the coding region of TIMP-3 (Weber et al. 1994). Amyotrophic lateral sclerosis (ALS) patients present an abnormally high amount of MMP-9 in the motor cortex as well as in the thoracic and lumbar cord tissue. It is hypothesized that the release of MMP-9 at the synapse may destroy the structural integrity of the surrounding matrix and contribute to the loss of motor function (Lim et al. 1996).

MMPs have also been associated with multiple sclerosis (MS) since MMP-9 activity was detected in the cerebrospinal fluid of patients suffering from the disease (Gijbels et al. 1992), as well as in animal models of experimental autoimmune encephalomyelitis (EAE) (Gijbels et al. 1993). More recently, in rats with EAE, Clements et al. (1997) detected a five-fold increase in MMP-9 and a striking 500-fold increase in MMP-7 mRNA levels at the onset of clinical signs. MMP-7 was immunohistochemically localized to the invading macrophages within the spinal cord, suggesting this enzyme is involved in the pathological processes. The demonstration that MMP-9 (Gijbels et al. 1993) and other MMPs, in particular MMP-2 (Chandler et al. 1995), can cleave myelin basic protein in vitro provides a possible mechanism of action for MMPs in demyelination. MMPs could participate in the in situ immuno-reaction by converting inactive TNF-α precursor into active TNF-α (Gearing et al. 1994). TNF-α has been implicated in inflammatory processes and pathologic changes associated with multiple sclerosis, brain trauma, cerebral ischemia, and epilepsy (Feuerstein et al. 1994). However, its precise role is yet to be defined and caution is required when assigning an exclusively neu-rotoxic role to this cytokine, since experimental evidence indicates that it may also play a neuroprotective role in excitotoxicity (Cheng et al. 1994; Nawashiro et al. 1997) and against amyloid-β protein toxicity (Barger et al. 1995). MMPs may contribute to neuroinflammatory diseases by facilitating leukocyte migration into the CNS through a weakened blood-brain barrier (BBB). Experimental evidence for this contingency was provided by the pio-neering work of Rosenberg et al. (1992), demonstrating that intracerebral injections of MMP-2 provoked the opening of the BBB, and that the asso-ciated tissue damage was reduced by TIMP-2. The same authors reported later that hemorrhagic injury activates MMP-9 in the brain (Rosenberg et al. 1994).

Cancer research has been at the forefront of MMP and TIMP research because alteration in their balance is important for the migration of cancer cells through the extracellular environment and for the formation of metas-tasis. In the brain, the most common form of malignant tumors are gliomas. MMP and TIMP activity and expression have been detected in cultured tumoral cells (Halaka et al. 1983; Apodaca et al. 1990) and in human brain tumors (Nakagawa et al. 1994). The activation of MMP-2 has been corre-lated with the invasive potential of gliomas in cooperation with u-PA, which activates pro-MMPs in these cells (Reith and Rucklidge 1992), highlighting the role of proteolytic cascades in tumor progression. It is also possible that MMPs contribute not only to cancer dissemination but also to the genera-tion of primary tumors, as has been inferred from observations in mice lack-ing MMP-7 (Wilson et al. 1997). Conversely, downregulation of both TIMP-1 and TIMP-2 contribute to the invasive potential of human glio-blastoma multiforme and anaplastic astrocytomas (Mohanam et al. 1995). Accordingly, astrocytoma cells transfected with TIMP-1 present a reduced invasiveness in vitro (Matsuzawa et al. 1996). Finally, as mitogens, TIMPs could act in some situations as tumor inducers rather than tumor suppressors (Soloway et al. 1996).

Human retroviral infections are frequently associated with neurological disturbances. In human T-cell leukemia/lymphoma virus type I (HTLV-I)– associated myelopathy (TSP/HAM), infected human primitive neuroecto-dermal cells express high levels of MMP-9, MMP-3, and TIMP-3 (Giraudon et al. 1995, 1997). According to these authors, the pathogenesis of TSP/

HAM may be related to the degradation of the BBB, myelin constituent cleavage, and conversion of inactive TNF-α precursor to its active form.

Direct or indirect evidence that MMPs and TIMPs may play a role in different forms of neurodegeneration is further supported by experiments in which broad-spectrum hydroxamic acid–based MMP inhibitors can substantially reduce the clinical signs and weight loss in an acute EAE model in Lewis rats (Clements et al. 1997) or block edema in intracerebral hemorrhage in the rat (Rosenberg and Navratil 1997). These results suggest that MMPs can be therapeutic targets of primary importance, not only in peripheral tissues but also in the CNS.

FUTURE DIRECTIONS AND CONCLUDING REMARKS

We are just beginning to appreciate the complexity of the interactions between MMPs and TIMPs, as well as their interactions with other molecules. It is reasonable to infer that MMPs and TIMPs will play an important role in the CNS, as is evidenced from their roles in the physiopathology of peripheral tissues and from the works reviewed in this chapter. The growing number of MMPs and TIMPs identified in the CNS, their complex regulation at the transcriptional and post-translational level, and their potential interactions with multiple substrates, provide the basis for an emerging field in neuronal plasticity and pathology. Among the challenging questions that need to be addressed are the following: What is the expression of MMPs and TIMPs at the cellular level and how do they contribute to the crosstalk between neurons and glial cells? What are the specific matrix and nonmatrix substrates for MMPs and TIMPs in the CNS? What are the multifunctional roles of TIMPs in the CNS? Do MMPs and TIMPs influence neuronal plasticity and, conversely, does plasticity modulate their activity? Can drugs that control MMP and TIMP balance be used as modulators of neuronal plasticity and as therapeutic agents in neurological disorders? There is no doubt that within the next few years, new data will shed light on the role of MMPs and TIMPs in the CNS, thus contributing to a better understanding of neuronal plasticity and pathology.

ACKNOWLEDGMENTS

We thank Dr. Yezekiel Ben-Ari for helpful discussions, Drs. Patrick Bassand, Alfonso Represa, and Maureen Miller for critically reading the manuscript, and Jérôme Jourquin for his help in preparing the figures. This work was supported by INSERM and by AFM grants to M.K. S.R. was a recipient of fellowships from Sidaction and from the Fyssen Foundation.

REFERENCES

Adams, J. C., and Watt, F. M. (1993). Regulation of development and differentiation by the extracellular matrix. *Development* 117: 1183–1198.

Akiyama, S. K. (1996). Integrins in cell adhesion and signaling. *Hum. Cell* 9: 181–186.

Alexander, C. M., Howard, E. W., Bissell, M. J., and Werb, Z. (1996). Rescue of mammary epithelial cell apoptosis and entactin degradation by a tissue inhibitor of metalloproteinases-1 transgene. *J. Cell Biol.* 135: 1669–1677.

An, G., Lin, T. N., Liu, J. S., Xue, J. J., He, Y. Y., and Hsu, C. Y. (1993). Expression of *c-fos* and *c-jun* family genes after focal cerebral ischemia. *Ann. Neurol.* 33: 457–464.

Apodaca, G., Rutka, J. T., Bouhana, K., Berens, M. E., Giblin, J. R., Rosenblum, M. L., McKerrow, J. H., and Banda, M. J. (1990). Expression of metalloproteinases and metalloproteinase inhibitors by fetal astrocytes and glioma cells. *Cancer Res.* 50: 2322–2329.

Arribas, J., Coodly, L., Vollmer, P., Kishimoto, T. K., Rose-John, S., and Massagué, J. (1996). Diverse cell surface protein ectodomains are shed by a system sensitive to metalloproteinase inhibitors. *J. Biol. Chem.* 271: 11376–11382.

Backstrom, J. R., and Tökes, Z. A. (1995). The 84–kDa form of human matrix metalloproteinase-9 degrades substance P and gelatine. *J. Neurochem.* 64: 1312–1318.

Backstrom, J. R., Lim, G. P., Cullen, M. J., and Tökés, Z. A. (1996). Matrix metalloproteinase-9 (MMP9) is synthesized in neurons of the human hippocampus and is capable of degrading the amyloid-β peptide (1–40). *J. Neurosci.* 16: 7910–7919.

Bahr, B. A., Staubli, U., Xiao, P., Chun, D., Ji, Z. X., Esteban, E. T., and Lynch, G. (1997). Arg-Gly-Asp-Ser-selective adhesion and the stabilization of long-term potentiation: pharmacological studies and the characterization of a candidate matrix receptor. *J. Neurosci.* 17: 1320–1329.

Barger, S. W., Horster, D., Furukawa, K., Goodman, Y., Krieglstein, J., and Mattson M. P. (1995). Tumor necrosis factors alpha and beta protect neurons against amyloid beta-peptide toxicity: evidence for involvement of a kappa B-binding factor and attenuation of peroxide and Ca^{2+} accumulation. *Proc. Natl. Acad. Sci. USA* 92: 9328–9332.

Barth, A. I., Nathke, I. S., and Nelson, W. J. (1997). Cadherins, catenins and APC protein: interplay between cytoskeletal complexes and signaling pathways. *Curr. Opin. Cell. Biol.* 9: 683–690.

Bazan, N. G., Ershov, A. V., and DeCoster, M. A. (1997). Significance of MMPs in the CNS: Introduction. Matrix metalloproteinases and the central nervous system. Presented at Satellite Symposium of the Society for Neuroscience, New Orleans, October 30–31, p. 9.

Begovac, P. C., and Shur, B. D. (1990). Cell surface galactosyltransferase mediates the initiation of neurite outgrowth from PC12 cells on laminin. *J. Cell Biol.* 110: 461–470.

Ben-Ari, Y. (1985). Limbic seizure and brain damage produced by kainic acid: mechanisms and relevance to human temporal lobe epilepsy. *Neuroscience* 14: 375–403.

Ben-Ari, Y., and Represa, A. (1990). Brief seizure episodes induce long-term potentiation and mossy fibre sprouting in the hippocampus. *Trends Neurosci.* 13: 312–318.

Bertolotto, A., Manzardo, E., and Guglielmone, R. (1996). Immunohistochemical mapping of perineuronal nets containing chondroitin unsulfated proteoglycan in the rat central nervous system. *Cell Tissue Res.* 283: 283–295.

Bi, X., Chang, V., Molnar, E., McIlhinney, R. A., and Baudry, M. (1996). The C-terminal domain of glutamate receptor subunit 1 is a target for calpain-mediated proteolysis. *Neuroscience* 73: 903–906.

Bi, X., Chen, J., Dang, S., Wenthold, R. J., Tocco, G., and Baudry, M. (1997). Characterization of calpain-mediated proteolysis of GluR1 subunits of alpha-amino-3–hydroxy-5–methylisoxazole-4–propionate receptors in rat brain. *J. Neurochem.* 68: 1484–1494.

Bignami, A., Perides, G., and Rahemtulla, F. (1993). Versican, a hyaluronate-binding proteoglycan of embryonal precartilaginous mesenchyma, is mainly expressed postnatally in rat brain. J. Neurosci. Res. 34: 97–106.

Bigmami, A., LeBlanc, A., and Perides, G. (1994). A role for extracellular matrix degradation and matrix metalloproteinases in senile dementia? Acta Neuropathol. 87: 308–312.

Biroc, S. L., Payan, D. G., and Fisher, J. M. (1993). Isoforms of agrin are widely expressed in the developing rat and may function as protease inhibitors. Brain Res. Dev. Brain Res. 75: 119–129.

Black, R. A., Rauch, C. T., Kozlosky, C. J., Peschon, J. J., Slack, J. L., Wolfson, M. F., Castner, B. J., Stocking, K. L., Reddy, P., Srinivasan, S., Nelson, N., Boiani, N., Schooley, K. A., Gerhart, M., Davis, R., Fitzner, J. N., Johnson, R. S., Paxton, R. J., March, C. J., and Cerretti, D. P. (1997). A metalloproteinase disintegrin that releases tumour-necrosis factor-α from cells. Nature 385: 729–732.

Borden, P., and Heller, R. A. (1997). Transcriptional control of matrix metalloproteinases and the tissue inhibitors of matrix metalloproteinases. Crit. Rev. Eukaryot. Gene Expr. 7: 159–178.

Boudreau, N., Sympson, C. J., Werb, Z., and Bissell, M. N. (1995). Supression of ICE and apoptosis in mammary epithelial cells by extracellular matrix. Science 267: 891–893.

Brittis, P. A., Canning, D. R., and Silver, J. (1992). Chondroitin sulfate as a regulator of neuronal patterning in the retina. Science 255: 733–736.

Bronner-Fraser, M. (1994). Neural crest cell formation and migration in the developing embryo. FASEB J. 8: 699–706.

Brooks, P. C., Strömblad, S., Sanders, L. C., von Schalscha, T. L., Aimes, R. T., Stetler-Stevenson, W. G., Quigley, J. P., and Cheresh, D. A. (1996). Localization of matrix metalloproteinase MMP-2 to the surface of invasive cells by interaction with integrin alpha-v-beta-3. Cell 85: 683–693.

Bugno, M., Graeve, L., Gatsios, P., Koj, A., Heinrich, P. C., Travis, J., and Kordula, T. (1995). Identification of the interleukin-6/oncostatin M response element in the rat tissue inhibitor of metalloproteinases-1 (TIMP-1) promoter. Nucleic Acids Res. 23: 5041–5047.

Bugra, K., Pollard, H., Charton, G., Moreau, J., Ben-Ari, Y., and Khrestchatisky, M. (1994). α FGF, β FGF and flg mRNAs show distinct patterns of induction in the hippocampus following kainate-induced seizures. Eur. J. Neurosci. 6: 58–66.

Castrén, E., Zafra, F., Thoenen, H., and Lindholm, D. (1992). Light regulates expression of brain-derived neurotrophic factor mRNA in rat visual cortex. Proc. Natl. Acad. Sci. USA 89: 9444–9448.

Chamak, B., Dobbertin, A., and Mallat, M. (1995). Immunohistochemical detection of thrombospondin in microglia in the developing rat brain. Neuroscience 69: 177–187.

Chandler, S., Coates, R., Gearing, A., Lury, J., Wells, G., and Bone, E. (1995). Matrix metalloproteinases degrade myelin basic protein. Neurosci. Lett. 201: 223–226.

Charriaut-Marlangue, C., Aggoun-Zouaoui, D., Represa, A., and Ben-Ari, Y. (1996). Apoptotic features of selective neuronal death in ischemia, epilepsy and gp 120 toxicity. Trends Neurosci. 19: 109–114.

Chen, Z. L., and Strickland, S. (1997). Neuronal death in the hippocampus is promoted by plasmin-catalyzed degradation of laminin. Cell 91: 917–925.

Cheng, B., Christakos, S., and Mattson, M. P. (1994). Tumor necrosis factors protect neurons against metabolic-excitotoxic insults and promote maintenance of calcium homeostasis. Neuron 12: 139–153.

Chernousov, M. A., and Carey, D. J. (1993). *N*-syndecan (syndecan 3) from neonatal rat brain binds basic fibroblast growth factor. *J. Biol. Chem.* 268: 16810–16814.

Clements, J. M., Cossins, J. A., Wells, G. M., Corkill, D. J., Helfrich, K., Wood, L. M., Pigott, R., Stabler, G., Ward, G. A., Gearing, A. J., and Miller, K. M. (1997). Matrix metalloproteinase expression during experimental autoimmune encephalomyelitis and effects of a combined matrix metalloproteinase and tumour necrosis factor-alpha inhibitor. *J. Neuroimmunol.* 74: 85–94.

Collingridge, G. L., Kehl, S. J., and McLennan, H. (1983). Excitatory amino acids in synaptic transmission in the Schaeffer-commissural pathway of the rat hippocampus. *J. Physiol.* 334: 33–46.

Crowe, P. D., Walter, B. N., Mohler, K. M., Otten-Evans, C., Black, R. A., and Ware, C. F. (1995). A metalloprotease inhibitor blocks shedding of the 80–kD TNF receptor and TNF processing in T lymphocytes. *Exp. Med.* 181: 1205–1210.

Deb, S., and Gottschall, P. E. (1996). Increased production of matrix metalloproteinases in enriched astrocyte and mixed hippocampal cultures treated with β-amyloid peptides. *J. Neurochem.* 66: 1641–1647.

Dragunow, M. (1996). A role for immediate-early transcription factors in learning and memory. *Behav. Genet.* 26: 293–299.

Dragunow, M., Beilharz, E., Mason, B., Lawlor, P., Abraham, W., and P. G. (1993). Brain-derived neurotrophic factor expression after long-term potentiation. *Neurosci. Lett.* 160: 232–236.

Dugich-Djordjevic, M. M., Tocco, G., Lapchak, P. A., Pasinetti, G. M., Najm, I., Baudry, M., and Hefti, F. (1992). Regionally specific and rapid increases in brain-derived neurotrophic factor messenger RNA in the adult rat brain following seizures induced by systemic administration of kainic acid. *Neuroscience* 47: 303–315.

Eddleston, M., and Mucke, L. (1993). Molecular profile of reactive astrocytes—implications for their role in neurologic disease. *Neuroscience* 54: 15–36.

Edwards, D. R., Beaudry, P. P., Laing, T. D., Kowal, V., Leco, K. J., Leco, P. A., and Lim, M. S. (1996). The roles of tissue inhibitors of metalloproteinases in tissue remodelling and cell growth. *Int. J. Obesity* 20: S9–S15.

Einheber, S., Schnapp, L. M., Salzer, J. L., Cappiello, Z. B., and Milner, T. A. (1996). Regional and ultrastructural distribution of the alpha 8 integrin subunit in developing and adult rat brain suggests a role in synaptic function. *J. Comp. Neurol.* 370: 105–134.

Estus, S., Zaks, W. J., Freeman, R. S., Gruda, M., Bravo, R., and Johnson, E. M. (1994). Altered gene expression in neurons during programmed cell death: identification of c-jun as necessary for neuronal apoptosis. *J. Cell Biol.* 127: 1717–1727.

Estus, S., Tucker, H. M., van Rooyen, C., Wright, S., Brigham, E. F., Wogulis, M., and Rydel, R. E. (1997). Aggregated amyloid-β protein induces cortical neuron apoptosis and concomitant "apoptotic" pattern of gene induction. *J. Neurosci.* 17: 7736–7745.

Fazeli, M. S., Breen, K., Errington, M. L., and Bliss, T. V. (1994). Increase in extracellular NCAM and amyloid precursor protein following induction of long-term potentiation in the dentate gyrus of anaesthetized rats. *Neurosci. Lett.* 169: 77–80.

Ferhat, L., Chevassus-Au-Louis, N., Khrestchatisky, M., Ben-Ari, Y., and Represa, A. (1996). Seizures induce tenascin-C mRNA expression in neurons. *J. Neurocytol.* 25: 535–546.

Feuerstein, G. Z., Liu, T., and Barone, F. C. (1994). Cytokines, inflammation, and brain injury: role of tumor necrosis factor-α. *Cerebrovasc. Brain Metab. Rev.* 6: 341–360.

Fowlkes, J. L., Enghild, J. J., Suzuki, K., and Nagase, H. (1994). Matrix metalloproteinases degrade insulin-like growth factor–binding protein-3 in dermal fibroblast cultures. *J. Biol. Chem.* 269: 25742–25746.

Frey, U., Muller, M., and Kuhl, D. (1996). A different form of long-lasting potentiation revealed in tissue plasminogen activator mutant mice. *J. Neurosci.* 16: 2057–2063.

Friedlander, D. R., Milev, P., Karthikeyan, L., Margolis, R. K., Margolis, R. U., and Grumet, M. (1994). The neuronal chondroitin sulfate proteoglycan neurocan binds to the neural cell adhesion molecules Ng-CAM/L1/NILE and N-CAM, and inhibits neuronal adhesion and neurite outgrowth. *J. Cell Biol.* 125: 669–680.

Frisch, S. M., and Ruoslahti, E. (1997). Integrins and anoikis. *Curr. Opin. Cell Biol.* 9: 701–706.

Frisen, J. (1997). Determinants of axonal regeneration. *Histol. Histopathol.* 12: 857–868.

Fukamauchi, F., Mataga, N., Wang, Y. J., Sato, S., Youshiki, A., and Kusakabe, M. (1996). Abnormal behavior and neurotransmissions of tenascin gene knockout mouse. *Biochem. Biophys. Res. Commun.* 221: 151–156.

Fuxe, K., Chadi, G., Tinner, B., Agnati, L. F., Pettersson, R., and David, G. (1994). On the regional distribution of heparan sulfate proteoglycan immunoreactivity in the rat brain. *Brain Res.* 636: 131–138.

Gall C., and Isackson, P. J. (1989). Limbic seizures increase neuronal production of mRNA for nerve growth factor. *Science* 245: 758–760.

Gall, C., Berschauer, B., and Isackson, P. (1994). Basic fibroblast growth factor mRNA is increased in forebrain neurons and glia following recurrent limbic seizures. *Mol. Brain. Res.* 21: 190–205.

Gearing, A. J. H., Beckett, P., Christodoulou, M., Churchill, M., Clements, J., Davidson, A. H., Drummond, A. H., Galloway, W. A., Gilbert, R., Gordon, J. L., Leber, T. M., Mangan, M., Miller, K., Nayee, P., Owen, K., Patel, S., Thomas, W., Wells, G., Wood, L. M., and Wooley, K. (1994). Processing of tumour necrosis factor-α precursor by metalloproteinases. *Nature* 370: 555–557.

Gearing, AJ, Beckett, P, Christodoulou, M, Churchill, M, Clements, JM, Crimmin, M, Davidson, AH, Drummond, AH, Galloway, WA, and Gilbert, R, et al. (1995). Matrix metalloproteinases and processing of pro-TNF-alpha. *J. Leukoc. Biol.* 57: 774–777.

Gijbels, K., Masure, S., Carton, H., and Opdenakker, G. (1992). Gelatinase in the cerebrospinal fluid of patients with multiple sclerosis and other inflammatory neurological disorders. *J. Neuroimmunol.* 41: 29–34.

Gijbels, K., Proost, P., Masure, S., Carton, H., Billiau, A., and Opdenakker, G. (1993). Gelatinase B is present in the cerebrospinal fluid during experimental autoimmune encephalomyelitis and cleaves myelin basic protein. *J. Neurosci. Res.* 36: 432–440.

Giraudon, P., Thomasset, N., Bernard, A., Verrier, B., and Belin, M. F. (1995). Induction of MMP9 (92 kDA gelatinase) activity and expression of tissue inhibitor of metalloproteinases-2 mRNA (TIMP-2) in primitive neuroectodermal cells infected with retrovirus HTLV-1. *Eur. J. Neurosci.* 7: 841–848.

Giraudon, P., Buart, S., Bernard, A., and Belin, M.-F. (1997). Cytokines secreted by glial cells infected with HTLV-1 modulate the expression of matrix metalloproteinases (MMPs) and their natural inhibitor (TIMPs): possible involvement in neurodegenerative processes. *Mol. Psychiatry* 2: 107–110.

Golgi, C. (1889). On the structure of nerve cells. *J. Microsc.* 155: 3–7.

Gottschall, P. E., and Yu, X. (1995). Cytokines regulate gelatinase A and B (matrix metalloproteinase 2 and 9) activity in cultured rat astrocytes. *J. Neurochem.* 64: 1513–1520.

Gottschall, P. E., Yu, X., and Bing, B. (1995). Increased production of gelatinase B (matrix metalloproteinase-9) and interleukin-6 by activated rat microglia in culture. *J. Neurosci. Res.* 42: 335–342.

Greene, J., Wang, M., Liu, Y. E., Raymond, L. A., Rosen, C., and Shi, Y. E. (1996). Molecular cloning and characterization of human tissue inhibitor of metalloproteinase 4. *J. Biol. Chem.* 29: 30375–30380.

Grotewiel, M. S., Beck, C. D. O., Hang Wu, K., Zhu, X. R., and Davis, R. L. (1998). Integrin-mediated short-term memory in *Drosophila. Nature* 391: 455–460.

Gum, R., Lengyel, E., Juarez, J., Chen, H. J., Sato, H., Seiki, M., and Boyd, D. (1996). Stimulation of 92–kD[a] gelatinase B promoter activity by ras is mitogen-activated protein kinase kinase 1–independent and requires multiple transcription factor binding sites including closely spaced PEA3/ets and AP-1 sequences. *J. Biol. Chem.* 271: 10672–10680.

Halaka, A. N., Bunning, R. A. D., Bird, C. C., Gibson, M., and Reynolds, J. J. (1983). Production of collagenase and inhibitor (TIMP) by intracranial tumors and dura in vitro. *J. Neurosurg.* 59: 461–466.

Ham, J., Babij, C., Whitfield, J., Pfarr, C. M., Lallemand, D., Yanivm, M., and Rubin, L. L. (1995). A c-Jun dominant negative mutant protects sympathetic neurons against programmed cell death. *Neuron* 14: 927–939.

Hammond, C., Crépel, V., Gozlan, H., and Ben-Ari, Y. (1994). Anoxic LTP sheds light on the mutiple facets of NMDA receptors. *Trends Neurosci.* 17: 497–503.

Hell, J. W., Westenbroek, R. E., Breeze, L. J., Wang, K. K., Chavkin, C., and Catterall, W. A. (1996). N-methyl-D-aspartate receptor–induced proteolytic conversion of postsynaptic class C L-type calcium channels in hippocampal neurons. *Proc. Natl. Acad. Sci. USA* 93: 3362–3367.

Herrmann, J. L., Menter, D. G., Hamada, J., Marchetti, D., Nakajima, M., and Nicolson, G. L. (1993). Mediation of NGF-stimulated extracellular matrix invasion by the human melanoma low-affinity p75 neurotrophin receptor: melanoma p57 functions independently of trkA. *Mol. Biol. Cell.* 4: 1205–1216.

Hoffman, J. R., Dixit, V. M., and O'Shea, K. S. (1994). Expression of thrombospondin in the adult nervous system. *J. Comp. Neurol.* 340: 126–139.

Hynes, R. O. (1992). Integrins: versatility, modulation, and signaling in cell adhesion. *Cell* 69: 11–25.

Ichtchenko, K., Hata, Y., Nguyen, T., Ullrich, B., Missler, M., Moomaw, C., and Sudhof, T. C. (1995). Neuroligin 1: a splice site-specific ligand for beta-neurexins. *Cell* 81: 435–443.

Ichtchenko, K., Nguyen, T., and Sudhof, T. C. (1996). Structures, alternative splicing, and neurexin binding of multiple neuroligins. *J. Biol. Chem.* 271: 2676–2682.

Imai, K., Yokohama, Y., Nakanishi, I., Ohuchi, E., Fujii, Y., Nakai, N., and Okada, Y. (1995). Matrix metalloproteinase 7 (matrilysin) from human rectal carcinoma cells. Activation of the precursor, interaction with other matrix metalloproteinases and enzymic properties. *J. Biol. Chem.* 270: 6691–6697.

Irie, M., Hata, Y., Takeuchi, M., Ichtchenko, K., Toyoda, A., Hirao, K., Takai, Y., Rosahl, T. W., and Sudhof, T. C. (1997). Binding of neuroligins to PSD-95. *Science* 277: 1511–1515.

Iruela-Arispe, M. L., Liska, D. J., Sage, E. H., and Bornstein, P. (1993). Differential expression of thrombospondin 1, 2, and 3 during murine development. *Dev. Dyn.* 197: 40–56.

Isackson, P. J., Murray, K., Huntsman, M., and Gall, C. M. (1991). BDNF mRNA expression is increased in adult rat forebrain after limbic seizures: temporal patterns of induction distinct from NGF. *Neuron* 6: 937–948.

Ito, A., Mukaiyama, A., Itoh, Y., Nagase, H., Thogersen, I. B., Enghild, J. J., Sasaguri, Y., and Mori, Y. (1996). Degradation of interleukin 1β by matrix metalloproteinases. *J. Biol. Chem.* 271: 14657–14660.

Itoh, T., Ikeda, T., Gomi, H., Nakao, S., Suzuki, T., and Itohara, S. (1997). Unaltered secretion of beta-amyloid precursor protein in gelatinase A (matrix metalloproteinase 2)–deficient mice. *J. Biol. Chem.* 272: 22389–22392.

Jomary, C., Neal, M. J., and Jones, S. E. (1995). Increased expression of retinal TIMP3 mRNA in simplex retinitis pigmentosa is localized to photoreceptor-retaining regions. *J. Neurochem.* 64: 2370–2373.

Jones, S. E., Jomary, C., and Neal, M. J. (1994). Expression of TIMP3 mRNA is elevated in retinas affected by simplex retinitis pigmentosa. *FEBS Lett.* 352: 171–174.

Kennedy, M. B. (1997). The postsynaptic density at glutamatergic synapses. *Trends Neurosci.* 20: 264–268.

Khrestchatisky, M., Ferhat, L., Charton, G., Bernard, A., Pollard, H., Represa, A., and Ben-Ari, Y. (1995). Molecular correlates between reactive and developmental plasticity in the rat hippo-campus. *J. Neurobiol.* 26: 426–436.

Khrestchatisky, M., Timsit, S., Rivera, S., Tremblay, E., and Ben-Ari, Y. (1996). *Neuronal Death and Damage Repair: Roles of Proto-Oncogenes and Cell Cycle–Related Proteins,* pp 41–56. ed. Stuttgart, Medpharm.

Kleiner, D. E., and Stetler-Stevenson, W. G. (1993). Structural biochemistry and activation of matrix metalloproteases. *Curr. Opin. Cell Biol.* 5: 891–897.

Knauper, V., Wilhelm, S. M., Seperack, P. K., DeClerck, Y. A., Langley, K. E., Osthues, A., and Tschesche, H. (1993). Direct activation of human neutrophil procollagenase by recombinant stromelysin. *Biochem. J.* 295: 581–586.

Koppe, G., Bruckner, G., Hartig, W., Delpech, B., and Bigl, V. (1997). Characterization of proteo-glycan-containing perineuronal nets by enzymatic treatments of rat brain sections. *Histochem. J.* 29: 11–20.

Kornau, H. C., Schenker, L. T., Kennedy, M. B., and Seeburg, P. H. (1995). Domain interaction between NMDA receptor subunits and the postsynaptic density protein PSD-95. *Science* 269: 1737–1740.

Korzus, E., Nagase, H., Rydell, R., and Travis, J. (1997). The mitogen-activated protein kinase and JAK-STAT signaling pathways are required for an oncostatin M-responsive element-mediated activation of matrix metalloproteinase 1 gene expression. *J. Biol. Chem.* 272: 1188–1196.

Krystosek, A., and Seeds, N. W. (1984). Peripheral neurons and Schwann cells secrete plami-nogen activator. *J. Cell Biol.* 98: 773–776.

La Fleur, M., Underwood, J. L., Rappolee, D. A., and Werb, Z. (1996). Basement membrane and repair of injury to peripheral nerve: defining a potential role for macrophages, matrix metal-loproteinases, and tissue inhibitor of metalloproteinases-1. *J. Exp. Med.* 184: 2311–2326.

Lauterborn, J. C., Rivera, S., Stinis, C. T., Hayes, V. Y., Isackson, P. J., and Gall, C. M. (1996). Differential effects of protein synthesis inhibition on the activity-dependent expression of BDNF transcripts: Evidence for immediate-early gene responses from specific promoters. *J. Neurosci.* 16: 7428–7436.

Letourneau, P. C., Condic, M. L., and Snow, D. M. (1994). Interactions of developing neurons with the extracellular matrix. *J. Neurosci.* 14: 915–928.

Levi, E., Fridman, R., Miao, H.-Q., Ma, Y.-S., Yayon, A., and Vlodavsky, I. (1996). Matrix metal-loproteinase 2 releases active soluble ectodomain of fibroblast growth factor receptor I. *Proc. Natl. Acad. Sci. USA* 93: 7069–7074.

Lim, G. P., Backstrom, J. R., Cullen, M. J., Miller, C. A., Atkinson, R. D., and Tokés, Z. A. (1996). Matrix metalloproteinases in the neocortex and spinal cord of amyotrophic lateral sclerosis patients. *J. Neurochem.* 67: 251–259.

Lim, G. P., Russell, M. J., Cullen, M. J., and Tokes, Z. A. (1997). Matrix metalloproteinases in dog brains exhibiting Alzheimer-like characteristics. *J. Neurochem.* 68: 1606–1611.

Lindvall, O., Ernfors, P., Bengzon, J., Kokaia, Z., Siesjö, B. K., and Persson, H. (1992). Differential regulation of mRNAs for nerve growth factor, brain-derived neurotrophic factor, and neurotrophin 3 in the adult rat brain following cerebral ischemia and hypoglycemic coma. *Proc. Natl. Acad. Sci. USA* 89: 648–652.

Lochter, A., Vaughan, L., Kaplony, A., Prochiantz, A., Schachner, M., and Faissner, A. (1991). J1/tenascin in substrate-bound and soluble form displays contrary effects on neurite outgrowth. *J. Cell Biol.* 113: 1159–1171.

Lochter, A., Taylor, J., Fuss, B., and Schachner, M. (1994). The extracellular matrix molecule janusin regulates neuronal morphology in a substrate- and culture time-dependent manner. *Eur. J. Neurosci.* 6: 597–606.

Logan, A., and Berry, M. (1993). Transforming growth factor-$\beta 1$ and basic fibroblast growth factor in the injured CNS. *Trends Pharmacol. Sci.* 14: 337–343.

Logan, S. K., Garebedian, M. J., Campbell, C. E., and Werb, Z. (1996). Synergetic transcriptional activation of the tissue inhibitor of metalloproteinases-1 promoter via functional interaction of AP-1 and Ets-1 transcription factors. *J. Biol. Chem.* 271: 774–782.

Lu, B., and Figurov, A. (1997). Role of neurotrophins in synapse development and plasticity. *Rev. Neurosci.* 8: 1–12.

Lüthi, A., van der Putten, H., Botteri, F. M., Mansuy, I. M., Meins, M., Frey, U., Sansig, G., Portet, C., Schmutz, M., Schröder, M., Nitsch, C., Laurent, J. P., and Monard, D. (1997). Endogenous serine protease inhibitor modulates epileptic activity and hippocampal long-term potentiation. *J. Neurosci.* 17: 4688–4699.

Lynch, G., Larson, J., and Baudry, M. (1986). Proteases, neuronal stability, and brain aging: a hypothesis. In *Treatment and Development Strategies for Alzheimer's Disease*, ed. Crook, R. Bartus, S. Ferris, and S. Gershon, eds., pp. 119–139. Madison, CT, Mark Powley.

Lyons, P. D., and Benveniste, E. N. (1998). Cleavage of membrane-associated ICAM-1 from astrocytes: involvement of a metalloprotease. *Glia* 22: 103–112.

Machida, C. M., Rodland, K. D., Matrisian, L., Magun, B. E., and Ciment, G. (1989). NGF induction of the gene encoding the protease transin accompanies neuronal differentiation in PC12. *Neuron* 2: 1587–1596.

Matsuzawa, K., Fukuyama, K., Hubbard, S. L., Dirks, P. B., and Rutka, J. T. (1996). Transfection of an invasive human astrocytoma cell line with a TIMP-1 cDNA : modulation of astrocytoma invasive potential. *J. Neuropathol. Exp. Neurol.* 55: 88–96.

McDonnell, S. E., Kerer, L. D., and Matrisian, L. M. (1990). Epidermal growth factor stimulation of stromelysin mRNA in rat fibroblasts requires induction of proto-oncogenes c-fos and c-jun and activation of protein kinase C. *Mol. Cell Biol.* 10: 4284–4293.

Meiri, N., Masos, T., Rosenblum, K., Miskin, R., and Dudai, Y. (1994). Overexpression of urokinase-type plasminogen activator in transgenic mice is correlated with impaired learning. *Proc. Natl. Acad. Sci. USA* 91: 3196–3200.

Meredith, J. E., Jr, Fazeli, B., and Schwartz, M. A. (1993). The extracellular matrix as a cell survival factor. *Mol. Biol. Cell* 4: 953–961.

Milev, P., Fischer, D., Haring, M., Schulthess, T., Margolis, R. K., Chiquet-Ehrismann, R., and Margolis, R. U. (1997). The fibrinogen-like globe of tenascin-C mediates its interactions with neurocan and phosphacan/protein-tyrosine phosphatase-zeta/beta. *J. Biol. Chem.* 272: 15501–15509.

Minami, M., Kuraishi, Y., Yamaguchi, T., Nakai, S., Hirai, Y., and Satoh, M. (1990). Convulsants induce interleukin-1 beta messenger RNA in rat brain. *Biochem. Biophys. Res. Commun.* 171: 832–837.

Minami, M., Kuraishi, Y., Yabuuchi, K., Yamazaki, A., and Satoh, M. (1992). Induction of interleukin-1 beta mRNA in rat brain after transient forebrain ischemia. *J. Neurochem.* 58: 390–392.

Miyazaki, K., Hasegawa, M., Funahashi, K., and Umeda, M. (1993). A metalloproteinase inhibitor domain in Alzheimer amyloid protein precursor. *Nature* 362: 839–841.

Mohanam, S., Wang, S. W., Rayford, A., Yamamoto, M., Sawaya, R., Nakajima, M., Liotta, L. A., Nicolson, G. L., Stetler-Stevenson, W. G., and Rao, J. S. (1995). Expression of tissue inhibitors of metalloproteinases: negative regulators of human glioblastoma invasion *in vivo*. *Clin. Exp. Metastasis* 13: 57–62.

Monard, D. (1988). Cell-derived proteases and protease inhibitors as regulators of neurite outgrowth. *Trends Neurosci.* 11: 541–544.

Moss, M. L., Jin, S.-L. C., Milla, M. E., Burkhart, W., Carter, H. L., Chen, W.-J., Clay, W. C., Didsbury, J. R., Hassier, D., Hoffman, C. R., Kost, T. A., Lambert, M. H., Leesnitzer, M. A., McCauley, P., McGeehan, G., Mitchell, J., Moyer, M., Pahel, G., Rocque, W., Overton, L. K., Schoenen, F., Seaton, T., Su, J.-L., Warner, J., Willard, D., and Becherer, D. (1997). Cloning of a disintegrin metalloproteinase that processes precursor tumour-necrosis factor-α. *Nature* 385: 733–736.

Muir, D. (1994). Metalloproteinase-dependent neurite outgrowth within a synthetic extracellular matrix is induced by nerve growth factor. *Exp. Cell Res.* 210: 243–252.

Muir, D., and Manthorpe, M. (1992). Stromelysin generates a fibronectin fragment that inhibits Schwann cell proliferation. *J. Cell Biol.* 116: 177–185.

Mullberg, J., Durie, F. H., Otten-Evans, C., Alderson, M. R., Rose-John, S., Cosman, D., Black, R. A., and Mohler, K. M. (1995). A metalloprotease inhibitor blocks shedding of the IL-6 receptor and the p60 TNF receptor. *J. Immunol.* 155: 5198–5205.

Muller, U., Cristina, N., Li, Z. W., Wolfer, D. P., Lipp, H. P., Rulicke, T., Brandner, S., Aguzzi, A., and Weissmann, C. (1994). Behavioral and anatomical deficits in mice homozygous for a modified beta-amyloid precursor protein gene. *Cell* 79: 755–765.

Murphy, G., Cockett, M. I., Stephens, P. E., Smith, B. J., and Docherty, A. J. (1987). Stromelysin is an activator of procollagenase. A study with natural and recombinant enzymes. *Biochem. J.* 248: 265–268.

Nakagawa, T., Kubota, T., Kabuto, M., Sato, K., Kawano, H., Hayakawa, T., and Okada, Y. (1994). Production of matrix metalloproteinases and tissue inhibitor of metalloproteinases-1 by human brain tumors. *J. Neurosurg.* 81: 69–77.

Nakic, M., Mitrovic, N., Sperk, G., and Schachner, M. (1996). Kainic acid activates transient expression of tenascin-C in the adult rat hippocampus. *J. Neurosci. Res.* 44: 355–362.

Nawashiro, H., Tasaki, K., Ruetzler, C. A., and Hallenbeck, J. M. (1997). TNF-alpha pretreatment induces protective effects against focal cerebral ischemia in mice. *J. Cereb. Blood Flow Metab.* 17: 483–490.

Nedivi, E., Hevroni, D., Naot, D., Israeli, D., and Citri, Y. (1993). Numerous candidate plasticity-related genes revealed by differential cDNA cloning. *Nature* 363: 718–722.

Niquet, J., Jorquera, I., Ben-Ari, Y., and Represa, A. (1994). Proliferative astrocytes may express fibronectin-like protein in the hippocampus of epileptic rats. *Neurosci. Lett.* 180: 13–16.

Niquet, J., Gillian, A., Ben-Ari, Y., and Represa, A. (1996). Reactive glial cells express a vitronectin-like protein in the hippocampus of epileptic rats. *Glia* 16: 359–367.

Nitecka, L., Tremblay, E., Charton, G., Bouillot, J. P., Berger, M. L., and Ben-Ari, Y. (1984). Maturation of kainic acid seizure–brain damage syndrome in the rat II. Histopathological sequelae. *Neuroscience* 13: 1073–1094.

Ogata, Y., Enghild, J. J., and Nagase, H. (1992). Matrix metalloproteinase 3 (stromelysin) activates the precursor for the human matrix metalloproteinase 9. *J. Biol. Chem.* 267: 3581–3584.

Ohta, K., Mizutani, A., Kawakami, A., Murakami, Y., Kasuya, Y., Takagi, S., Tanaka H., and Fujisawa, H. (1995). Plexin: a novel neuronal cell surface molecule that mediates cell adhesion via a homophilic binding mechanism in the presence of calcium ions. *Neuron* 14: 1189–1199.

Ohuchi, E., Imai, K., Fujii, Y., Sato, H., Seiki, M., and Okada, Y. (1977). Membrane type 1 matrix metalloproteinase digests interstitial collagens and other extracellular matrix macromolecules. *J. Biol. Chem.* 272: 2446–2451.

Okamoto, M., Mori, S., and Endo, H. (1994). A protective action of chondroitin sulfate proteoglycans against neuronal cell death induced by glutamate. *Brain Res.* 637: 57–67.

Pangalos, M. N., Shioi, J., Efthimiopoulos, S., Wu, A., and Robakis, N. K. (1996). Characterization of appican, the chondroitin sulfate proteoglycan form of the Alzheimer amyloid precursor protein. *Neurodegeneration* 5: 445–451.

Pei, D., and Weiss, S. J. (1995). Furin-dependent intracellular activation of the human stromelysin-3 zymogen. *Nature* 375: 244–247.

Peress, N., Perillo, E., and Zucker, S. (1995). Localization of tissue inhibitor of matrix metalloproteinases in Alzheimer's disease and normal brain. *J. Neuropathol. Exp. Neurol.* 54: 16–22.

Perides, G., Asher, R. A., Lark, M. W., Lane, W. S., Robinson, R. A., and Bignami, A. (1995). Glial hyaluronate-binding protein: a product of metalloproteinase digestion of versican? *Biochem. J.* 312: 377–384.

Perris, R. (1997). The extracellular matrix in neutral crest-cell migration. *Trends Neurosci.* 20: 23–31.

Pesheva, P., Gloor, S., Schachner, M., and Probstmeier, R. (1997). Tenascin-R is an intrinsic autocrine factor for oligodendrocyte differentiation and promotes cell adhesion by a sulfatide-mediated mechanism [erratum appears in *J. Neurosci.* (1997) 17: 6021]. *J. Neurosci.* 17: 4642–4651.

Pittman, R. N. (1985). Release of a plasminogen activator and a calcium-dependent metalloprotease from cultured sympathetic and sensory neurons. *Dev. Biol.* 110: 91–101.

Pittman, R. N., and Williams, A. G. (1988). Neurite penetration into collagen gels requires Ca^{2+} dependent metalloproteinase activity. *Dev. Neurosci.* 11: 41–51.

Planas, A. M., Soriano, M. A., Berruezo, M., Justicia, C., Estrada, A., Pitarch, S., and Ferrer, I. (1996). Induction of Stat3, a signal transducer and transcription factor, in reactive microglia following transient focal cerebral ischemia. *Eur. J. Neurosci.* 8: 2612–2618.

Planas, A. M., Justicia, C., and Ferrer, I. (1997). Stat1 in developing and adult rat brain. Induction after transient focal ischemia. *Neuroreport* 8: 1359–1362.

Qian, Z., Gilbert, M. E., Colicos, M. A., Kandel, E. R., and Kuhl, D. (1993). Tissue-plasminogen activator is induced as an immediate-early gene during seizure, kindling and long-term potentiation. *Nature* 361: 453–457.

Rajan, P., Stewart, C. L., and Fink, S. J. (1995) LIF-mediated activation of stat proteins after neuronal injury *in vivo. Neuroreport* 6: 2240–2244.

Raulo, E., Chernousov, M. A., Carey, D. J., Nolo, R., and Rauvala, H. (1994). Isolation of a neuronal cell surface receptor of heparin binding growth- associated molecule (HB-GAM). Identification as *N*-syndecan (syndecan-3). *J. Biol. Chem.* 269: 12999–3004.

Rauvala, H., and Peng, H. B. (1997). HB-GAM (heparin-binding growth-associated molecule) and heparin-type glycans in the development and plasticity of neuron-target contacts. *Prog. Neurobiol.* 52: 127–144.

Reeben, M., Abratova, J., Riekkinen, P., and Saarma, M. (1996). Role of a calcium-activated metalloprotease stromelysin-1 (transin) in the brain damage during epileptic seizures. *J. Neurochem.* 66: S56.

Reith, A., and Rucklidge, G. J. (1992). Invasion of brain tissue by primary glioma: evidence for the involvement of urokinase-type plasminogen activator as an activator of type IV collagenase. *Biochem. Biophys. Res. Commun.* 186: 348–354.

Represa, A., Niquet, J., Pollard, H., Khrestchatisky, M., and Ben-Ari, Y. (1994). From seizures to neo-synaptogenesis : intrinsic and extrinsic determinants of mossy fiber sprouting in the adult hippocampus. *Hippocampus* 4: 270–274.

Represa, A., Niquet, J., Pollard, H., and Ben-Ari, Y. (1995). Cell death, gliosis, and synaptic remodeling in the hippocampus of epileptic rats. *J. Neurobiol.* 26: 413–425.

Rivera, S., Timsit, S., Tremblay, E., Prats, E., Ouaghi, P., Ben-Ari, Y., and Khrestchatisky, M. (1996). Tissue inhibitor of metalloproteases 1 (TIMP-1) is an immediate early gene upregulated in epilepsy and ischemia. *Soc. Neurosci. Abstr.* 22: 1480.

Rivera, S., Tremblay, E., Timsit, S., Canals, O., Ben-Ari, Y., and Khrestchatisky, M. (1997). Tissue inhibitor of metalloproteinases-1 (TIMP-1) is differentially induced in neurons and astrocytes after seizures: evidence for developmental, immediate early gene, and lesion response. *J. Neurosci.* 17: 4223–4235.

Roher, A. E., Kasunic, T. C., Woods, A. S., Cotter, R. J., Ball, M. J., and Fridman, R. (1994). Proteolysis of A beta peptide from Alzheimer disease brain by gelatinase A. *Biochem. Biophys. Res. Commun.* 205: 1755–1761.

Romanic, A. M., and Madri, J. A. (1994). Extracellular matrix-degrading proteinases in the nervous system. *Brain Pathol.* 4: 145–156.

Rosenberg, G. A., and Navratil, M. (1997). Metalloproteinase inhibition blocks edema in intracerebral hemorrhage in the rat. *Neurology* 48: 921–926.

Rosenberg, G. A., Kornfeld, M., Estrada, E., Kelley, R. O., Liotta, L. A., and Stetler-Stevenson, W. G. (1992). TIMP-2 reduces proteolytic opening of blood-brain barrier by type IV collagenase. *Brain Res.* 576: 203–207.

Rosenberg, G. A., Dencoff, J. E., McGuire, P. G., Liotta, L. A., and Stetler-Stevenson, W. G. (1994). Injury-induced 92–kilodalton gelatinase and urokinase expression in rat brain. *Lab. Invest.* 71: 417–422.

Rosenberg, G. A., Navratil, L., Barone, F., and Feurstein, G. (1996). Proteolytic cascade enzymes increase in focal cerebral ischemia in rat. *J. Cereb. Blood Flow Metab.* 16: 360–366.

Rothman, S. M., and Olney, J. W. (1986). Glutamate and the pathophysiology of hypoxic-ischemic brain damage. *Ann. Neurol.* 19: 105–111.

Rothwell, N. J., and Hopkins, S. (1995). Cytokines and the nervous system II: actions and mechanisms of action. *Trends Neurosci.* 18: 130–136.

Rutishauser, U., and Landmesser, L. (1996). Polysialic acid in the vertebrate nervous system: a promoter of plasticity in cell-cell interactions. *Trends Neurosci.* 19: 422–427.

Sang, Q. A., Bodden, M. K., and Windsor, L. J. (1996). Activation of human progelatinase A by collagenase and matrilysin: activation of procollagenase by matrilysin. *J. Protein Chem.* 15: 243–253.

Sato, H., Kinoshita, T., Takino, T., Nakayama, K., and Seiki, M. (1996). Activation of a recombinant membrane type 1–matrix metalloproteinase (MT1–MMP) by furin and its interaction with tissue inhibitor of metalloproteinases (TIMP)-2. *FEBS Lett.* 393: 101–104.

Schachner, M. (1997). Neural recognition molecules and synaptic plasticity. *Curr. Opin. Cell. Biol.* 9: 627–634.

Schindler, C., and Darnell, J. E. (1995). Transcriptional responses to polypeptide ligands: the Jak-Stat pathway. *Annu. Rev. Biochem.* 64: 621–651.

Schwartz, N. B., Domowicz, M., Krueger, R. C., Jr., Li, H., and Mangoura, D. (1996). Brain aggrecan. *Perspect. Dev. Neurobiol.* 3: 291–306.

Seeds, N., Williams, B. L., and Bickford, P. C. (1995). Tissue plasminogen activator induction in Purkinje neurons after cerebellar motor learning. *Science* 270: 1992–1994.

Sheng, M., and Wyszynski, M. (1997). Ion channel targeting in neurons. *Bioessays* 19: 847–853.

Smeyne, R. J., Vendrell, M., Hayward, M., Baker, S. J., Miao, G. G., Schilling, K., Robertson, L. M., Curran, T., and Morgan, J. I. (1993). Continuous c-fos expression precedes programmed cell death in vivo. *Nature* 363: 166–169.

Snow, D. M., Lemmon, V., Carrino, D. A., Caplan, A. I., and Silver J. (1990). Sulfated proteoglycans in astroglial barriers inhibit neurite outgrowth in vitro. *Exp. Neurol.* 109: 111–130.

Soloway, P. D., Alexander, C. M., Werb, Z., and Jaenisch, R. (1996). Targeted mutagenesis of TIMP-1 reveals that lung tumor invasion is influenced by TIMP-1 genotype of the tumor but not by that of the host. *Oncogene* 13: 2307–2314.

Sonderegger, P., and Rathjen, F. G. (1992). Regulation of axonal growth in the vertebrate nervous system by interactions between glycoproteins belonging to two subgroups of the immunoglobulin superfamily. *J. Cell Biol.* 119: 1387–1394.

Stipp, C. S., Litwack, E. D., and Lander, A. D. (1994). Cerebroglycan: an integral membrane heparan sulfate proteoglycan that is unique to the developing nervous system and expressed specifically during neuronal differentiation. *J. Cell Biol.* 124: 149–160.

Takahashi, S., Sato, T., Ito, A., Ojima, Y., Hosono, T., Nagase, H., and Mori, Y. (1993). Involvement of protein kinase C in the interleukin 1 alpha-induced gene expression of matrix metalloproteinases and tissue inhibitor-1 of metalloproteinases (TIMP-1) in human uterine cervical fibroblasts. *Biochim. Biophys. Acta* 1220: 57–65.

Takino, T., Sato, H., Shinagawa, A., and Seiki, M. (1995). Identification of the second membrane-type matrix metalloproteinase (MT- MMP-2) gene from a human placenta cDNA library. MT-MMPs form a unique membrane-type subclass in the MMP family. *J. Biol. Chem.* 270: 23013–23020.

Tchelingerian, J.-L., Quinonero, J., Booss, J., and Jacque, C. (1993). Localization of TNF-α and IL-1α immunoreactivities in striatal neurons after surgical injury to the hippocampus. *Neuron* 10: 213–224.

Tremblay, E., Nitecka, L., Berger, M. L., and Ben-Ari, Y. (1984). Maturation of kainic acid seizure–brain damage syndrome in the rat I. Clinical, electrographic and matabolic observations. *Neuroscience* 13: 1051–1072.

Tsen, G., Halfter, W., Kroger, S., and Cole, G. J. (1995). Agrin is a heparan sulfate proteoglycan. *J. Biol. Chem.* 270: 3392–3399.

Tsirka, S. E., Gualandris, A., Amaral, D. G., and Strickland, S. (1995). Excitotoxin-induced neuronal degeneration and seizure are mediated by tissue plasminogen activator. *Nature* 377: 340–344.

Tsirka, S. E., Rogove, A. D., Bugge, T. H., Degen, J. L., and Strickland, S. (1997). An extracellular proteolytic cascade promotes neuronal degeneration in the mouse hippocampus. *J. Neurosci.* 15: 543–552.

Turgeon, V. L., and Houenou, L. J. (1997). The role of thrombin-like (serine) proteases in the development, plasticity and pathology of the nervous system. *Brain Res. Brain Res. Rev.* 25: 85–95.

Uemura, Y., Kowall, N. W., and Moskowitz, M. A. (1991). Focal ischemia in rats causes time-dependent expression of c-fos protein immunoreactivity in widespread regions of ipsilateral cortex. *Brain Res.* 552: 99–105.

Ushkaryov, Y. A., Petrenko, A. G., Geppert, M., and Sudhof, T. C. (1992). Neurexins: synaptic cell surface proteins related to the alpha-latrotoxin receptor and laminin. *Science* 257: 50–56.

Vallet, V., Chraibi, A., Gaeggeler, H. P., Horisberger, J. D., and Rossier, B. C. (1997). An epithelial serine protease activates the amiloride-sensitive sodium channel. *Nature* 389: 607–610.

Varnum-Finney, B., Venstrom, K., Muller, U., Kypta, R., Backus, C., Chiquet, M., and Reichardt, L. F. (1995). The integrin receptor alpha 8 beta 1 mediates interactions of embryonic chick motor and sensory neurons with tenascin-C. *Neuron* 14: 1213–1222.

Wang, X., Yue, T., White, R. F., Barone, F. C., and Feuerstein, G. Z. (1995). Transforming growth factor-β1 exhibits delayed gene expression following focal cerebral ischemia. *Brain Res. Bull.* 36: 607–609.

Weber, B. H., Vogt, G., Pruett, R. C., Stohr, H. and Felbor, U. (1994). Mutations in the tissue inhibitor of metalloproteinases-3 (TIMP3) in patients with Sorsby's fundus dystrophy. *Nat. Genet.* 8: 352–356.

Werb, Z. (1997). ECM and cell surface proteolysis: regulating cellular ecology. *Cell* 91: 439–442.

Werb, Z., Mainardi, C. L., Vater, C. A., and Harris, E. D. (1977). Endogenous activiation of latent collagenase by rheumatoid synovial cells. Evidence for a role of plasminogen activator. *N. Engl. J. Med.* 296: 1017–1023.

Wessel, T. C., Joh, T. H., and Volpe, B. T. (1991). *In situ* hybridization analysis of c-fos and c-jun expression in the rat brain following transient forebrain ischemia. *Brain Res.* 567: 231–240.

Williams, L. M., Gibbons, D. L., Gearing, A., Maini, R. N., Feldmann, M., and Brennan, F. M. (1996). Paradoxical effects of a synthetic metalloproteinase inhibitor that blocks both p55 and p75 TNF receptor shedding and TNF alpha processing in RA synovial membrane cell cultures. *J. Clin. Invest.* 97: 2833–2841.

Wilson, C. L., Heppner, K. J., Labosky, P. A., Hogan, B. L., and Matrisian, L. M. (1997). Intestinal tumorigenesis is suppressed in mice lacking the metalloproteinase matrilysin. *Proc. Natl. Acad. Sci. USA* 94: 1402–1407.

Wu, A., Pangalos, M. N., Efthimiopoulos, S., Shioi, J., and Robakis, N. K. (1997). Appican expression induces morphological changes in C6 glioma cells and promotes adhesion of neural cells to the extracellular matrix. *J. Neurosci.* 17: 4987–4993.

Yamada, H., Fredette, B., Shitara, K., Hagihara, K., Miura, R., Ranscht, B., Stallcup, W. B., and Yamaguchi, Y. (1997). The brain chondroitin sulfate proteoglycan brevican associates with astrocytes ensheathing cerebellar glomeruli and inhibits neurite outgrowth from granule neurons. *J. Neurosci.* 17: 7784–7795.

Yamaguchi, Y. (1996). Brevican: a major proteoglycan in adult brain. *Perspect. Dev. Neurobiol.* 3: 307–317.

Zucker, S., Conner, C., DiMassmo, B. I., Ende, H., Drews, M., Seiki, M., and Bahou, W. F. (1995). Thrombin induces activation of progelatinase A in vascular endothelial cells. Physiological regulation of agiogenesis. *J. Biol. Chem.* 270: 23730–23738.

Rivera and Khrestchatisky

4 Long-Term Potentiation: From Molecular Mechanisms to Structural Changes

Dominique Muller, Nicolas Toni, and Pierre-Alain Buchs

Long-term potentiation (LTP) remains without doubt one of the most fascinating properties expressed by central excitatory synapses. The reproducibility of the phenomenon, as well as its stability, has brought about an unprecedented amount of work that, surprisingly, has so far failed to provide a clear understanding of the mechanisms underlying this property. Covalent modifications of proteins or receptors, activation of enzymes, second messenger cascades, retrograde messengers, involvement of growth factors, adhesion molecules, activation of gene expression and plasticity programs, structural reorganization of synapses, formation of new synaptic connections —all have been proposed to contribute to LTP. The variety of these mechanisms clearly indicates that a complex interplay of molecular and biochemical events is likely to participate in LTP. The aim of this chapter is to summarize some of these recent results and propose the idea that LTP could represent more than a simple way to modify synaptic strength. It is argued that many of the events that have been reported to contribute to LTP are consistent with the idea that LTP could, at least in part, be associated with a remodeling of synaptic contacts and the formation of new synapses. According to this view, LTP could be part of a more general mechanism that would be important during development, as in adult life, in promoting the formation and stabilizing the existence of appropriate synapses.

ROLE OF PROTEIN PHOSPHORYLATION IN LTP

Activation of protein kinases by the rise in calcium occurring during induction of LTP was one of the first biochemical events to be postulated to contribute to the increase in synaptic strength. Originally, this proposition was based on the results of pharmacological studies showing that various antagonists of protein kinases were capable of blocking induction of LTP, while exogenous activation could result in an enhancement of synaptic transmission (Malenka et al. 1986; Malinow et al. 1988; Lovinger et al. 1987). Consistent with this interpretation, several kinases have been reported to be activated by high-frequency stimulation. This includes protein kinase C (PKC) (Akers et al. 1986; Klann et al. 1991), calcium-calmodulin–dependent protein kinase II (CaMKII) (Fukunaga et al. 1993), cyclic adenosine monophosphate (AMP)–dependent kinase (Roberson et al. 1996), and casein kinase (Chariault-Marlangue et al. 1991). While the precise contribution of these enzymes still remains unclear for most of them, a large body of evidence has accumulated suggesting a major role for CaMKII. This kinase is of particular interest not only because it is highly enriched in postsynaptic density (PSD) fractions (Kennedy et al. 1983) but also because of specific properties concerning its mode of activation. Calcium and calmodulin are the triggering signals that activate the enzyme. In addition, activity of CaMKII is also modulated by phosphorylation in such a way that autophosphorylated CaMKII remains active in a calcium-independent fashion (Miller and Kennedy 1986).

The idea was thus proposed that CaMKII could work as a kind of molecular switch that would be activated by calcium and calmodulin during high-frequency stimulation and then maintain its high level of activity for a prolonged period of time through an autophosphorylation process (Lisman 1994). In support of this interpretation, it was found that postsynaptic blockade of CaMKII prevents LTP induction (Malinow et al. 1989; Malenka et al. 1989), that genetic manipulations that disrupt the expression of CaMKII also result in a deficient LTP (Silva et al. 1992), that induction of LTP results in a D-AP5–sensitive, long-lasting increase in the calcium-independent activity of CaMKII (Fukunaga et al. 1993), and that this activation is correlated with an increased autophosphorylation of the kinase as measured by ^{32}P incorporation into the protein (Fukunaga et al. 1995). This result was recently confirmed not only by measuring ^{32}P incorporation in the kinase but also by analyzing immunoblots using a phosphospecific antibody and measuring the amount of the protein phosphorylated on the threonine (Thr)286 site responsible for the calcium-independent activity of the enzyme (Barria et al. 1997).

Another interesting result about this enzyme concerns the possibility that LTP induction is not only associated with an increase in the activity and level of autophosphorylation of the enzyme but also with an increased expression of the protein. The experiments in which the activity of CaMKII was measured before and after LTP induction showed an increase in the total activity of the enzyme that could not be explained by a different distribution among subcellular fractions (Fukunaga et al. 1993, 1995). Furthermore, analysis of gene expression after LTP induction reproducibly concluded that the gene coding for the α-subunit of CaMKII was a likely candidate for a plasticity gene, since its expression was enhanced by LTP induction (Nedivi et al. 1993). Finally, a recent study provided evidence using immunocytochemistry for an increase in the amount of the protein and of its autophosphorylation in the dendrites following LTP induction (Ouyang et al. 1997). One can conclude from these studies that the patterns of stimulation that produce LTP and result in a postsynaptic rise in calcium not only activate the kinase but probably also enhance the expression of the gene and translation of the protein.

What then, could be the function of the kinase? Answers to this question still remain conjectural. Substrates of the enzyme have started to be identified and one important target could be postsynaptic glutamate receptors of the α-amino-3-hydroxy-5-methylisoxazole-4-propionic acid (AMPA) type. Recent experiments carried out following immunoprecipitation of AMPA receptors using antibodies against the GluR1 subunit revealed a progressive and lasting increase in the level of ^{32}P incorporation in the GluR1 subunit following LTP induction (Barria et al. 1997). Phosphorylation of the AMPA receptor was found to be D-AP5 sensitive and could be blocked by pre-incubation with the CaMKII inhibitor, KN-62. Furthermore, peptide mapping experiments showed that the phosphorylation of the GluR1 subunit found after LTP induction was comparable to that observed in HEK293 cells by coexpression of GluR1 and an active form of CaMKII (Barria et al. 1997). Thus phosphorylation of the AMPA receptor on GluR1 is likely to be due to the activation of CaMKII. This cascade of events involving calcium entry in the postsynaptic spine, activation and autophosphorylation of CaMKII, and phosphorylation of the AMPA receptor may therefore represent a major biochemical process associated with LTP induction. This possibility is so much more attractive that phosphorylation of the AMPA receptor has been shown to result in an enhancement of AMPA responses. This was demonstrated in HEK-293 cells by coexpression of the GluR1 subunit and an active form of CaMKII (McGlade-McCulloh et al. 1993). Similar results were also obtained in hippocampal pyramidal neurons either by injection of a phosphatase inhibitor or of calmodulin, which activates CaMKII (Figurov et al. 1993; Wang et Kelly, 1995), or by direct injection of an active form of the kinase (Lledo et al. 1995). This effect seems to be due, as suggested by recent experiments, to an increase in the number of available channels (Shirke and Malinow, 1997). This potentiation of AMPA responses has been reported, in some cases, to be occluded by prior induction of LTP. This could suggest that at least part of the synaptic potentiation that characterizes LTP may result from a phosphorylation of the AMPA receptor and associated changes in receptor properties.

There is, however, one piece of evidence that does not perfectly fit with this hypothesis. If LTP were simply to be explained by an activation of CaMKII and the phosphorylation of AMPA receptors, then blockade of the kinase after induction should reverse synaptic potentiation. Experiments carried out by several groups, including recent intracellular perfusion studies in which CaMKII antagonists were used, showed that these treatments do not reverse established LTP (Malinow et al. 1989; Ito et al. 1991; Otmakov et al. 1997). One possible explanation for this result could be that the CaMKII cascade is necessary but not sufficient for generating LTP. Activation of other kinases (PKC, prokininogenase, tyrosine kinases), other enzymes, or transcription factor cascades might also be required. Phosphorylation mechanisms might thus contribute to LTP not only through covalent modifications of proteins but also as a means to signal where in the dendritic tree, in which synapse, more profound modifications may have to take place. The phosphorylation of the AMPA receptor reported above, as well as the phosphorylation of other substrates, could represent a way to locally modify more complex processes such as the turnover of proteins, insertion of new proteins in the membrane, remodeling of synaptic structures, and modifications of PSD. The observation that insertion and distribution of N-methyl-D-aspartate (NMDA) receptors on the cell surface can be regulated by protein phosphorylation is in this respect particularly interesting (Ehlers et al. 1995). The phosphorylation cascade involving CaMKII and AMPA receptors should therefore be considered not only in terms of the covalent modifications that this cascade produces on the receptor itself but probably also in the context of the other changes that have been reported to occur at the synapse.

LONG-TERM POTENTIATION AND ULTRASTRUCTURAL MODIFICATIONS OF SYNAPSES

Among changes that have repeatedly been associated with the induction of synaptic potentiation and learning are structural modifications of the synapse. At the beginning of this century, Ramón y Cajal, based on his observations of the complexity of neuronal and synaptic networks, proposed that remodeling of synaptic connections could represent a mechanism underlying learning in the brain. Later, when LTP was discovered by Bliss and colleagues (Bliss and Lømo, 1973), one of the first mechanisms that was considered involved morphological changes. In a series of studies, Fifkova and Van Harreveld (1977) and Fifkova and Anderson (1981) reported an increase in the size of spine heads and an enlargement and a decrease in the length of spine necks following high-frequency stimulation. By contributing to a reduction of the resistance to synaptic currents, the changes in spine necks could have accounted for an increase in synaptic strength as proposed by modeling studies (Rall 1978). However, changes in size of spine necks were not detected in later studies and physiological tests of the possible role of spine neck enlargement in LTP concluded in a negative result (Jung et al. 1991; Svoboda et al. 1996).

Numerous studies were then undertaken which all concluded that LTP was associated with some kind of morphological changes (Lee et al. 1980, 1981; Desmond and Levy 1986a,b 1988; Chang and Greenough, 1984; Schuster et al. 1990; Trommald et al. 1990, 1997; Chang et al. 1991; Geinisman et al. 1989, 1991, 1996; Geinisman 1993; Buchs and Muller 1996). While there are clearly discrepancies between the different results of these studies, there seem to be two major types of changes that emerge. On the one hand there are modifications of the synaptic zones and particularly an increase in the proportion of synapses with perforated PSDs (Schuster et al. 1990; Geinisman et al. 1989, 1991, 1993; Buchs and Muller 1996). Secondly, changes were also observed in the density of synapses and particularly in the number of specific types of synapses (Lee et al. 1980, 1981; Chang et al. 1991; Trommald et al. 1990, 1997; Rusakov et al. 1996; Geinisman et al. 1996).

Modifications of the PSDs, and more specifically changes in the number of synapses exhibiting perforated PSDs, probably represent one of the most robust and reproducible morphological alterations that have been found to correlate with synaptic plasticity (Greenough et al. 1978; Calverley and Jones 1990). Perforated synapses are defined by the presence of a clear interruption of the PSD. Usually, perforations are quite heterogeneous and may vary greatly from a simple, short discontinuity of the PSD to the presence of multiple segmentations (see figure 4.3). Sometimes also, PSDs are completely partitioned and separated by a small invagination of the postsynaptic membrane into the presynaptic terminal called a spinule (Routtenberg and Tarrant 1975). It is of interest to note that in most of the cases where the perforation is associated with a small spinule, it is possible to observe in the presynaptic terminal that the synaptic vesicles accumulate in apparently two distinct groups as if the synapse were made of two separate functional units.

Geinisman et al. (1989) and Schuster et al. (1990) were the first to describe an increase in the proportion of perforated synapses in the dentate gyrus following LTP induction. Later, Geinisman and colleagues confirmed and extended these observations. Using unbiased, stereological methods they found in in vivo experiments that a strong LTP stimulation paradigm induced a significant and marked increase in the proportion of perforated synapses with multiple, completely partitioned transmission zones (Geinisman et al. 1991, 1992; Geinisman 1993). We recently confirmed this result using a quite different approach. Taking advantage of slice cultures and a precipitation technique that allowed us to reveal the presence of calcium accumulated in subcellular structures under the form of a fine precipitate (Buchs et al. 1994), we were able to identify a subset of synapses that could represent activated synapses (Buchs and Muller 1996). We found that application of high-frequency burst stimulation to these cultures resulted in a marked increase in the number of postsynaptic spines that contained the precipitates. This accumulation occurred only with stimulation paradigms that induced LTP and required NMDA receptor activation. The approach used therefore allowed identification of a subset of synapses in which calcium had accumulated in the postsynaptic spine through activated NMDA receptors (figure 4.1). Comparison of the ultrastructural characteristics of labeled and presumably potentiated synapses with naive and nonlabeled synaptic contacts revealed a dramatic increase in the proportion of perforated synapses (figure 4.2). Calculations suggested that among the simple synapses activated by high-frequency stimulation, about 60% to 80% of them exhibited perforated PSDs after LTP induction. Although these numbers may have to be taken with caution, since the analysis was not carried out using unbiased stereological methods, the magnitude of the change strongly supported the hypothesis that LTP induction in this model was associated with the formation of synapses with perforated PSDs.

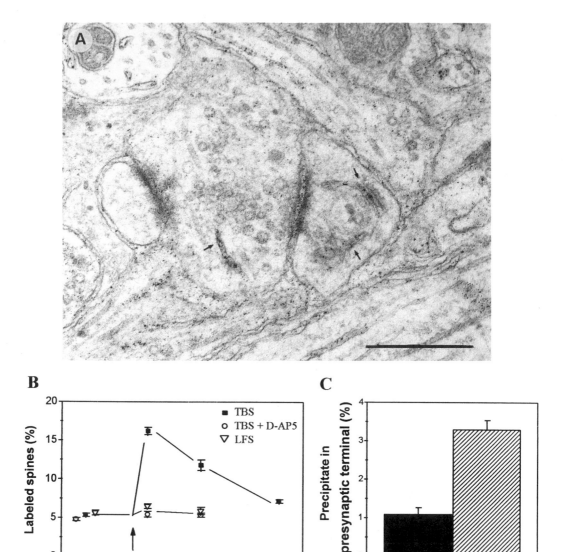

Figure 4.1 Labeling of a subset of synapses activated by high-frequency stimulation was achieved through the use of a precipitation method that reveals the accumulation of calcium in subcellular organelles under the form of a fine, electron-dense precipitate. A, Illustration of a spine profile obtained from a slice culture fixed five minutes after long-term potentiation (LTP) induction using a theta burst stimulation paradigm. Note the presence of dense precipitates in reticulum-like tubules in the postsynaptic spine. B, Changes in the proportion of spine profiles that contained precipitates in cultures fixed before, two, seven, and fifteen minutes after high-frequency stimulation. The increase in labelled spine profiles observed after theta burst stimulation (TBS, black squares) was prevented by pretreatment with D-AP5, an antagonist of N-methyl-D-aspartate (NMDA) receptors (open circles), or by application of stimulation trains (10 Hz) that did not induce LTP (open triangles). C, Stimulation of slice cultures resulted in a concomitant increase in the accumulation of calcium precipitate in presynaptic terminal profiles.

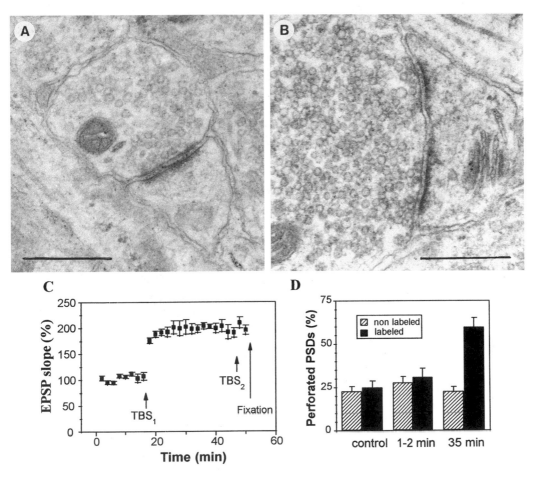

Figure 4.2 Morphological analysis of labeled spine profiles revealed a dramatic increase in the proportion of perforated synapses thirty minutes after LTP induction. (A) Illustration of a non-labeled spine profile found in a stimulated hippocampal slice culture. (B) Illustration of a labeled perforated spine profile observed in a slice culture thirty minutes after LTP induction. (C) Graph illustrating the changes in synaptic efficacy recorded in the six slice cultures in which morphological analyses were carried out. (D) Changes in the proportion of perforated spine profiles found in labeled and unlabeled synapses in fourteen slice cultures before, two minutes, and thirty-five minutes after LTP induction. Note that the increase in perforated synapses occurs 35 minutes, but not 2 minutes, after stimulation.

Another remarkable feature observed in these studies was that the synapses with perforated PSDs did not occur immediately. Analysis of labeled synapses two to five minutes after stimulation showed no changes in the proportion of perforated contacts. Then the proportion of synapses with perforated PSDs gradually increased over time to reach a maximum at about thirty minutes after LTP induction (see figure 4.2). Control experiments carried out under conditions where LTP was blocked prevented the occurrence of these morphological changes (unpublished data). These results therefore strengthen the possibility of a direct link between the induction of synaptic plasticity and a structural remodeling of the PSD.

What could be the role of synapses with perforated PSDs? One of the first ideas to be proposed was that perforated synapses could contribute to synaptic plasticity, to the formation and elimination of synapses, and thus to the turnover of synapses (Carlin and Siekevitz 1983). Perforated synapses were indeed found to be increased during development and synapse maturation (Dyson and Jones 1984; Itarat and Jones 1992), as well as in animals raised in a complex environment or subjected to visual training (Greenough et al. 1978). Furthermore, perforated synapses were reported to increase transiently in a model of synapse turnover produced by entorhinal lesions (Nieto-Sampedro et al. 1982) and were also associated with kindling in the dentate gyrus (Geinisman et al. 1992). All these observations led therefore to the concept that perforated synapses could represent an intermediate step in spine division. According to this hypothesis, synaptic activity might result in the incorporation of material in the PSD of a simple synapse and thereby an increase in length of the PSD and the appearance of perforations. As the synapse enlarges, a spinule could develop resulting in the formation of a completely partitioned synapse. Ultimately, the dendritic spine could then split in two or be reorganized so as to produce two new distinct simple synapses, which should be visualized, at least at some point, as double synapses where the same terminal makes a synaptic contact with two adjacent spines.

It still remains unclear whether this scheme represents more than a simple hypothesis and whether changes of this type may also occur following induction of LTP. Suggestive images can indeed be found in organotypic hippocampal cultures after high-frequency stimulation (figure 4.3). Also, the results of several studies suggest that the late phases of LTP could rather be associated with an increase in the total number of synapses. Trommald et al. (1990) found an increase in the number of bifurcating spines after LTP. Using confocal analyses Hosokawa et al. (1995) reported changes in the orientation and density of spines. Recently, Geinisman and colleagues (1996) carried out an analysis using unbiased stereological methods thirteen days following in vivo induction of LTP. The essential result of this study is the observation of an increase in the number of asymmetrical axodendritic synapses with no differences in the number of perforated synapses or other types of spine synapses. It seems not unlikely therefore that the late phases of LTP could rather be associated with changes in the total number of synapses.

Increases in synapse number could occur in different ways and, as already mentioned, could involve perforated synapses as an intermediate step. A splitting mechanism should result in a sequence of events involving multiple-synapse boutons in which a single terminal should contact two neighboring spines on the same dendrite. Preliminary experiments carried out using the calcium precipitation method to identify activated synapses indeed suggest

Muller, Toni, and Buchs

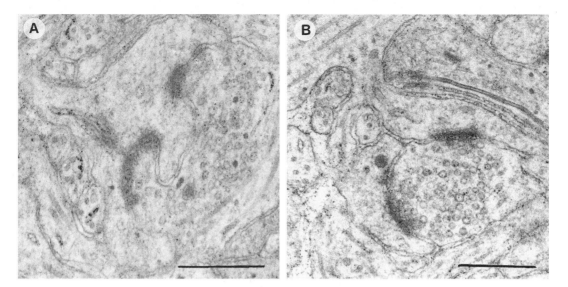

Figure 4.3 Illustration of synaptic profiles found in hippocampal organotypic cultures after induction of LTP and that are consistent with the idea that perforated synapses could represent an intermediate step in spine division. (A) Illustration of a spine profile exhibiting a perforated postsynaptic density (PSD) separated by a prominent spinule. Note also the presence of labeled membranous tubular structures in the postsynaptic spine. (B) Illustration of an example of a double synapse in which the same terminal makes synaptic contacts with two, possibly adjacent spines.

that perforated synapses might not be a stable morphological change and that multiple synaptic boutons can indeed be observed (see figure 4.3). However, little information is yet available on the frequency of these synapses following LTP induction. It should also be noted that a recent study carried out following three-dimensional-reconstruction of a few bifurcating spines concluded that a splitting mechanism seems unlikely, since the twin spine heads in these cases rarely shared the same presynaptic terminal (Trommald et al. 1997). Another possibility is that perforated synapses relax or retract into axodendritic synapses. This could be consistent with the result of several studies, including the recent study by Geinisman et al. (1996) showing that the only detectable morphological change observed thirteen days after in vivo LTP induction was an increase in the proportion of axodendritic synapses. Because of their direct apposition to a dendritic shaft, axodendritic synapses could be expected to express a high level of synaptic efficacy. It remains, however, to be demonstrated that axodendritic synapses contribute significantly to the late phases of LTP. Important information is still missing with regard to the various steps involved in synapse remodeling to be able to understand precisely whether the morphological changes observed following LTP induction fit into a more general hypothesis stating that LTP could represent a mechanism by which new synapses are formed.

MOLECULAR ASPECTS OF LTP

In addition to the morphological evidence supporting the idea of a structural remodeling of the synapse following LTP induction, several recent studies have also implicated molecules, such as adhesion molecules, extracellular proteases, or growth factors, that are known to contribute to intercellular communication and structural plasticity. In a recent study carried out using antibodies and various peptides that interfered with the homo- and heterophilic binding of the adhesion molecules L1 and nerve cell adhesion molecules (N-CAMs), it was possible to show that these molecules are involved in LTP induction (Lüthi et al. 1994). More recently, we found additional evidence for a role of the adult and embryonic forms of the NCAM molecule in this form of synaptic plasticity. The embryonic form of the NCAM molecule is characterized by the presence of long chains of $\alpha2$–8-polysialic acid (PSA) bound to the molecule and referred to as PSA-NCAM. This embryonic form of NCAM is highly expressed during development and is believed to confer antiadhesive properties to cellular membrane. Accordingly, the upregulation of PSA-NCAM expression at the cell surface in various models of plasticity has been proposed to reduce NCAM-dependent membrane interactions and facilitate membrane remodeling (Kiss and Rougon 1997). By studying the role of PSA-NCAM in the hippocampus, we found that this molecule is directly expressed at synapses and that its expression is under the control of neuronal and synaptic activity (Muller et al. 1996). Thus trains of high-frequency stimulation could represent a means to increase the level of expression of the molecule in synaptic membranes. Furthermore, elimination of PSA-NCAM by a specific endoneuraminidase was found to prevent LTP induction (Muller et al. 1996). Since these experiments were carried out in slice cultures, it was possible, after the enzymatic elimination of PSA, to wash out the enzyme and wait for reexpression of PSA-NCAM. Interestingly, these experiments showed that the reexpression of the molecule in the synaptic field, as detected by immunocytochemistry, coincided with a recovery in the capacity to induce LTP. These results therefore clearly indicated that PSA-NCAM is required for the induction of synaptic potentiation.

How adhesion molecules contribute to LTP remains unclear. One possibility is that these molecules act through a modulation of second messenger cascades that are critical for inducing synaptic plasticity. As mentioned above, phosphorylation mechanisms are involved in this form of plasticity and modifications of hetero- and homophilic interactions between adhesion molecules could indirectly affect such mechanisms. It is, however, also possible that the contribution of adhesion molecules to LTP is to participate in the remodeling of synaptic structures by modifying the interactions between pre- and postsynaptic membranes. A similar argument has been made with regard to tissue plasminogen activator. This secreted extracellular protease is expressed in the central nervous system (CNS), transcription of its gene is under the control of neuronal activity (Qian et al. 1993), and experiments demonstrating that transgenic animals that do not express the protease also lack stable LTP (Huang et al. 1996) suggest that it contributes to induction of synaptic plasticity. In the same way, LTP-inducing activity enhances the transcription of genes for growth factors and in particular brain-derived neurotrophic factor (BDNF). This growth factor modulates synaptic transmission and facilitates induction of LTP (Figurov et al. 1996). Transgenic animals that are deficient in the *BDNF* gene lack stable potentiation and this deficit can be rescued by exogenous application of BDNF (Korte et al. 1995; Patterson et al. 1996). Taken together, these recent data indicate that morphoregulatory molecules, which have an overt implication in various aspects of neuronal development, also play a significant role in properties of synaptic plasticity and have an expression that is under the control of neuronal activity. This suggests that they could represent a link between activity-induced changes in synaptic strength and ultrastructural modifications of synapses and the remodeling of synaptic networks that may be associated.

CONCLUSION

The molecular and morphological results described in this chapter make it extremely tempting to propose that LTP may be part of an ensemble of mechanisms that allow translation of neuronal activity into modifications in the function and structural organization of synaptic networks. Despite discrepancies among studies, the vast majority of morphological analyses have demonstrated the existence of structural changes associated with the induction of LTP. Among these, one of the best-documented modifications involves the formation of perforated synapses. Interestingly, it is also at the level of the PSD that some of the major biochemical events believed to contribute to LTP take place, namely the activation and autophosphorylation of CaMKII and the phosphorylation of AMPA receptors. Several other molecules could also be involved, including adhesion molecules such as PSA-NCAM, which are expressed at the synapse in an activity-dependent manner, and could participate in the structural changes accompanying LTP. One of the critical issues, however, that remains to be answered is whether these morphological changes associated with LTP are purely coincidental or whether they directly account for the lasting functional changes in synaptic strength that characterizes LTP. Answers to this question will require analysis of the contribution of molecules important for the increase in synaptic strength in the morphological changes. It is likely that the recent developments in gene technology that allow selective modification of the expression of specific proteins, in particular brain areas, combined with the exciting advances made in two-photon confocal microscopy that make it possible to visualize cellular structures such as spines within living tissue will open new avenues for investigating and testing this hypothesis.

ACKNOWLEDGMENT

This work was supported by the Swiss National Science Foundation.

REFERENCES

Akers, R. F., Lovinger, D. M., Colley, P. A., Linden, D. J., and Routtenberg, A. (1986). Translocation of protein kinase C activity may mediate hippocampal long-term potentiation. *Science* 231: 587–589.

Barria, A., Muller, D., Derkach, V., Griffith, L. C., and Soderling, T. R. (1997). Regulatory phosphorylation of AMPA-type glutamate receptors by CaM-KII during long-term potentiation. *Science.* 276: 2042–2045.

Bliss, T. V. P., and Lømo, T. (1973). Long-lasting potentiation of synaptic transmission in the dentate area of anaesthetized rabbit following stimulation of the perforant path. *J. Physiol. (Lond.)* 232: 331–356.

Buchs, P.-A., Stoppini, L., Parducz, A., Siklos, L., and Muller, D. (1994) A new cytochemical method for the ultrastructural localization of calcium in the central nervous system. *J. Neurosci. Methods* 54: 83–93.

Buchs, P.-A., and Muller, D. (1996). LTP induction is associated with major ultrastructural changes of activated synapses. *Proc. Natl. Acad. Sci. USA* 96: 8040–8045.

Calverley, R. K., and Jones, D. G. (1990). Contributions of dendritic spines and perforated synapses to synaptic plasticity. *Brain Res. Brain Res. Rev.* 15: 215–249.

Carlin, R. K., and Siekevitz, P. (1983). Plasticity in the central nervous system: do synapses divide? *Proc. Natl. Acad. Sci. USA* 80: 3517–3521.

Chang, F-L. F., and Greenough, W. T. (1984). Transient and enduring morphological correlates of synaptic activity and efficacy change in the rat hippocampal slice. *Brain Res.* 309: 35–46.

Chang, P. L., Isaacs, K. R., and Greenough, W. T. (1991). Synapse formation occurs in association with the induction of long-term potentiation in two-year-old rat hippocampus in vitro. *Neurobiol. Aging* 12: 517–522.

Charriaut-Marlangue, C., Otani, S., Creuzet, C., Ben-Ari, Y., and Loeb, J. (1991). Rapid activation of hippocampal casein kinase II during long-term potentiation. *Proc. Natl. Acad. Sci. USA* 88: 10232–10236.

Desmond, N. L., and Levy, W. B. (1986a). Changes in the numerical density of synaptic contacts with long-term potentiation in the hippocampal dentate gyrus. *J. Comp. Neurol.* 253: 466–475.

Desmond, N. L., and Levy, W. B. (1986b). Changes in the postsynaptic density with long-term potentiation in the dentate gyrus. *J. Comp. Neurol.* 253: 476–482.

Desmond, N. L., and Levy, W. B. (1988). Synaptic interface surface area increases with long-term potentiation in the hippocampal dentate gyrus. *Brain Res.* 453: 308–314.

Dyson, S. E., and Jones, D. G. (1984). Synaptic remodelling during development and maturation: junction differentiation and splitting as a mechanism for modifying connectivity. *Dev. Brain Res.* 13: 125–137.

Ehlers, M. D., Tingley, W. G., and Huganir, R. L. (1995). Regulated subcellular distribution of the NR1 subunit of the NMDA receptor. *Science* 269: 1734–1737.

Fifkova, E., and Anderson, C. L. (1981). Stimulation-induced changes in dimensions of stalks of dendritic spines in the dentate molecular layer. *Exp. Neurol.* 74: 621–627.

Fifkova, E., and Van Harreveld, A. (1977). Long-lasting morphological changes in dendritic spines of dentate granular cells following stimulation of the entorhinal area. *J. Neurocytol.* 6: 211–230.

Figurov, A., Boddeke, H., and Muller, D. (1993). Enhancement of AMPA-mediated synaptic transmission by the protein phosphatase inhibitor calyculin A in rat hippocampal slices. *Eur. J. Neurosci.* 5: 1035–1041.

Figurov, A., Pozzo Miller, L. D., Olafsson, P., Wang, T., and Lu, B. (1996). Regulation of synaptic responses to high-frequency stimulation and LTP by neurotrophins in the hippocampus. *Nature* 381: 706–709.

Fukunaga, K., Stoppini, L., Miyamoto, E., and Muller, D. (1993). Long-term potentiation is associated with an increased activity of calcium/calmodulin-dependent protein kinase II. *J. Biol. Chem.* 268: 7863–7867.

Fukunaga, K., Muller, D., and Miyamoto, E. (1995). Increased phosphorylation of Ca2+/calmodulin-dependent protein kinase II and its endogenous substrates in the induction of long-term potentiation. *J. Biol. Chem.* 270: 6119–6124.

Geinisman, Y. (1993). Perforated axospinous synapses with multiple, completely partitioned transmission zones: probable structural intermediates in synaptic plasticity. *Hippocampus* 3: 417–434.

Geinisman, Y., deToledo Morrell, L., and Morrell, F. (1991). Induction of long-term potentiation is associated with an increase in the number of axospinous synapses with segmented postsynaptic densities. *Brain Res.* 566: 77–88.

Geinisman, Y., Morrell, F., and de Toledo-Morrell, L. (1989). Perforated synapses on double-headed dendritic spines: a possible structural substrate of synaptic plasticity. *Brain Res.* 480: 326–329.

Geinisman, Y., Morrell, F., and deToledo Morrell, L. (1992). Increase in the number of axospinous synapses with segmented postsynaptic densities following hippocampal kindling. *Brain Res.* 569: 341–347.

Geinisman, Y., DeToledo-Morrell, L., Morrell, F., Persina, I. S., and Beatty, M. A. (1996). Synapse restructuring associated with the maintenance phase of hippocampal long-term potentiation. *J. Comp. Neurol.* 368: 413–423.

Greenough, W. T., West, R. W., and DeVoogd, T. J. (1978). Subsynaptic plate perforations: changes with age and experience in the rat. *Science* 202: 1096–1098.

Hosokawa, T., Rusakov, D. A., Bliss, T. V., and Fine, A. (1995). Repeated confocal imaging of individual dendritic spines in the living hippocampal slice: evidence for changes in length and orientation associated with chemically induced LTP. *J. Neurosci.* 15: 5560–5573.

Huang, Y. Y., Bach, M. E., Lipp, H. P., Zhuo, M., Wolfer, D. P., Hawkins, R. D., Schoonjans, L., Kandel, E. R., Godfraind, J. M., Mulligan, R., Collen, D., and Carmeliet, P. (1996). Mice lacking the gene encoding tissue-type plasminogen activator show a selective interference with late-phase long-term potentiation in both Schaffer collateral and mossy fiber pathways. *Proc. Natl. Acad. Sci. USA* 93: 8699–7004.

Itarat, W., and Jones, D. G. (1992). Perforated synapses are present during synaptogenesis in rat neocortex. *Synapse* 11: 279–286.

Ito, I., Hidaka, H., and Sugiyama, H. (1991). Effects of KN-62, a specific inhibitor of calcium/calmodulin-dependent protein kinase II, on long-term potentiation in the rat hippocampus. *Neurosci. Lett.* 121: 119–121.

Jung, M. W., Larson, J., and Lynch, G. (1991). Evidence that changes in spine neck resistance are not responsible for expression of LTP. *Synapse* 7: 216–220.

Kennedy, M. B., Bennett, M. K., and Erondu, N. E. (1983). Biochemical and immunochemical evidence that the major postsynaptic density protein is a subunit of a calmodulin-dependent protein kinase. *Proc. Natl. Acad. Sci. USA* 80: 7357–7361.

Kiss, J. Z., and Rougon, G. (1997). Cell biology of polysialic acid. *Curr. Opin. Neurobiol.* 7: 640–646.

Klann, E., Chen, S.-J., and Sweatt, J. D. (1991). Persistent protein kinase activation in the maintenance phase of long-term potentiation. *J. Biol. Chem.* 266: 24253–24256.

Korte, M., Carroll, P., Wolf, E., Brem, G., Thoenen, H., and Bonhoeffer, T. (1995). Hippocampal long-term potentiation is impaired in mice lacking brain-derived neurotrophic factor. *Proc. Natl. Acad. Sci. USA* 92: 8856–8860.

Lee, K., Schottler, F., Oliver, M., and Lynch, G. (1980). Brief bursts of high frequency stimulation produce two types of structural changes in rat hippocampus. *J. Neurophysiol.* 44: 247–258.

Lee, K., Oliver, M., Schottler, F., and Lynch, G. 1981, Electron microscopic studies of brain slices: the effects of high frequency stimulation on dendritic ultrastructure. In *Electrical Activity in Isolated Mammalian C. N. S. Preparations*, G. Kerkut and H. V. Wheal, eds., pp. 189–212. New York, Academis Press.

Lisman, J. (1994). The CaM kinase II hypothesis for the storage of synaptic memory. *Trends Neurosci.* 17: 406–412.

Lledo, P. M., Hjelmstad, G. O., Mukherji, S., Soderling, T. R., Malenka, R. C., and Nicoll, R. A. (1995). Calcium calmodulin–dependent kinase II and long-term potentiation enhance synaptic transmission by the same mechanism. *Proc. Natl. Acad. Sci. USA* 92: 11175–11179.

Lovinger, D. M., Wong, K. L., Murakami, K., and Routtenberg, A. (1987). Protein kinase C inhibitors eliminate hippocampal long-term potentiation. *Brain Res.* 436: 177–183.

Lüthi, A., Laurent, J. P., Figurov, A., Muller, D., and Schachner, M. (1994). Hippocampal long-term potentiation and neural cell adhesion molecules L1 and NCAM. *Nature* 372: 777–779.

Malenka, R. C., Madison, D. V., and Nicoll, R. A. (1986). Potentiation of synaptic transmission in the hippocampus by phorbol esters. *Nature* 321: 175–177.

Malenka, R. C., Kauer, J. A., Perkel, D. J., Mauk, M. D., Kelly, P. T., Nicoll, R. A., and Waxham, M. N. (1989). An essential role for postsynaptic calmodulin and protein kinase activity in long-term potentiation. *Nature* 340: 554–557.

Malinow, R., Madison, D. V., and Tsien, R. W. (1988). Persistent protein kinase activity underlying long-term potentiation. *Nature* 335: 820–824.

Malinow, R., Schulman, H., and Tsien, R. W. (1989). Inhibition of postsynaptic PKC or CaMKII blocks induction but not expression of LTP. *Science* 245: 862–866.

McGlade-McCulloh, E., Yamamoto, H., Tan, S. E., Brickey, D. A., and Soderling, T. R. (1993). Phosphorylation and regulation of glutamate receptors by calcium/calmodulin-dependent protein kinase II. *Nature* 362: 640–642.

Miller, S. G., and Kennedy, M. B. (1986). Regulation of brain type II Ca/calmodulin-dependent protein kinase by autophosphorylation: a Ca-triggered molecular switch. *Cell* 44: 861–870.

Muller, D., Wang, C., Skibo, G., Toni, N., Cremer, H., Calaora, V., Rougon, G., and Kiss, J. Z. (1996). PSA-NCAM is required for activity-induced synaptic plasticity. *Neuron* 17: 413–422.

Nedivi, E., Hevroni, D., Naot, D., Israeli, D., and Citri, Y. (1993). Numerous candidate plasticity-related genes revealed by differential cDNA cloning. *Nature* 363: 718–722.

Nieto-Sampedro, M., Bussineau, C. M., and Cotman, C. W. (1982). Turnover of brain post-synaptic densities after selective deafferentation: detection by means of an antibody to antigen PSD-95. *Brain Res.* 251: 211–220.

Otmakhov, N., Griffith, L. C., and Lisman, J. E. (1997). Postsynaptic inhibitors of calcium/calmodulin-dependent protein kinase type II block induction but not maintenance of pairing-induced long-term potentiation. *J. Neurosci.* 17: 5357–5365.

Ouyang, Y., Kantor, D., Harris, K. M., Schuman, E., and Kennedy, M. B. (1997) Visualization of the distribution of the autophosphorylated calcium/calmodulin-dependent protein kinase II after tetanic stimulation in the area CA1 of the hippocampus. *J. Neurosci.* 17: 5416–5427.

Patterson, S. L., Abel, T., Deuel, T. A., Martin, K. C., Rose, J. C., and Kandel, E. R. (1996). Recombinant BDNF rescues deficits in basal synaptic transmission and hippocampal LTP in BDNF knockout mice. *Neuron* 16: 1137–1145.

Qian, Z., Gilbert, M. E., Colicos, M. A., Kandel, E. R., and Kuhl, D. (1993). Tissue-plasminogen activator is induced as an immediate- early gene during seizure, kindling and long-term potentiation. *Nature* 361: 453–457.

Rall, W. (1978). Dendritic spines and synaptic potency. In: *Studies in Neurophysiology*, R. Porter, ed., pp. 203–209. Cambridge: Cambridge University Press.

Roberson, E. D., and Sweatt, J. D. (1996). Transient activation of cyclic AMP–dependent protein kinase during hippocampal long-term potentiation. *J. Biol. Chem.* 271: 30436–30441.

Routtenberg, A., and Tarrant, S. (1975). The extended spinule complex: dendritic spine invagination of presynaptic terminals. *Anat. Rec.* 181: 467–473.

Rusakov, D. A., Stewart, M. G., and Korogod, S. M. (1996). Branching of active dendritic spines as a mechanism for controlling synaptic efficacy. *Neuroscience* 75: 315–323.

Schuster, T., Krug, M., and Wenzel, J. (1990). Spinules in axospinous synapses of the rat dentate gyrus: changes in density following long-term potentiation. *Brain Res.* 523: 171–174.

Shirke, A. M., and Malinow, R. (1997). Mechanisms of potentiation by calcium/calmodulin kinase II of postsynaptic sensitivity in rat hippocampal CA1 neurons. *J. Neurophysiol.* 78: 2682–2692.

Silva, A. J., Stevens, C. F., Tonegawa, S., and Wang, Y. (1992). Deficient hippocampal long-term potentiation in calcium-calmodulin kinase II mutant mice. *Science* 257: 201–206.

Svoboda, K., Denk, W., Knox, W., and Tsuda, S. (1996). Direct measurement of coupling between dendritic spines and shaft. *Science* 272: 716–719.

Trommald, M., and Hulleberg, G. (1997). Dimensions and density of dendritic spines from rat dentate granule cells based on reconstructions from serial electron micrographs. *J. Comp. Neurol.* 377: 15–28.

Trommald, M., Vaaland, J. L., Blackstad, T. W., and Andersen, P. (1990). Dendritic spine changes in rat dentate granule cells associated with long-term potentiation. In *Neurotoxicity of Excitatory Amino Acids*, pp. 163–174. Guidotti A, ed, Raven Press.

Wang, J. H., and Kelly, P. T. (1995). Postsynaptic injection of Ca2+/CaM induces synaptic potentiation requiring CaMKII and PKC activity. *Neuron* 15: 443–452.

5 Role of Synaptic Geometry in the Dynamics and Efficacy of Synaptic Transmission

Jim-Shih Liaw, Xiaping Xie, Taraneh Ghaffari, Michel Baudry, Gilbert A. Chauvet, and Theodore W. Berger

Changes in synaptic morphology consistently have been observed as a consequence of a variety of experimental manipulations, including associative learning (Black et al. 1990; Federmeier et al. 1994; Kleim et al. 1994, 1997), environmental rearing conditions (Bhide and Bedi 1984; Diamond et al. 1964; Globus et al. 1973; Turner and Greenough 1983, 1985; Volkmar and Greenough 1972), and increased synaptic "use" induced by direct electrical stimulation (Buchs and Muller 1996; Desmond and Levy 1983, 1988; Geinisman et al. 1993; Wojtowicz et al. 1989), as well as in relation to the processes of normal development and aging (De Groot and Bierman 1983; Dyson and Jones 1984; Harris et al. 1992). Structural characteristics identified as "plastic," or susceptible to environmental and experiential influence, include size and shape of the postsynaptic spine head, length of the postsynaptic spine neck, length and thickness of the postsynaptic density (PSD), and changes in the number of presynaptic vesicles and presynaptic active zones, among others. In addition to such alterations in subsynaptic features, changes in the incidence of other morphological profiles corresponding to "perforated" or "partitioned" synapses suggest a more global restructuring. A defining property of perforated and partitioned synapses is the finger-like formations of postsynaptic membrane and cytoplasm enveloped by presynaptic membrane and cytoplasm at single or multiple locations along the synaptic cleft. The pre- and postsynaptic specializations are correspondingly discontinuous, resulting in multiple, compartmentalized synaptic zones within the same end-terminal region.

These various forms of experience-dependent morphological synaptic plasticity are frequently interpreted in terms of an anatomical substrate for representational and memory capacity, premotor regulation of skilled behaviors, and stimulation-induced enhancement of synaptic excitation, for example, long-term potentiation (LTP). Although compelling arguments can be made to support these hypotheses, the functional relevance of differences in synaptic morphology remains unclear and largely unexplored due to the technical barriers to conducting both morphological and physiological analyses at the subcellular level. Differences in parameters of the PSD, for example, could reflect alteration in any number of regulatory molecules, in addition to differences in postsynaptic receptor-channel number or properties. It is particularly difficult to interpret the global synaptic restructuring characteristic of perforated and partitioned synapses because of the irregular geometry of the terminal and synaptic membrane, though clearly there are implications of membrane geometry for the spatiotemporal distribution of substances transported by diffusion, and thus the many synaptic processes that depend critically on local ions and neurotransmitters. It is precisely within the domain of investigating issues of fundamental importance that lie beyond the reach of current technologies, however, that mathematical modeling can contribute uniquely to the advancement of neuroscience.

In this chapter, we present results of three studies in which mathematical models of a synapse incorporate both known dynamics of synaptic mechanisms and morphological parameters to analyze the impact of alterations in morphology on synaptic transmission and plasticity. In the first analysis, the presynaptic terminal is modeled as a simple geometry (rectangle) to study specific spatial factors and molecular interactions involved in synaptic transmission. The model incorporates calcium channels, diffusion, pumping and buffering, and the kinetics of the interaction of calcium ions with vesicle proteins which is critical in the regulation of the release process. The objective is to account for two hallmark characteristics of neurotransmitter release, and accomplish it by using the simplified model. The first characteristic is the highly nonlinear relationship between the amount of neurotransmitter release and the concentration of calcium and the magnitude of presynaptic depolarization. Our modeling study shows that the kinetics of the interaction between calcium ions and the vesicle proteins is an important factor in accounting for such a nonlinearity. The second characteristic is the dissociation of the amount of release and the time course of release: while the amount of release may be changed by three orders of magnitude, the time course remains constant. Simulation of our model demonstrates that the distance between the release site and calcium channel plays a critical role in determining the time course of release. In particular, a constant time course consistent with experimental data can be obtained when the distance between the release site and calcium channel is less than 30 nm.

Second, the model is extended to include complex geometry conforming to the shape of a partitioned hippocampal synapse following the induction of LTP as revealed by electron microscopy (EM) (Geinisman 1993; Geinisman et al. 1993). This detailed model is used to study the impact of the combination of various spatial factors on synaptic function. Simulations of this complex model demonstrate that the release sites associated with each compartment of the partitioned synapse exhibit different dynamics of neurotransmitter release. The complex dynamics emerge from the interplay of multiple structural features. Further investigation identifies several spatial features that influence calcium dynamics and neurotransmitter release, including the effect of compartmentalization, the distance between release site and the compartment membrane, the size of the compartment, and the width of the opening of the compartment.

Finally, an extension of the model that incorporates a representation of synaptic cleft and postsynaptic receptor channels is described. This comprehensive model of a synapse is used in an integrated experimental and modeling study of the cellular and molecular mechanisms mediating LTP. Results from our electrophysiological experiment reveal several differences in the response of alpha-amino-3-hydroxy-5-methylisoxazole-4-propionic acid (AMPA) and N-methyl-D-aspartate (NMDA) receptor channels after the induction of LTP. Specifically, while both the AMPA and NMDA receptor channel-mediated responses are increased by presynaptic stimulation, only the NMDA response is higher by focal application of their respective agonists. The inclusion of a representation of synaptic cleft and postsynaptic receptors in our model enables us to test a specific hypothesis that the aggregation of AMPA receptor channels is a mechanism underlying the expression of LTP.

MOLECULAR MECHANISMS UNDERLYING NEUROTRANSMITTER RELEASE

The release of neurotransmitter from nerve terminals occurs when vesicles docked to the presynaptic release sites fuse with the terminal membrane, allowing vesicle content to enter the synaptic cleft. The docking and fusion of synaptic vesicles are regulated by several membrane proteins, although their precise roles are not well understood. Release is triggered by an elevation in presynaptic calcium concentration ($[Ca^{2+}]_i$), and thus, the interaction between calcium and various proteins underlying vesicular docking and fusion must be critical in defining their respective contributions to the physiology of synaptic transmission. To this end, we have developed a mathematical model that incorporates the diffusion of Ca^{2+} and its interaction with vesicle proteins to study the kinetics of neurotransmitter release.

The classic hypothesis that elevated $[Ca^{2+}]_i$ plays a critical role in triggering the release process has been successful in explaining many characteristics of this process. However, the failure of earlier models based on the calcium hypothesis to reproduce the dissociation of the amount and the time course of neurotransmitter release has prompted alternative hypotheses. Most notably, it has been proposed that an additional voltage-dependent process regulates the time course of release (Dudel et al. 1983; Parnas and Parnas 1988). We address this issue by examining the effect of spatial arrangements of synaptic elements such as calcium channels and release sites on the time course of release since the movement of calcium ions depends on diffusion, a process that is highly sensitive to the spatial variations in the diffusion medium.

METHOD

General Structure of the Model

The model represents a planar cross section of a terminal bouton as a discretized two dimensional array (figure 5.1). The input of the model consists of depolarization steps such as those commonly used in voltage-clamp experiments, while the output is the amount of neurotransmitter released from the presynaptic terminal. Calcium channels and pumps are located on the synaptic membrane. Each calcium channel represents a population of channels to accommodate the required intracellular calcium concentration required for release. One neurotransmitter release site is associated with every calcium channel at a certain distance from the channel. Release sites are 100 nm apart, following the models of Parnas et al. (1989) and Yamada and Zucker (1992). One calcium pump is placed between every two release sites. Calcium buffers are distributed uniformly throughout the terminal. Parameter values of the model were obtained by fitting simulation results with experimental data on the time course of response to a pair of depolarizations delivered 5 ms apart (e.g., Parnas et al. 1989). This set of parameter values is used for all simulations presented in this section.

Calcium Diffusion

After entering the presynaptic terminal, free calcium ions diffuse into the intracellular space and are quickly bound to the calcium buffers. This process is simulated by solving the diffusion equation for calcium:

$$\frac{\partial c(x, y, t)}{\partial t} = D_c \cdot \frac{\partial c^2(x, y, t)}{\partial x \cdot \partial y} - B(t) \tag{1}$$

where $c(x, y, t)$ is the calcium concentration inside the diffusion medium at time t at location (x, y), D_c is the diffusion coefficient of free calcium ions $(6 \cdot 10^{-6} \text{ cm}^2/\text{s}$; (Hodgkin and Keynes 1957)), and $B(t)$ is the calcium buffering process which is assumed to be immobile and uniformly distributed in the cytoplasm. Given that the process of calcium binding to buffers occurs at a much faster time scale than the diffusion, local equilibrium is reached between free and bound calcium ions (Crank 1975) and therefore the above equation can be simplified to

$$\frac{\partial c(x, y, t)}{\partial t} = \frac{D_c}{1 + \beta} \cdot \frac{\partial c^2(x, y, t)}{\partial x \cdot \partial y} \tag{2}$$

where β is the ratio of bound to free calcium in the cytoplasm.

Calcium Current and Pumps

The calcium current in the model is determined by

$$I_{ca} = G \cdot j \tag{3}$$

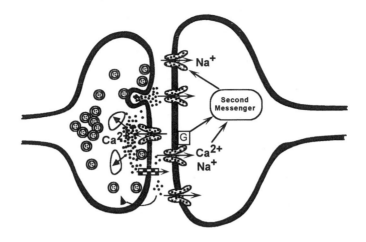

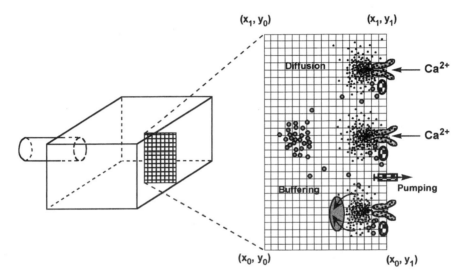

Figure 5.1 A model of the presynaptic terminal. The model represents a subspace of the terminal bouton as a discretized two-dimensional array consisting of 20×80 cells. Each cell is 10×10 nm in size which is the same as the smallest cells used in Yamada and Zucker (1992). The spatial resolution and the time steps (10 µs) used in our simulation are sufficient for the numerical method to yield results with reasonable accuracy (Crank 1975). The calcium channels, active zones, and calcium pumps are located along the boundary of $y = y_1$.

where G is the number of channels in the open state, and j is the rate of flow through a single channel as described by Llinás and colleagues (Llinás et al. 1981). G and j are functions of membrane potential, V, and temperature, T, as described below.

$$G = G_0 \cdot \left\{ \frac{k_1}{k_1 + k_2} \cdot (1 - e^{-(k_1+k_2)\cdot t}) \right\}^n \tag{4}$$

$$j = \frac{\beta_1 K[c_0 \cdot e^{-80V} - c_i]}{1 + Kc_0 e^{-80V}} \tag{5}$$

Parameter values in the above equations are the same as those indicated by Llinás et al., unless specified otherwise. Calcium current, as obtained in Eq. (1), is converted to the number of calcium particles that enter the cell per unit of time and incorporated into the boundary condition at the appropriate boundary element to model calcium channels. Since calcium current changes with time, the boundary conditions are reevaluated and updated at every time step. An additional step is taken in which $k_{pump} \cdot C(x_p, y_0, t)$ is subtracted ($k_{pump} = 0.001$, x_p are the boundary elements along the face of the membrane, y_0, where calcium pumps are located).

Neurotransmitter Release

The process of neurotransmitter release and its time course is described by a set of equations governing the interaction of calcium and certain vesicle proteins:

$$Ca^{2+} + X\_V \underset{k_{-1}}{\overset{k_1}{\longleftrightarrow}} CaX\_V + Ca^{2+} \underset{k_{-2}}{\overset{k_2}{\longleftrightarrow}} Ca_2X\_V \tag{6}$$

$$n(Ca_2X)\_V \overset{k_3}{\longrightarrow} n(Ca_2X)\_V^* \underset{k_{-4}}{\overset{k_4}{\longleftrightarrow}} I \tag{7}$$

where X is the vesicle protein, V is the synaptic vesicle, $n(Ca_2X)\_V^*$ is the number of vesicles in the open state allowing neurotransmitter release, and I is the insensitive state of the fusion pore. The kinetic parameters in Eq. (6) and (7) are obtained by fitting simulation results with experimental data on the time course of response to a pair of depolarization steps delivered at 5 ms apart (Parnas et al. 1989).

RESULTS

Calcium-and Voltage Dependency of Neurotransmitter Release

Quantitative data obtained from various experiments show a highly nonlinear calcium dependency of the probability of neurotransmitter release. For example, Dodge and Rahamimoff (1967) found that the release of neurotransmitter at the frog neuromuscular junction during an action potential

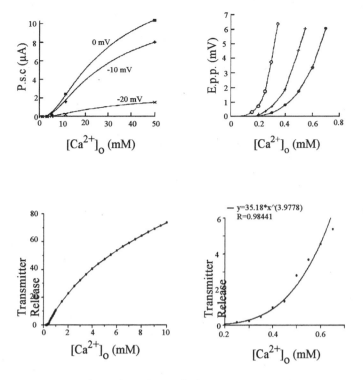

Figure 5.2 Calcium dependency of release. The amount of neurotransmitter release is related to $[Ca^{2+}]_0$ in a highly nonlinear fashion. The top left graph shows changes in neurotransmitter release indicated by the postsynaptic current (Psc) measured from squid giant synapse by Augustine et al. (1985). Psc's are recorded with three different levels of depolarization, while $[Ca^{2+}]_0$ is varied up to 50 mM. The bottom left graph shows simulations in which $[Ca^{2+}]_0$ is varied from 0.2 mM to 10 mM with depolarization from −70 to 0 mV. The two graphs on the right illustrates the "power of 4" relationship between $[Ca^{2+}]_0$ and the amount of release which occurs at low calcium concentrations. The top graph is an experimental record obtained from frog neuromuscular junction by Dodge and Rahamimoff (1967). The bottom graph shows the initial part of the graph of simulation result on the left.

increases as the fourth power of $[Ca^{2+}]_0$. Katz and Miledi (1968) postulated that Ca^{2+} entering the terminal interacts with intracellular receptors. Several such receptors cooperatively control the release of one vesicle, thus giving rise to a high order of calcium dependency. However, it is not clear how many such molecules are involved in triggering release. We simulate $n = 1, 2, 3$, and 4 in Eq. (11), along with the classic formulation that the amount of release $R = ([Ca^{2+}]_i)^4$. Our simulation shows that n = 2 produces the best fit with data in terms of the 4th power dependency (figure 5.2).

The amplitude of I_{ca} depends on the magnitude of presynaptic depolarization, and therefore, the amount of neurotransmitter released also should show a similar voltage dependency. However, there are several subtle points. First, though the curves of both I_{ca} and neurotransmitter release as a function of voltage are bell-shaped, the latter shows a much steeper voltage

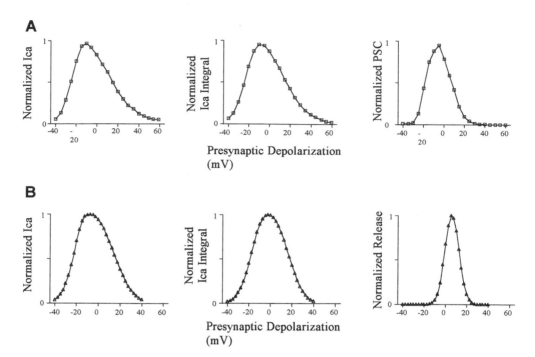

Figure 5.3. I_{ca} and the amount of release as a function of presynaptic depolarization. (A) Presynaptic calcium current (I_{ca}, left), normalized I_{ca} (middle), and postsynaptic currents (PSC, right) measured from squid giant synapse at different level of depolarizations. (Redrawn from Augustine et al. 1985.) (B) Simulations based on our model under the same conditions. In both the experimental and simulation results, the curves of both I_{ca} and neurotransmitter release are bell-shaped, with the latter showing a much steeper voltage dependency. No measurable neurotransmitter release occurs at low or high levels of depolarization, despite the presence of I_{ca}. The voltage dependency is steeper in the simulated I_{ca}, which is magnified in the simulated amount of release. The peak of the curve of neurotransmitter release is shifted towards higher depolarization relative to that of I_{ca}.

dependency. Second, no measurable neurotransmitter release occurs at low or high levels of depolarization, despite the presence of I_{ca}. Third, the peak of the curve of neurotransmitter release occurs at a higher depolarization compared to that of I_{ca}. Our model shows all these subtle features (figure 5.3). Furthermore, the shape of individual release waveform matches well with the experimental data.

Time Course of Neurotransmitter Release

The time course of neurotransmitter release also has a characteristic phenomenology. It begins about 1 ms after activation of I_{ca} and rises rapidly until about 1 to 2 ms after the end of I_{ca}, then starts to decay back to baseline in 5 to 10 ms (figure 5.4A; Augustine et al. 1985; Parnas et al. 1989). Though the amount of neurotransmitter released is highly sensitive to $[Ca^{2+}]_0$ and the magnitude of depolarization, the time course is independent of both of these factors (Kloot 1988; Parnas et al. 1989). The time course of release in response to a pair of 1-ms depolarizations delivered 5 ms apart has been used as the primary criterion for judging the performance of previous models (Parnas et al. 1989; Yamada and Zucker 1992). We have used this input condition (specifically, a pair of 1-ms depolarizations from -70 to 0 mV, with a 5-ms interval and 2 mM $[Ca^{2+}]_0$ at 27 °C), to constrain the parameters of our model (figure 5.4B). An additional constraint of a low affinity for the calcium receptor has been suggested based on the rapid decay time course such that the bound Ca^{2+} can be freed from the receptor quickly (Almers 1994; Augustine and Neher 1992). The set of parameter values that produces the best fit for this condition is used in all simulations presented here unless otherwise specified.

Results of simulations revealed that the model reproduces the characteristic features of the time course of neurotransmitter release observed experimentally. The time course of release is independent of the magnitude of presynaptic depolarization as shown in figure 5.5. Even though the peak amplitude of neurotransmitter release nearly triples with greater depolarization, the time course is almost identical. Furthermore, only a slight increase occurs in the time course of release evoked by the second depolarization compared to that evoked by the first depolarization, consistent with experimental observations (Kloot 1988; Parnas et al. 1989). The same characteristic is seen when $[Ca^{2+}]_0$ is varied (figure 5.6). The time courses of release for different $[Ca^{2+}]_0$ are virtually indistinguishable even when the peak amplitude is more than six times greater at higher $[Ca^{2+}]_0$. Again, only a slight increase in the time course is seen in response to the second depolarization.

Distance Between Calcium Channel and Release Site

The time course of diffusion is a function of space. The farther away from the point of particle injection, the slower the time course becomes. Since $[Ca^{2+}]_i$ plays an essential role in regulating neurotransmitter release, the time course of release should depend on the distance between the calcium channel and the release site. To study the significance of this spatial relationship, we carry out a series of simulations in which the distance between the calcium channel and the release site is varied. Figure 5.7 shows the result when $[Ca^{2+}]_i$ is measured at a point 10, 20, ..., 50 nm away from the calcium channel. As expected, the rate of change in $[Ca^{2+}]_i$ decreases as the distance from the channel increases, leading to a decrease in the magnitude and a slower release time course. Moreover, as a result of slower change in $[Ca^{2+}]_i$, the residual calcium is higher at distant locations resulting in a greater facilitated response to the second stimulation.

Simulations of our simplified model highlight the importance of spatial factors in the regulation of synaptic transmission. In the next section, our model is extended to include a specific morphology of a partitioned synapse

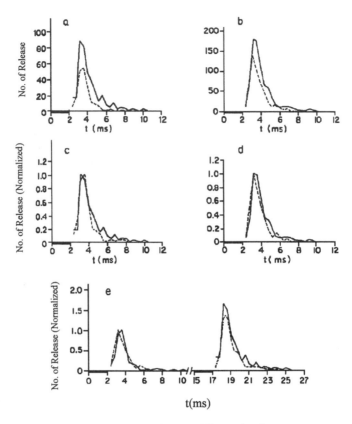

Figure 5.4 Time course of release at different depolarizations. (A) Experimental record taken from Parnas et al. (1989) showing data obtained in lobster neuromuscular junction. (a) The number of release elicited by the first (dashed line) and second (solid line) 2-ms pulses of depolarizations with −0.8 µA. (b) As in a, but for −1.0 µA. The traces in (a) and (b) are normalized to their peak amplitudes in (c) and (d), respectively. (e) On the left side, the first pulses of the −0.8 µA (solid line) and −1.0 µA (dashed line) are normalized with respect to their peak amplitude. On the right side, the second pulse of the depolarizations is normalized to the peak amplitude of its first pulse. Note that the lower depolarization (solid line) shows higher facilitation. (B, top) The time course of release at 0 mV and −5 mV are superimposed. Middle, The first (solid line) and second (dashed line) responses elicited by depolarizations to 0 mV (left) and −5 mV (right) are normalized to their peak amplitudes. (Bottom). The two traces in the middle panel are normalized to their first peak amplitudes. Note that the lower depolarization (solid line) shows higher facilitation, similar to experimental recording shown in A.

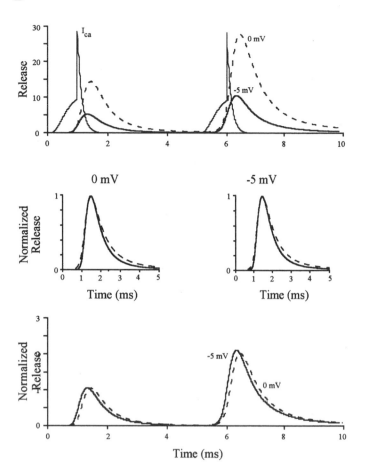

Figure 5.4 (continued)

as revealed by EM study for a thorough investigation of the impact of structural modification on synaptic function.

IMPACT OF MORPHOLOGY ON SYNAPTIC DYNAMICS

Structural modifications, particularly perforated synapses, have been consistently reported after electrophysiological stimulation, changes in the external or internal environment, development, and aging. Several studies have identified an increase in the number of perforations in the PSD of the rat dentate gyrus following a lesion in entorhinal cortex (Nieto-Sampedro et al. 1982). Similar findings have been reported in the visual cortex of rabbits following light/dark rearing (Muller et al. 1981), the visual cortex of rats following prolonged exposure to a visually enriched environment (Greenough et al. 1979; Schwartz and Rothblat 1980), and the motor and visual cortices of

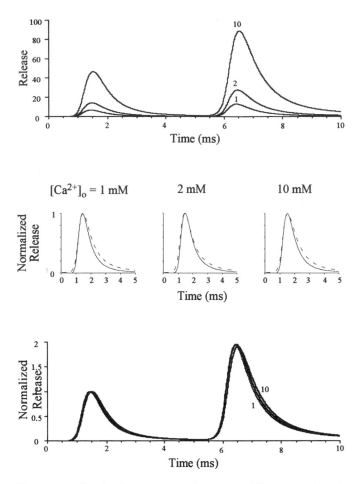

Figure 5.5 Simulated time course of release at different $[Ca^{2+}]_o$. The simulation results are presented in the same way as in figure 5.4B.

mature rabbits during development (Muller et al. 1981; Vrensen et al. 1980). Geinisman and co-workers identified a novel synaptic subtype that exhibited partitioned PSDs (Geinisman 1993), and reported an increase in the number of these perforated and partitioned synapses, one hour after induction of LTP in the rat dentate gyrus (Geinisman et al. 1993). Despite the compelling evidence relating structural modification to synaptic plasticity, the mechanisms by which perforated and partitioned synapses contribute to synaptic plasticity remain unknown. Given the sensitivity of diffusion to changes in the geometric boundary of diffusion medium, an accurate structural representation in a synapse model can help elucidate the relevance of partitioning in synaptic plasticity.

In this section, we illustrate the impact of structural modifications on neurotransmitter release and synaptic dynamics using a mathematical model of partitioned synapses. Specifically, a serial section electron micrograph of a

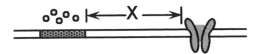

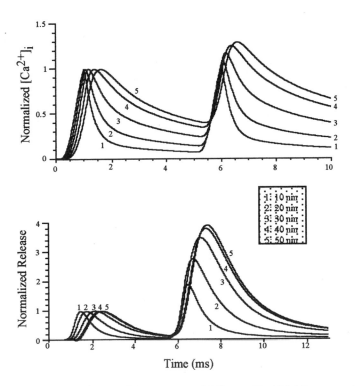

Figure 5.6 The spatial characteristic of diffusion. (Top) $[Ca^{2+}]_i$ measured at different distances away from the calcium channel (10, 20, 30, 40, and 50 nm) after two 1-ms depolarizations to 0 mV 5 ms apart are normalized to their peak concentrations after the first depolarization. (Bottom). The time course of release when the assumed distance between calcium channel and release site is varied. All traces are normalized to the peak of their first response.

hippocampal partitioned synapse (figure 5.7A) (Geinisman et al. 1993) after high-frequency stimulation was used to specify the geometry of the model (figure 5.7B). The effect of morphological alterations on neurotransmitter release is examined with the extended computational capabilities to simulate calcium diffusion in complex geometries.

METHOD

Due to the difficulty of solving partial differential equations for diffusion with time-varying boundary conditions over a highly irregular geometry, most models of transmitter release, including the model described in the first section, assume a regular domain, that is, rectangle, circular disk, and so on (Bertram 1997; Bertram et al. 1996; Kruk et al. 1997; Wahl et al. 1996). The

A

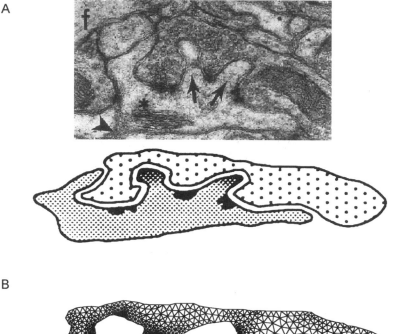

B

Figure 5.7 Partitioned synapse: electron microscope (EM) data and the model. (A) The EM picture of a partitioned synapse used to specify the geometry of the model (From "Perforated axospinous synapses with multiple, completely partitioned transmission zones: probable structural intermediates in synaptic plasticity," Yuri Geinisman, *Hippocampus* 3 (1993) 417–434, Copyright © 1993 Wiley-Liss, Inc. Reprinted by permission of Wiley-Liss, Inc., a subsidiary of John Wiley & Sons, Inc.). (B) The model of the partitioned synapse, showing the triangular mesh and location of calcium channel release site complexes labeled as R1, R2, and R3.

general structure of our extended model of the axon terminal, however, consists of finite element representation of any two-dimensional geometry, such as that of a partitioned presynaptic terminal. The geometric representation of the model is developed using MATLAB with the "constructive solid geometry" modeling paradigm. The two-dimensional geometry is then discretized by generating a triangular mesh. The mesh is refined until the smallest boundary element is just smaller than 0.5 nm wide in order to minimize the approximation error. After the terminal boundary is accurately specified, calcium channels, and neurotransmitter release sites are assigned as time-varying boundary conditions. We have extended the mathematical functionality such that boundary conditions can be specified at any location on the boundary. In the case of the partitioned synapse, the calcium channels and release sites are placed (10 nm apart) at positions corresponding to the location of PSDs in the EM picture. An additional step is taken to refine the mesh such that the triangles near the calcium channels and release sites are higher in number and smaller in size to increase the accuracy of the solution (figure 5.7B). The kinetics of calcium conductance and neurotransmitter release are the same as described in the previous section. The diffusion coefficient is specified to include the appropriate rate of calcium buffering. Given the discretized mesh representation of the terminal, the boundary and initial conditions, and the coefficients of the diffusion equation, a numerical solution of the diffusion equation is obtained using the MATLAB partial differential equation toolbox (The MathWorks 1995).

RESULT

A series of computer simulations are conducted to test the hypothesis that local structure in the partitioned synapse affects calcium diffusion and distribution, and hence the probability of neurotransmitter release. In the first set of simulations, a rectangular model of a symmetric presynaptic terminal is used as the control for comparison with the partitioned synapse model. There are three equally spaced calcium channel release sites in the control case (figure 5.8A). Simulations of the symmetric model show an equal release probability for all of the release sites, for both a single depolarization step and a train of random inputs (i.e., a sequence of depolarization steps over 200 ms shown in the bottom of figure 5.8B and C). The same input patterns will be used in all the simulations described in this section, unless specified otherwise.

Differential Probability of Release in the "Partitioned Synapse"

Simulations of the partitioned synapse model (see figure 5.7B) in response to a single depolarization step show that the probability of release is different for the three release sites. The peak amplitude of release probability for site 1 is 32% higher than that of site 2 and 19% higher than that of site 3 (figure 5.9A). The result indicates that the differences in the release probability within the time course of a single response are a consequence of unequal morphological partitioning.

Next, we simulate the partitioned synapse model with the random train of inputs. The peak response of site 1 to a sequence of depolarization steps (figure 5.9B) varied with respect to site 3. For example, site 3's peak response was higher than that of site 1 in response to the group of six consecutive pulses beginning with the second pulse (at 15 ms). However, the relative peak amplitudes of the two sites reverses from the eighth pulse to the end of the input train, revealing different temporal dynamics within a single synapse.

A

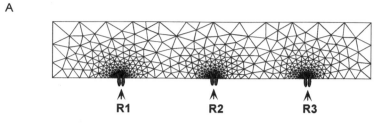

B

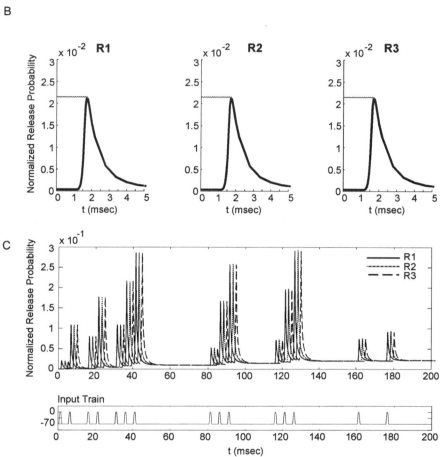

Figure 5.8 Equal release probability in a symmetrical terminal. (A) Model of a symmetrical axon terminal with three equally spaced calcium channel-release sites. (B) The three release sites exhibit equal probability of release in response to a single depolarization step (from −70 to 0 mV, 1 ms long, starting at 0.5 ms). (C) Equal probability of release in response to a random sequence of depolarization steps (bottom panel) for the three release sites was obtained.

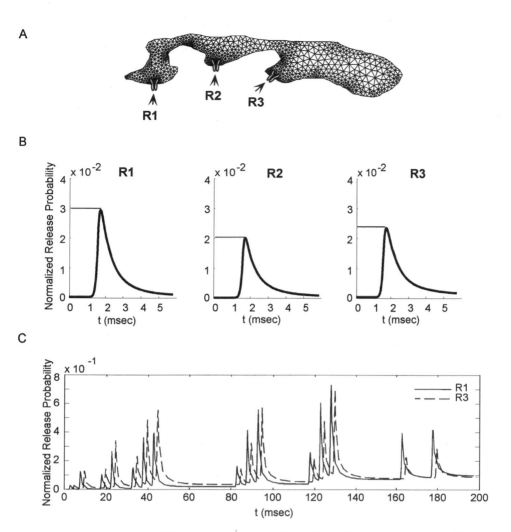

Figure 5.9 Differential release probability in the partitioned synapse. (A) A differential release probability was exhibited in the partitioned synapse among the three release sites (see figure 5.7B) in response to a single depolarization step. (B) Normalized release probability of R1 and R3 in the partitioned synapse. The two curves were superimposed on the same graph for comparison. The input sequence was the same as shown in figure 5.8C. There was a shift in the dominant release probability from R3 to R1 around 80 ms (reversal of release probability).

Geometric Features Influential in Calcium Dynamics

To isolate morphologic features that account for changes in synaptic dynamics, a model with simple rectangular geometry is used to systematically investigate the effect of individual spatial features.

The first set of simulations is designed to test the influence of the partitioning membrane wall on calcium dynamics by varying the distance between the release site from the wall (figure 5.10). Three distances are simulated,

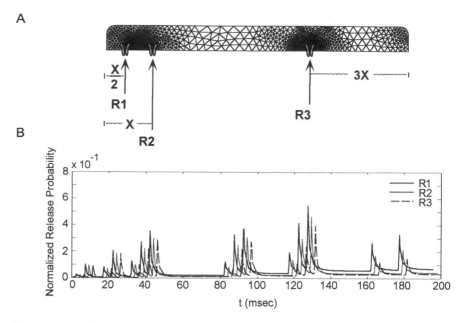

Figure 5.10 Effect of proximity to adjacent membrane wall on release probability. (A) Symmetrical terminal used in several simulation while the distance between the calcium channel-release site and the adjacent membrane wall was varied. The distances used in the simulations were X/2, X, and 2X. (B) Comparison of release probability between release sites at different distances from the nearby membrane wall. R1 had the smallest distance to the nearby membrane wall (X/2), resulting in the highest peak amplitudes in probability of release. On the other hand, R3 had the largest distance from the nearby membrane wall (3X), resulting in the lowest peak amplitudes in probability of release.

namely, 1/2, 1, and 3 units from the wall where a unit is roughly 235 nm. Comparison of the release probability curves indicates that the release site closest to the wall has the highest probability of neurotransmitter release.

The second set of simulations examines the effect of compartmentalization by dividing the terminal into two compartments. Calcium channel release site complexes were placed in each compartment, as shown in figure 5.11a. The result shows that the release probability is higher for release site 1 when it is confined in the small compartment (figure 5.11B). However, there is no change for release site 2 as a result of compartmentalization (data not shown). A further investigation of the effect of compartmentalization on release is carried out by varying the local volume of the compartment (figure 5.12A). As shown in figure 12B, the probability of release is higher when the size of the compartment is decreased.

An important issue with respect to compartmentalization is the size of the "neck," that is, the opening though which the small pocket is connected to the rest of the terminal (figure 5.13A). This issue is examined by simulating the model while varying the size of the neck. The result shows that the release probability is higher when the neck size is decreased (figure 5.13B).

A

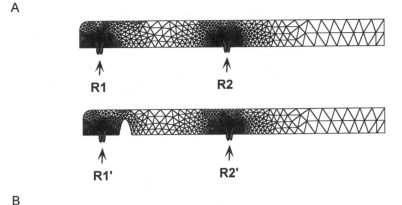

B

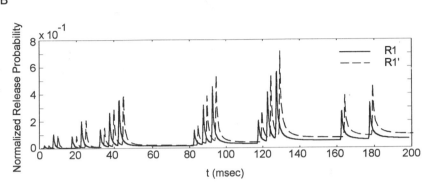

Figure 5.11 Effect of compartmentalization on release probability. (A) A partition was placed in the bottom panel to create a compartment around R1'. (B) Comparison of the simulation results show that R1' (in a compartment) had a higher release probability than R1 (not in a compartment). Input sequence was the same as shown in bottom panel of figure 5.8C.

Spatial Features in the Partitioned Synapse

The differential release probability observed in the partitioned synapse (see figure 5.9) is a consequence of one, or a combination, of the above spatial features. In order to verify this hypothesis, a series of simulations of the partitioned synapse are carried out in which the morphology is altered to eliminate one or more of these spatial features.

First, to eliminate the influence of the partitioning wall, the release site 3 in the partitioned synapse is moved approximately 300 nm to the right (figure 5.14A). As seen in figure 5.14B, comparison of the new release probability for site 3 at the new location to its original release probability shows a decrease in magnitude. Furthermore, the reversal of the relative peak amplitudes between release sites 1 and 3 as seen in figure 5.9B is eliminated. Instead, the probability of release is always higher in release site 1 than release site 3 at the new location.

The effect of local volume and partitioning is demonstrated by modifying the boundary of the Geinisman geometry (figure 5.15A). By removing the

A

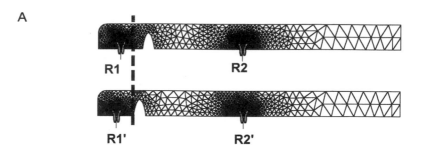

B

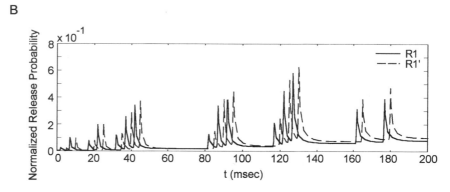

Figure 5.12 Effect of the compartment size on release probability. (A) The size of the compartment in the terminal was varied as shown. (B) Comparison of the simulation results show that R1 (in the large compartment) had a lower release probability than R1' (in the small compartment). Therefore, the decrease in compartment size resulted in an increase in the probability of release.

compartmentalization in the terminal, the reversal of the relative peak amplitudes between release sites 1 and 3 disappears. In addition, the dynamics of the three release sites now resemble each other (figure 5.15B).

STRUCTURAL FEATURES UNDERLYING LONG-TERM POTENTIATION

LTP is a widely studied form of use-dependent synaptic plasticity expressed robustly by glutamatergic synapses of the hippocampus. Although there is a convergence of evidence concerning the cellular and molecular mechanisms mediating the induction of NMDA receptor-dependent STP (short-term potentiation) and LTP (Bliss and Collingridge 1993), there remains substantial debate as to whether the expression of potentiation reflects change in presynaptic release mechanisms or postsynaptic receptor-channel function. In this section, we present an integrated experimental and modeling study for testing a specific hypothesis of the cellular and molecular mechanisms underlying STP and LTP. In the electrophysiological experiments, we investigated the potential differential expression of STP by AMPA and NMDA recep-

A

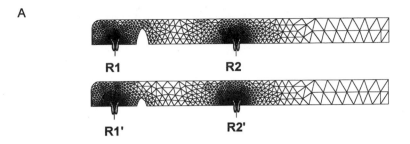

R1   **R2**

R1'   **R2'**

B

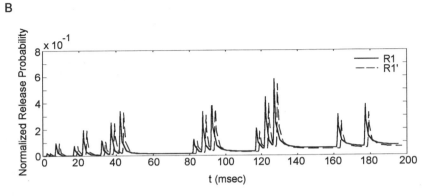

Figure 5.13 Effect of "neck" size on release probability. (A) The size of the opening of the compartment, or the neck, was varied as shown. (B) Comparison of the simulation results show that R1 (in the compartment with the narrow neck) had a higher release probability than R1' (in the compartment with the wide neck). Therefore, the increase in diameter of the neck resulted in a decrease in the probability of release.

tors, and found that the decay time course of STP is markedly different for AMPA and NMDA receptor-mediated EPSPs. Furthermore, during both STP and LTP, we found evidence of a differential responsivity of AMPA and NMDA receptors to focal application of their respective agonists. These results are strongly supportive of a postsynaptic expression mechanism of STP and LTP.

We extend our previous model to incorporate parameters for the synaptic space, the kinetic properties of AMPA and NMDA receptor channels, and the relative locations of the two receptor channel subtypes. A series of computer simulations is conducted to investigate several specific hypotheses regarding STP and LTP. Results suggest a unique expression mechanism not previously proposed, namely, receptor channel relocalization in the postsynaptic membrane. Our findings demonstrate that this hypothesis is sufficient to explain both STP and LTP of the AMPA receptor channel though not of the NMDA receptor channel, and moreover, it can explain experimental observations which cannot be accounted for by previously hypothesized mechanisms.

A

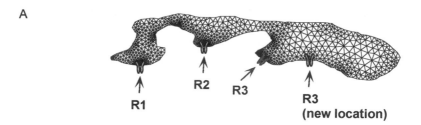

B

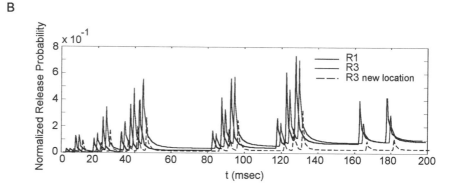

Figure 5.14 Simple spatial variation in the partitioned synapse. (A) R3 in the partitioned synapse was moved to a new location to examine the effect of absence of nearby *partitioning* membrane (from Geinisman 1993). (B) Comparison of the release probability for R3 at the new location to the release probability for R3 at its original location not only shows a significant decrease in the peak amplitudes but also exhibits no reversal of the release probability, as seen previously in figure 5.9B.

METHOD

Experimental Protocols

Standard techniques (Xie et al. 1992) were used to prepare transverse hippocampal slices from male New Zealand white rabbits and to evoke and record extracellular excitatory postsynaptic potentials (EPSPs) and whole cell excitatory postsynaptic currents (EPSCs) from dentate gyrus. Perfusing medium included reduced Mg^{2+} (0.1 mM) and picrotoxin (50 μM) to enhance NMDA receptor gated conductance (Mayer and Westbrook 1987; Nowak et al. 1984). CNQX (10 μM, Tocris Neuramin), an AMPA receptor antagonist (Drejer and Honore 1988), was added as indicated. In some experiments, the AMPA receptor agonist, AMPA (500 μM), or the NMDA receptor agonist, NMDA (500 μM), were microejected into the middle third dendritic region of the granule cell (single pulse, 5 psi, 100 ms in duration, pH 7.3) via a multibarrel pipette. Whole cell EPSCs were recorded from dentate granule cell soma. The pipettes were filled with (in millimolar): 120 cesium gluconate; 5 KCl; 2 $MgSO_4$; 10 HEPES; 0.1 $CaCl_2$; 1 BAPTA; 3 ATP-Mg. The membrane potential of the recorded cells (n = 20) was held at −80 mV except

A

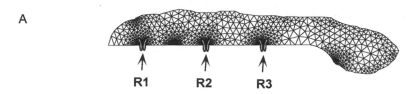

B

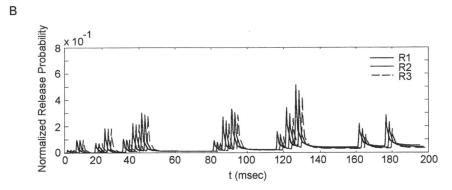

Figure 5.15 Elimination of compartments of the partitioned synapse. (A) The compartments of the partitioned synapse were eliminated in the model. The location of the calcium channel-release site complexes are kept at the same x-location. (B) Unlike the partitioned synapse, the simulated release probability for this modified terminal shows no significant differences among the three release sites. However, it should be noted that the small differences in peak amplitudes were due to asymmetry of the terminal and the relative location of the release sites with respect to each other and the terminal.

during high frequency stimulations (HFSs) at which the membrane potential was reduced to between -40 and -20 mV.

Synaptic Cleft Model

The mathematical model of a synaptic cleft includes the representations of a synaptic cleft as discretized two dimensional array where the neurotransmitter release sites are located at the upper boundary and the postsynaptic receptor channels are located at the lower boundary. The diffusion of neurotransmitter (glutamate) in the cleft is described by the following equation:

$$\frac{\partial N(x, y, t)}{\partial t} = D_N \frac{\partial N^2(x, y, t)}{\partial x \cdot \partial y} \tag{8}$$

where $N(x, y, t)$ denotes the concentration of neurotransmitter molecules at the point (x, y) at time t and $D_N = 7.6 \times 10^{-6}$ cm^2/second (Longsworth 1953).

Kinetic Model of Postsynaptic Receptor Channels

The EPSCs were computed from kinetic models of AMPA and NMDA receptor channels. The kinetic model of the AMPA receptor channel was adopted from (Ambros-Ingerson and Lynch 1993) while that of the NMDA receptor channel followed the model developed by Lester and Jahr (1992). The AMPA model includes one glutamate binding site, whereas the NMDA model assumes two binding sites.

DIFFERENTIAL EXPRESSION OF STP BY AMPA AND NMDA RECEPTORS

The first experiments examined the possibility of a differential expression of STP by AMPA and NMDA receptors. The magnitude of the NMDA response was enhanced by reducing $[Mg^{2+}]_0$ to 0.1 mM (figure 5.16A) and NMDA receptor-mediated EPSPs were pharmacologically isolated by blocking AMPA receptors using the specific antagonist, CNQX (10 μM). In reduced $[Mg^{2+}]_0$, a negative slope conductance is still clearly present in the I-V curve (figure 5.16B), and thus the receptor channel still behaves in a physiological manner characteristic of higher concentrations of $[Mg^{2+}]_0$ (Nowak et al. 1984). Under these conditions, HFS induced both NMDA STP and LTP (figure 5.16C). The decay time courses were fitted with a single exponential curve and the averaged STP decay time constant for NMDA STP was found to be 1.2 ± 0.20 minutes (mean ± sem, $n = 8$).

In the absence of CNQX and in the presence of 1.0 mM $[Mg^{2+}]_0$, EPSPs recorded in response to 0.1-Hz synaptic activation were almost exclusively AMPA receptor-mediated (figure 5.16A). HFS induced both STP and LTP of the AMPA response (figure 5.16D, open circles), though the decay time constant of STP was found to be substantially longer than for NMDA receptor-mediated EPSPs (6.39 ± 0.86 minutes, $n = 12$). The difference in STP decay time constants for AMPA and NMDA responses was not due to the differences in $[Mg^{2+}]_0$. When AMPA STP was examined in 0.1 mM $[Mg^{2+}]_0$, the averaged decay time constant was found to be 6.30 ± 0.86 minutes ($n = 11$) (figure 5.16D, solid circles), virtually identical to that observed in the presence of 1.0 mM $[Mg^{2+}]_0$.

An increase in the response of the AMPA receptor-mediated EPSP, with much less change in the response of the NMDA receptor-mediated EPSP, is classically interpreted as indicating a postsynaptic locus of expression. However, it has been argued that the expression of STP still might be due to increased presynaptic transmitter release, even if NMDA and AMPA receptor responses show different changes since they have different kinetic properties. To test this hypothesis, we conducted a series of simulations by systematically varying the quantal content within reported physiological range. Our model, which takes into account the different kinetics of the NMDA and AMPA receptor channels, predicts that the decay time course of STP of the NMDA component is longer than that of the AMPA component, contrary to our experimental finding. This is additional evidence supporting that STP results from modifications in the postsynaptic mechanisms.

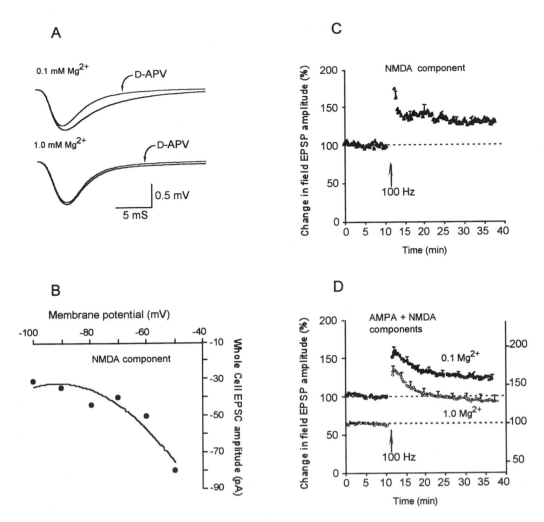

Figure 5.16 NMDA STP decays faster than AMPA STP. (A) Before (black traces) and after (gray traces) D-APV (50 μM) at 0.1 mM Mg^{2+}(upper) and 1.0 mM Mg^{2+} (lower). (B) I–V curve of NMDA receptor-mediated EPSC at 0.1 Mg^{2+} (in the presence of CNQX). (C) STP and LTP expressed by NMDA-mediated EPSPs (in the presence of CNQX). (D) STP and LTP expressed by AMPA-mediated EPSPs (in the absence of CNQX).

Differential Responsivity to Agonist by AMPA and NMDA Receptors During STP and LTP Expression

The above results strongly suggest that the expression mechanism for STP is postsynaptic in origin and as a consequence we examined whether or not receptor responsivity was increased during STP. A multibarrel pipette was placed in the dendritic region of the recorded granule cell and membrane conductance changes elicited by focal application of AMPA or NMDA were measured before and after induction of LTP (figure 5.17). Conductance

A

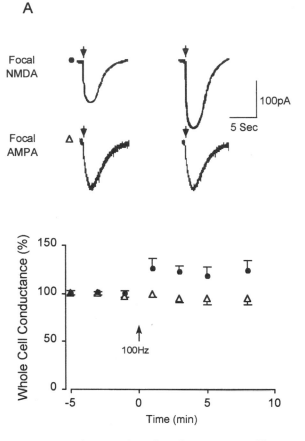

Figure 5.17 Change in channel conductance activated by AMPA and NMDA. (A) Membrane conductance in response to microapplication of NMDA, but *not* AMPA, is increased during STP. Insets: the upper two are responses induced by pressure ejection of NMDA at the moments indicated by downward arrowheads, (500 μM, 100 ms in duration); the lower two are responses induced by AMPA (500 μM, 100 ms in duration); before (left) and after induction of LTP (right). (B) STP was expressed by whole-cell EPSCs in both experimental groups. Insets: the upper two EPSCs are obtained from the same hippocampal slice as the one shown in A for focal application of NMDA; the lower two are from that for focal application of AMPA before (left) and during STP (right).

change was not altered in response to AMPA ($-0.7 \pm 3.5\%$; $p > .20$, $n = 8$); however, membrane conductance change elicited by NMDA was found to be enhanced ($24.1 \pm 7.2\%$; $p < .02$, $n = 7$) after LTP was induced. These results demonstrate that during LTP, NMDA receptor-mediated EPSCs are increased both in response to focal application of NMDA and perforant path stimulation. In contrast, AMPA receptor-mediated synaptic responses are increased, but AMPA receptor-mediated responses to focal application of agonist are unchanged.

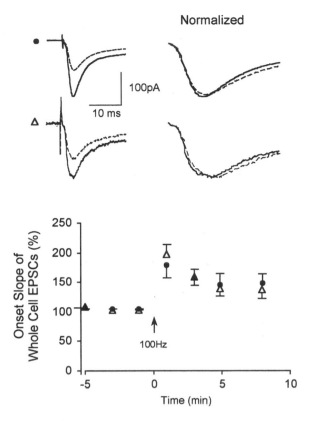

B

Figure 5.17 (continued)

Simulation Demonstrates a Novel Mechanism for AMPA Receptor STP Expression

Factors that could affect synaptic efficacy include changes in (1) mechanisms of presynaptic glutamate release, (2) number of postsynaptic receptors, (3) kinetic properties of postsynaptic receptors, and (4) the geometry of the synaptic junction. Because alteration of presynaptic release mechanisms would be expected to affect AMPA and NMDA receptor-mediated responses equivalently, the observed differences in expression of STP and LTP by the two receptor subtypes strongly suggest that the mechanisms are postsynaptic in origin. The fact that potentiation of the AMPA response is not observed during focal application of agonist further suggests that the mechanism of AMPA STP and LTP involves changes other than an increase in receptor responsivity or number. Because the contribution of changes in synaptic geometry is more difficult to evaluate, we conducted a series of computer simulations to investigate the possible consequences of changes in synaptic morphology.

Initial simulation studies revealed that the extreme narrowness of the synaptic cleft (20 nm) leads to a highly localized distribution of glutamate molecules along the postsynaptic membrane (figure 5.18A). As a consequence, we tested the hypothesis that the relative positions of the presynaptic release sites and postsynaptic receptor channels will be a significant factor in determining the magnitude and time course of the EPSCs. Specifically, we simulated AMPA and NMDA receptor-mediated EPSCs for different lateral displacements of release sites and receptor channels. Results showed that the AMPA receptor-mediated EPSC is 42% larger and the NMDA receptor-mediated EPSC is 17% larger in magnitude when the release sites and receptors are in complete alignment (a zero lateral displacement) compared to the EPSCs simulated for a 40-nm displacement (figure 5.18B and C). Furthermore, when release sites and receptors are in complete alignment, AMPA receptor–mediated EPSCs are characterized by a faster rate of onset and decay, in agreement with experimental findings (figures 5.17 and 5.18). The differential sensitivity of AMPA and NMDA receptors to the degree of "alignment" with presynaptic release sites can be explained by their different affinities to glutamate (30 mM for the AMPA receptor channel and 0.9 mM for the NMDA receptor channel in our model (see also Ambros-Ingerson and Lynch 1993; Lester and Jahr 1992; Patneau and Mayer 1990). Simulation results showed that due to its higher affinity, more than 98% of NMDA receptors are bound when a 40-nm displacement is assumed. As a consequence, change in the postsynaptic location of the NMDA receptors has little effect on the probability of binding with glutamate in changing the magnitude of the EPSC. In contrast, because only 23% of the AMPA receptors are liganded when a 40-nm displacement is assumed, lateral movement that increases alignment with the presynaptic release site will result in a higher proportion of bound receptors.

When glutamate is delivered to the synapse by means of perfusion, as during focal application of agonists, its distribution would be more uniform and the influence of receptor relocation should be reduced for both AMPA and NMDA receptor–mediated EPSCs. This condition was simulated by assuming that glutamate diffuses into the synaptic cleft from its perimeter: virtually no difference was seen in either AMPA or NMDA receptor–mediated EPSCs. To test the plausibility of changes in receptor channel kinetics accounting for STP and LTP of AMPA receptor–mediated responses, opening and closing rate were increased in magnitude as proposed by Ambros-Ingerson and Lynch (1993). Simulation results showed that the AMPA receptor–mediated response to focal application of agonist increases by 31%. These results strongly support the hypothesis that potentiation of AMPA receptor–mediated EPSCs reflects a relocation of the receptor channel in the postsynaptic membrane so as to become more aligned with presynaptic release sites. The same mechanism cannot account for STP or LTP of the NMDA receptor–mediated EPSP.

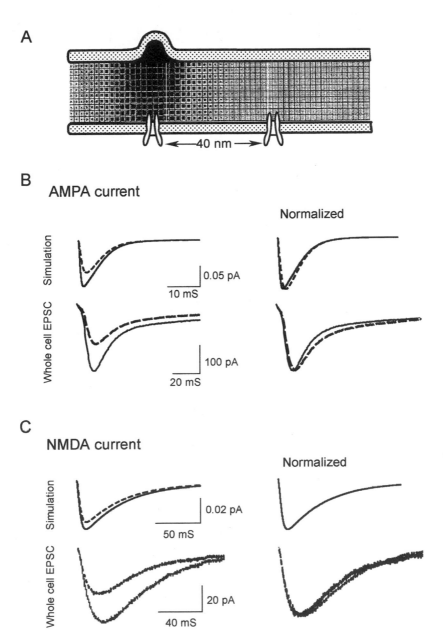

Figure 5.18 The effect of redistribution of receptors. (A) Simulation of neurotransmitter release from a vesicle into the synaptic cleft. Because the cleft is extremely narrow, the concentration of glutamate at the postsynaptic membrane is highly localized. (B) Simulated AMPA response (upper) and experimental whole cell EPSCs (lower). They exhibit a similar profile (note the normalized results). In simulation, the AMPA mediated current is 43% greater when the receptor is perfectly aligned with the release site than when they are 40 nm away (left). The two traces are normalized to show that the time course of the larger response (solid trace) is faster (right). (C) A smaller change is seen in the NMDA mediated EPSC (left) with virtually no change in its time course (right).

DISCUSSION

Molecular Interactions Underlying Neurotransmitter Release

We have presented a model of calcium dynamics in the presynaptic terminal and the interaction between calcium and vesicle proteins in regulating the process of neurotransmitter release. The parameter values for calcium dynamics, such as calcium channel kinetics, diffusion coefficient, and rate of calcium buffering and pumping, are based on experimental data and are consistent with those used in many existing models. The key assumptions made in developing the model described here are related to the underlying molecular interactions. One candidate molecule for binding with Ca^{2+} is a vesicle protein known as synaptotagmin. Two calcium binding sites are associated with synaptotagmin, and it has been postulated to be the presynaptic receptor for calcium ions (Brose et al. 1992; Perin et al. 1990; Petrenko et al. 1991; Wendland et al. 1991). Injection of peptides from the C2 domains of synaptotagmin into the squid giant presynaptic terminals rapidly and reversibly inhibits neurotransmitter release (Bommert et al. 1993). An increase in the number of vesicles docked under the presynaptic membrane is observed, indicating that the action of synaptotagmin takes place after docking but before fusion of the synaptic vesicles. Synaptotagmin also binds the docking-fusion complex, and vesicle fusion can be induced when such binding is replaced by competitive antagonists (Söllner et al. 1993).

With a representation of calcium current and calcium interaction with vesicle protein, our model accurately predicts the dependence of I_{ca} and the amount of release on the magnitude of presynaptic depolarization, including several subtle points (Augustine et al. 1985). These data have been interpreted as evidence for voltage dependency of the release process (Dudel et al. 1983; Parnas and Parnas 1988). Our simulation replicates this feature without assuming a voltage dependency. The shift in peak of release results from the combined effects of the kinetics of I_{ca} (it rises faster at higher depolarizations; see figure 5.18) and the interaction between Ca^{2+} and vesicle proteins.

Dissociation of the Amount of Neurotransmitter Release and Its Time Course

The dissociation of the amount of neurotransmitter release and the time course of release is a noted characteristic. A release time course consistent with experimental data has been achieved by the model of Yamada and Zucker (1992) when a step function representing the tail current of I_{ca} is included; the tail current also becomes the predominant factor for determining the amount and time course of release. Experimentally, however, the tail current appears to play a major role only for conditions associated with a small amount of neurotransmitter release, for example, at extremely low or high levels of depolarization (Augustine et al. 1985). Moreover, the release of neurotransmitter is triggered not only by the tail current but also by the initial, slower part of I_{ca}.

Our model produces a rapid time course incorporating a realistic I_{ca} with a spiking tail current. The major difference between the model presented here and previous models is the distance between the calcium channel and the release site. The distance is a critical factor in determining the distribution of Ca^{2+} due to diffusion. A more transient elevation and collapse of $[Ca^{2+}]_i$ would occur at locations closer to the source of calcium influx, resulting in a more rapid time course of release. A distance of 50 nm between the calcium channel and the release site was assumed in the models of Parnas et al. (1989) and Yamada and Zucker (1992). Simulations based on our model show that when the release sites are more than 30 nm away from a calcium channel, the time course of release becomes uncharacteristically slow (see figure 5.6). Recent estimates based on the interaction between the cysteine string protein and the calcium channel indicate that such distance should be less than 30 nm (Mastrogiacomo et al. 1994). Furthermore, synaptotagmin and the calcium channel have been implicated as part of a complex that mediates the docking-fusion process based on immunological studies (O'Connor et al. 1993). In this scheme, the distance between them would be extremely small.

Impacts of Morphology on Synaptic Dynamics

A systematic investigation of the impact of structural modifications on synaptic transmission is conducted by extending the model to include detailed, complex morphology. A series of computer simulations are conducted to test the hypothesis that local structure in the partitioned synapse affects calcium diffusion and distribution, and hence the probability of neurotransmitter release. We examine spatial features that are characteristic of a partitioned synapse, including proximity to adjacent partitioning membrane wall, compartmentalization, compartment size, and neck size.

The partitioning membrane wall acts as a barrier that blocks calcium diffusion and increases local calcium accumulation. Compartmentalization creates pockets in which calcium accumulates. The smaller the size of the pocket, the higher the local concentration of calcium. At a longer time scale, calcium diffuses away from the pockets through the opening (the neck), and the width of the neck determines the rate of outflux of calcium ions from the pocket. The increase in local calcium concentration caused by these spatial features gives rise to a higher release probability. These spatial features, when varied one at a time, alter release probability in a uniform way, for example, either all relative peak amplitudes increase or all peaks decrease in response to a train of input stimuli.

However, simulations of our model of the partitioned synapse reveal complex dynamics within a single axon terminal. The complex dynamics emerge from the interplay of multiple structural features. This concept is confirmed when some of the structural characteristics of the partitioned synapse are removed from the model in the experiments shown in figures 5.14 and 5.15.

Different Expression Mechanisms Underlie Potentiation of AMPA and NMDA Receptors

The major findings of our experimental study are that STP of the NMDA receptor exhibits a much shorter decay time course than that for the AMPA receptor. In addition, during the expression of both STP and LTP, only the postsynaptic response to microejection of NMDA is enhanced; the response to microejection of AMPA is unchanged. Thus, there are different mechanisms of expression for STP and LTP of AMPA and NMDA receptor channels. Assuming colocalization of the two glutamatergic receptor subtypes, these data also strongly argue that, for both AMPA and NMDA receptors, the expression of STP and LTP involves mechanisms that are postsynaptic in origin. Only the extremely rapid decay rate for NMDA STP suggests the possibility of a presynaptic mechanism, that is, that STP of the NMDA receptor channel reflects primarily post-tetanus potentiation (PTP). This hypothesis has been dealt with elsewhere (Xie et al. 1996). Results of our simulation studies showed that either sensitization of the NMDA receptor or an increase in the number of receptors is sufficient to account for the increased postsynaptic responsivity to agonist, and thus, the LTP expressed by the NMDA receptor. The failure of others to detect a similar change in NMDA receptor responsivity with focal application of glutamate (Lynch et al. 1976; Malgaroli and Tsien 1992; Murali and Sastry 1985; Taube and Schwartzkroin 1988) is most likely due to the use of high concentrations of Mg^{2+} in the perfusing media, suppressing NMDA channel opening.

Enhancement of synaptically evoked AMPA responses in the absence of increased responsivity to agonist further suggests that the expression mechanisms of AMPA STP and LTP involve changes other than an increase in number or sensitivity of the receptor. Because receptors and other membrane proteins can diffuse laterally in the plane of the cytoplasmic membrane (Alberts et al. 1994; Froehner 1993), the effects of changes in position of postsynaptic AMPA and NMDA receptors were investigated using computer simulations of a glutamatergic synapse. Results revealed that the relative positions of the presynaptic release site and the postsynaptic receptor can have a profound effect on the magnitude and time course of the EPSCs. Detailed studies found that properties of AMPA receptor-mediated STP and LTP were most consistent with the hypothesis that, in response to high-frequency stimulation, the receptor channel becomes relocalized in the postsynaptic membrane so as to be more closely aligned with the presynaptic release site.

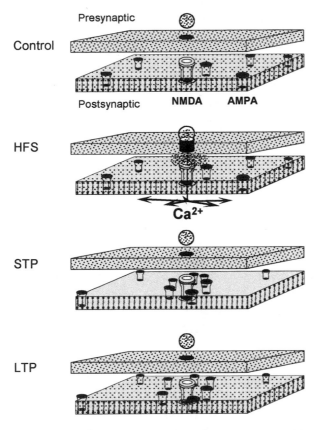

Figure 5.19 Schematic representation of our STP-LTP model. Control: patches of pre- and postsynaptic membrane in a nonpotentiated state. HFS: presynaptic LTP inducing pulses arrive which cause NMDA receptor channel activation and Ca^{2+} influx which in turn trigger the receptor attraction mechanism. STP: as a result, AMPA receptors are attracted toward the activated NMDA receptor channel which is aligned previously with the presynaptic release zone. LTP: depending on the effectiveness of the anchoring mechanism, all or part of the AMPA receptors will diffuse again. An electrophysiological observer then will interpret it as only STP or STP plus LTP correspondingly. Note that due to diffusion, AMPA receptors that used to be located farther away may enter this domain and can be utilized for further potentiation of synaptic strength.

Postsynaptic AMPA Receptor Realignment Model

Thus, we propose the following model for the mechanism of expression of NMDA receptor dependent STP and LTP of AMPA receptor—mediated synaptic responses (figure 5.19). NMDA receptor activation is known to be critical for glutamatergic synapse stabilization during development (Debski et al. 1990), and thus we assume that a close alignment of NMDA receptors and presynaptic release sites emerges from the process of synapse formation. For synapses in the unpotentiated state, we further assume that AMPA receptors have a wider spatial distribution, with many beyond the range of effective concentration of released neurotransmitter. Ca^{2+} influx through the NMDA receptor channel activates several calcium-dependent processes, among them, the calcium-dependent protease calpain (Vanderklish et al. 1995). Calpain-mediated degradation of cytoskeletal proteins has been shown to play an important role in the redistribution of cell surface receptors (Croall and Demartino 1991), and we postulate that it allows the lateral diffusion of AMPA receptors in synaptic membranes and their migration toward the region of recently activated NMDA receptor channels. This initial clustering of AMPA receptors in membrane locations more closely aligned with presynaptic release sites is the basis for STP.

As the mechanisms that promote receptor aggregation decay with time, AMPA receptors diffuse away from membrane locations proximal to the initially activated NMDA receptors (and thus to locations more displaced from the release site), and there is a corresponding time-dependent decay in the magnitude of the potentiated AMPA receptor–mediated response. Activation of other calcium-dependent processes and second messenger systems, including those related to adhesion molecules (Luthi et al. 1994; Xiao et al. 1991), have been shown to be required for the stabilization of STP into LTP. If AMPA receptors are "anchored" in their new position before relaxation of STP is complete, then the newly stabilized locations relative to the release sites leads to LTP. Without activation of the anchoring mechanisms, however, recently aggregated receptors will diffuse back to their original positions (or equivalently distant positions), with the resulting synaptic potentiation expressed only as STP. Thus, the magnitude of LTP is determined by the decay time course of the clustering process and the onset time course of the anchoring process.

The proposed model is consistent with previous conceptualizations of two parallel and independent processes for STP and LTP (Arai et al. 1990; Gustafsson et al. 1989; Nicoll and Malenka 1995), as well as numerous studies indicating that inhibition of second messenger pathways effectively blocks stabilization of LTP while having minimal effect on the magnitude of STP. In particular, the proposed model is consistent with our recent observation that STP can be induced repetitively in the presence of saturating levels of LTP (Xie et al. 1996). Saturation of LTP is presumed to represent the maximum density of receptors that can be anchored in the synaptic region. If the processes underlying clustering (increased receptor mobility and lateral displacement) are independent of the mechanisms underlying anchoring, then neither the magnitude of STP nor its repetitive induction should be altered by saturation of LTP.

Predictions of the Postsynaptic AMPA Realignment Model

A number of results can be predicted or explained by our model. First, increased responses to microejection of AMPA may occur during later phases of LTP. As shown in figure 5.19, receptor aggregation may cause an overall receptor redistribution on the membrane surface. This redistribution may serve as a signal for more receptors to be supplied to the membrane. As a result, the absolute number of AMPA receptors could gradually increase over time. Davies et al. (1989) observed such a progressive increase in AMPA responsivity, which started about 30 minutes after the induction of LTP with the peak magnitude appearing approximately 90 minutes later.

Second, if AMPA receptors are poorly aligned relative to the presynaptic site, the synapse can be functionally silent. Our simulation results showed that the amplitude of EPSP produced by an AMPA receptor channel displaced by 100 nm from the presynaptic release site is 32% of that generated by a receptor channel aligned with the release site, whereas a receptor channel displaced by 200 nm will generate an EPSP of only 6% in amplitude, making it almost undetectable. This prediction is consistent with reports that LTP arises from recruitment of inactive synapses or latent receptors (Andrew and Macvicar 1994; Edwards 1991; Kullmann 1994; Liao et al. 1992; Manabe et al. 1992). More recently, Liao et al. (1995) and Isaac et al. (1995) have confirmed that a high proportion of synapses in hippocampal area CA1 exhibits NMDA receptor–mediated transmission only, making these synapses effectively nonfunctional at normal resting potentials. These "silent" synapses acquire AMPA receptor-mediated response characteristics following LTP induction.

Third, our results show that the dynamics of neurotransmitter distribution in the synapse varies as a function of distance from the release site, namely, the greater the distance from the release site, the slower the variation in concentration of neurotransmitter. Because the model predicts that synaptic potentiation reflects the migration of AMPA receptors to positions closer to the release site, the rise and decay times of AMPA EPSCs should be more rapid during the expression of LTP, as found in the present and previous studies (Ambros-Ingerson et al. 1993). More generally, the location of AMPA receptor channels in the postsynaptic membrane should range from optimal alignment with the presynaptic release site to beyond the range of effective concentration of released neurotransmitter, that is, functionally "silent." Within this spectrum, the rise-fall time and peak amplitude of the AMPA EPSC waveform should correlate positively with proximity to the presynaptic release site.

Finally, the model predicts a nonuniform distribution of AMPA and NMDA receptors in the synapse. It is expected that NMDA receptors are at the most focal point opposite a given release site, with an "annulus" of more peripherally located AMPA receptors. The degree of nonuniformity should be more pronounced for potentiated synapses.

ACKNOWLEDGMENTS

This research was supported by the NIMH (MH51722 and MH00343), NCRR Biomedical Simulations Resource (P41 RR01861), the USC Brain

Project (NIMH, MH52194), ONR (N00014-98-1-0259), and the Human Frontiers Science Organization.

REFERENCES

Alberts, B., Bray, D., Lewis, J., Raff, M., Roberts, K., and Watson, J. D. (1994). *Membrane Structure*, Vol. 3. New York, Garland.

Almers, W. (1994). Synapses. How fast can you get? *Nature* 367: 682–683.

Ambros-Ingerson, J., and Lynch, G. (1993). Channel gating kinetics and synaptic efficacy: a hypothesis for expression of long-term potentiation. *Proc. Natl. Acad. Sci. U. S. A.* 90: 7903–7907.

Ambros-Ingerson, J., Xiao, P., Larson, J., and Lynch, G. (1993). Waveform analysis suggests that LTP alters the kinetics of synaptic receptor channels. *Brain Res.* 620: 237–244.

Andrew, R. D., and Macvicar, B. A. (1994). Imaging cell volume changes and neuronal excitation in the hippocampal slice. *Neuroscience* 62: 371–383.

Arai, A., Larson, J., and Lynch, G. (1990). Anoxia reveals a vulnerable period in the development of long-term potentiation. *Brain Res.* 511: 353–357.

Augustine, G. J., Charlton, M. P., and Smith, S. J. (1985). Calcium entry and transmitter release at voltage-clamped nerve terminals of squid. *J. Physiol. (Lond.)* 367: 163–181.

Augustine, G. J., and Neher, E. (1992). Neuronal Ca^{2+} signaling takes the local route. *Curr. Opin. Neurobiol.* 2: 302–307.

Bertram, R. (1997). A simple-model of transmitter release and facilitation. *Neural Computation* 9: 515–523.

Bertram, R., Sherman, A., and Stanley, E. F. (1996). Single-domain/bound calcium hypothesis of transmitter release and facilitation. *J. Neurophysiol.* 75: 1919–1931.

Bhide, P. G., and Bedi, K. S. (1984). The effects of a lengthy period of environmental diversity on well-fed and previously undernourished rats. II. Synapse-to-neuron ratios. *J. Comp. Neurol.* 227: 305–310.

Black, J. E., Isaacs, K. R., Anderson, B. J., Alcantara, A. A., and Greenough, W. T. (1990). Learning causes synaptogenesis, whereas motor activity causes angiogenesis, in cerebellar cortex of adult rats. *Proc. Natl. Acad. Sci. U. S. A.* 87: 5568–72.

Bliss, T. V. P., and Collingridge, G. L. (1993). A synaptic model of memory—long-term potentiation in the hippocampus. *Nature* 361: 31–39.

Bommert, K., Charlton, M. P., DeBello, W. M., Chin, G. J., Betz, H., and Augustine, G. J. (1993). Inhibition of neurotransmitter release by C2–domain peptides implicates synaptotagmin in exocytosis. *Nature* 363: 163–165.

Brose, N., Petrenko, A. G., Südhof, T. C., and Jahn, R. (1992). Synaptotagmin: a calcium sensor on the synaptic vesicle surface. *Science* 256: 1021–1025.

Buchs, P. A., and Muller, D. (1996). Induction of long-term potentiation is associated with major ultrastructural changes of activated synapses. *Proc. Natl. Acad. Sci. U. S. A.* 93: 8040–8045.

Crank, J. (1975). *The Mathematics of Diffusion*, (2d ed.). Oxford: Clarendon Press.

Croall, D. E., and Demartino, G. N. (1991). Calcium-activated neutral protease (calpain) system: structure, function, and regulation. *Physiol. Rev.* 71: 813–847.

Davies, S. N., Lester, R. A. J., Reymann, K. G., and Collingridge, G. L. (1989). Temporally distinct pre- and post-synaptic mechanisms maintain long-term potentiation. *Nature* 338: 500–503.

De Groot, D. M., and Bierman, E. P. (1983). The complex-shaped "perforated" synapse, a problem in quantitative stereology of the brain. *J. Microsc.* 131: 355–60.

Debski, E. A., Cline, H. T., and Constantine-Paton, M. (1990). Activity-dependent tuning and the NMDA receptor. *J. Neurobiol.* 21: 18–32.

Desmond, N. L., and Levy, W. B. (1983). Synaptic correlates of associative potentiation/depression: an ultrastructural study in the hippocampus. *Brain Res.* 265: 21–30.

Desmond, N. L., and Levy, W. B. (1988). Synaptic interface surface area increases with long-term potentiation in the hippocampal dentate gyrus. *Brain Res.* 453: 308–314.

Diamond, M. C., Krech, D., and Rosenzweig, M. R. (1964). The effects of an enriched environment on the histology of the rat cerebral cortex. *J. Comp. Neurol.* 123: 111–120.

Dodge, F. A., and Rahamimoff, R. (1967). Co-operative action of calcium ions in transmitter release at the neuromuscular junction. *J. Physiol. (Lond.)* 193: 419–432.

Drejer, J., and Honore, T. (1988). New quinoxalinediones show potent antagonism of quisqualate responses in cultured mouse cortical neurons. *Neurosci. Lett.* 87: 104–108.

Dudel, J., Parnas, I., and Parnas, H. (1983). Neurotransmitter release and facilitation in crayfish muscle. VI. Release determined in both intracellular calcium concentration and depolarization of the nerve terminal. *Pflügers Arch.* 339: 1–10.

Dyson, S. E., and Jones, D. G. (1984). Synaptic remodeling during development and maturation: junction differentiation and splitting as a mechanism for modifying connectivity. *Brain Res.* 315: 125–37.

Edwards, F. (1991). LTP is a long-term problem. *Nature* 350: 271–272.

Federmeier, K., Kleim, J. A., Anderson, B. J., and Greenough, W. T. (1994). Formation of double synapses in the cerebellar cortex of the rat following motor learning. *Soc. Neurosci. Abstr.* 20: 1435.

Froehner, S. C. (1993). Regulation of ion channel distribution at synapses. *Annu. Rev. Neurosci.* 16: 347–468.

Geinisman, Y. (1993). Perforated axospinous synapses with multiple, completely partitioned transmission zones: probable structural intermediates in synaptic plasticity. *Hippocampus* 3: 417–434.

Geinisman, Y., deToledo-Morrell, L., Morrell, F., Heller, R. E., Rossi, M., and Parshall, R. F. (1993). Structural synaptic correlate of long-term potentiation: formation of axospinous synapses with multiple, completely partitioned transmission zones. *Hippocampus* 3: 435–446.

Globus, A., Rosenzweig, M. R., Bennett, E. L., and Diamond, M. C. (1973). Effects of differential experience on dendritic spine counts in rat cerebral cortex. *J. Comp. Physiol. Psychol.* 82: 175–81.

Greenough, W. T., Juraska, J. M., and Volkmar, F. R. (1979). Maze training effects on dendritic branching in occipital cortex of adult rats. *Behav. Neural Biol.* 26: 287–97.

Gustafsson, B., Asztely, F., Hanse, E., and Wigström, H. (1989). Onset characteristics of long-term potentiation in the guinea-pig hippocampal CA1 region in vitro. *Eur. J. Neurosci.* 1: 382–394.

Harris, K. M., Jensen, F. E., and Tsao, B. (1992). 3-dimensional structure of dendritic spines and synapses in rat hippocampus %ca1< at postnatal day-15 and adult ages—implications for the maturation of synaptic physiology and long-term potentiation. *J. Neurosci.* 12: 2685–2705.

Hodgkin, A. L., and Keynes, R. D. (1957). Movement of labeled calcium in squid giant axons. *J. Physiol (Lond.)* 138: 253–281.

Isaac, J. T. R., Nicoll, R. A., and Malenka, R. C. (1995). Evidence for silent synapses: implications for the expression of LTP. *Neuron* 15: 427–434.

Katz, B., and Miledi, R. (1968). The role of calcium in neuromuscular facilitation. *J. Physiol. (Lond.)* 195: 481–492.

Kleim, J. A., Napper, R. M. A., Swain, R. A., Armstrong, K. E., Jones, T. A., and Greenough, W. T. (1994). Selective synaptic plasticity in the cerebellar cortex of the rat following complex motor learning. *Soc. Neurosci. Abstr.* 20: 1435.

Kleim, J. A., Vij, K., Ballard, D. H., and Greenough, W. T. (1997). Learning-dependent synaptic modifications in the cerebellar cortex of the adult rat persist for at least 4 weeks. *J. Neurosci.* 17: 717–721.

Kloot, V. d. (1988). The kinetics of quantal releases during end-plate currents at the frog neuro-muscular junction. *J. of Physiol. (Lond.)* 402: 605–626.

Kruk, P. J., Korn, H., and Faber, D. S. (1997). The effects of geometrical parameters on synaptic transmission: a Monte Carlo simulation study. *Biophys. J.* 73: 2874–2890.

Kullmann, D. M. (1994). Amplitude fluctuations of dual-component EPSCs in hippocampal pyramidal cells: implications for long-term potentiation. *Neuron* 12: 1111–1120.

Lester, R. A. J., and Jahr, C. E. (1992). NMDA channel behavior depends on agonist affinity. *J. Neurosci.* 12: 635–643.

Liao, D., Hessler, N. A., and Malinow, R. (1995). Activation of postsynaptically silent synapses during pairing-induced LTP in CA1 region of hippocampal slice. *Nature* 375: 400–404.

Liao, D., Jones, A., and Malinow, R. (1992). Direct measurement of quantal changes underlying long-term potentiation in CA1 hippocampus. *Neuron* 9: 1089–1097.

Llinás, R., Steinberg, I. Z., and Walton, K. (1981). Presynaptic calcium currents in squid giant synapse. *Biophys. J.* 33: 289–322.

Longsworth, L. G. (1953). Diffusion measurements at 25 C of aqueous solutions of amino acids, peptides and sugars. *J. Am. Chem. Soc.* 75: 5705–5709.

Luthi, A., Laurent, J. P., Figurov, A., Muller, D., and Schachner, M. (1994). Hippocampal long-term potentiation and pleural cell adhesion molecules L1 and NCAM. *Nature* 372: 777–779.

Lynch, G., Gribkoff, V., and Deadwyler, S. A. (1976). Long-term potentiation is accompanied by a reduction in dendritic responsiveness to glutamic acid. *Nature* 263: 151–153.

Malgaroli, A., and Tsien, R. W. (1992). Glutamate-induced long-term potentiation of the frequency of miniature synaptic currents in cultured hippocampal neurons. *Nature* 357: 134–139.

Manabe, T., Renner, P., and Nicoll, R. A. (1992). Postsynaptic contribution to long-term potentiation revealed by the analysis of miniature synaptic currents. *Nature* 355: 50–55.

Mastrogiacomo, A., Parsons, S. M., Zampighi, G. A., Jenden, D. J., Umbach, J. A., and Gundersen, C. B. (1994). Cysteine string proteins: a potential link between synaptic vesicles and presynaptic Ca^{2+} channels. *Science* 263: 981–982.

Mayer, M. L., and Westbrook, G. L. (1987). Permeation and block of N-methyl-D-aspartic acid receptor channels by divalent cations in mouse cultured central neurons. *J. Physiol.* 394: 501–527.

Muller, L., Pattiselanno, A., and Vrensen, G. (1981). The postnatal development of the presynaptic grid in the visual cortex of rabbits and the effect of dark-rearing. *Brain Res.* 205: 39–48.

Murali, M. P., and Sastry, B. R. (1985). Calcium and unit response decrement to locally applied glutamate on rat hippocampal CA1 neurons. *Eur. J. Pharmacol.* 114: 335–341.

Nicoll, R. A., and Malenka, R. C. (1995). Contrasting properties of two forms of long-term potentiation in the hippocampus. *Nature* 377: 115–118.

Nieto-Sampedro, M., Hoff, S. F., and Cotman, C. W. (1982). Perforated postsynaptic densities: probable intermediates in synapse turnover. *Proc. Natl. Acad. Sci. U. S. A.* 79: 5718–5722.

Nowak, L., Bregestovski, P., and Ascher, P. (1984). Magnesium gates glutamate-activated channels in mouse central neurons. *Nature* 307: 462–465.

O'Connor, V. M., Shamotienko, O., Grishin, E., and Betz, H. (1993). On the structure of the "synaptosecretosome." Evidence for a neurexin/synaptotagmin/syntaxin/Ca^{2+} channel complex. *FEBS Letters* 326: 255–260.

Parnas, H., Hovav, G., and Parnas, I. (1989). Effect of Ca^{2+} diffusion on the time course of neurotransmitter release. *Biophys. J.* 55: 859–874.

Parnas, I., and Parnas, H. (1988). The "Ca-voltage" hypothesis for neurotransmitter release. *Biophys. Chem.* 29: 85–93.

Patneau, D. K., and Mayer, M. L. (1990). Structure-activity relationships for amino acid transmitter candidates acting at N-methyl-D-aspartate and quisqualate receptors. *J. Neurosci.* 10: 2385–2399.

Perin, M. S., Fried, V. A., Mignery, G. A., Jahn, R., and Südhof, T. C. (1990). Phospholipid binding by a synaptic vesicle protein homologous to the regulatory region of protein kinase C. *Nature* 345: 260–263.

Petrenko, A. G., Perin, M. S., Davletov, B. A., Ushkaryov, Y. A., Geppert, M., and Südhof, T. C. (1991). Binding of synaptotagmin to the alpha-latrotoxin receptor implicates both in synaptic vesicle exocytosis. *Nature* 353: 65–68.

Schwartz, M. L., and Rothblat, L. A. (1980). Long-lasting behavioral and dendritic spine deficits in the monocularly deprived albino rat. *Exp. Neurol.* 68: 136–146.

Söllner, T., Whiteheart, S. W., Brunner, M., Erdjument, B. H., Geromanos, S., Tempst, P., and Rothman, J. E. (1993). SNAP receptors implicated in vesicle targeting and fusion. *Nature* 362: 318–324.

Taube, J. S., and Schwartzkroin, P. A. (1988). Mechanisms of long-term potentiation: EPSP/spike dissociation, intradendritic recordings, and glutamate sensitivity. *J. Neurosci.* 8: 1632–1644.

The MathWorks, I. (1995). *Partial Differential Equation Toolbox User's Guide.* The MathWorks, Inc.

Turner, A. M., and Greenough, W. T. (1983). Synapses per neuron and synaptic dimensions in occipital cortex of rats reared in complex, social or isolation housing. *Acta Stereol (Suppl.)* 2: 239–244.

Turner, A. M., and Greenough, W. T. (1985). Differential rearing effects on rat visual cortex synapses. I. Synaptic and neuronal density and synapses per neuron. *Brain Res.* 329: 195–203.

Vanderklish, P., Saido, T. C., Gall, C., and Lynch, G. (1995). Proteolysis of spectrin by calpain accompanies theta-burst stimulation in cultured hippocampal slices. *Mol. Brain Res.* 32: 25–35.

Volkmar, F. R., and Greenough, W. T. (1972). Rearing complexity affects branching of dendrites in the visual cortex of the rat. *Science* 176: 1145–7.

Vrensen, G., Cardozo, J. N., Muller, L., and van der Want, J. (1980). The presynaptic grid: a new approach. *Brain Res.* 184: 23–40.

Wahl, L. M., Pouzat, C., and Stratford, K. J. (1996). Monte Carlo simulation of fast excitatory synaptic transmission at a hippocampal synapse. *J. Neurophysiol.* 75: 597–608.

Wendland, B., Miller, K. G., Schilling, J., and Scheller, R. H. (1991). Differential expression of the p 65 gene family. *Neuron* 6: 993–1007.

Wojtowicz, J. M., Marin, L., and Atwood, H. L. (1989). Synaptic restructuring during long-term facilitation at the crayfish neuromuscular junction. *Can. J. Physiol. Pharmacol.* 67: 167–71.

Xiao, P., Bahr, B. A., Staubli, U., Vanderklish, P., and Lynch, G. (1991). Evidence that matrix recognition contributes to stabilization but not induction of LTP. *Neuroreport* 2: 461–464.

Xie, X., Barrionuevo, G., and Berger, T. W. (1996). Differential expression of short-term potentiation by AMPA and NMDA receptors in dentate gyrus. *Learning Memory* 3: 115–123.

Xie, X., Berger, T. W., and Barrionuevo, G. (1992). Isolated NMDA receptor–mediated synaptic responses express both LTP and LTD. *J. Neurophysiol.* 67: 1009–1013.

Yamada, W. M., and Zucker, R. S. (1992). Time course of transmitter release calculated from simulations of a calcium diffusion model. *Biophys. J.* 61: 671–82.

6 Neuron/Glia Signaling and Use-Dependent Modification of Synaptic Strength

David J. Linden

NEURON-GLIA SIGNALING

The historical view of glial physiology held that glial cells were the ubiquitous, silent partners of neurons. Initial microelectrode recordings from glial cells in the brain characterized glial membranes as being devoid of active voltage-gated responses, dominated by a large passive potassium conductance present at rest, and extensively coupled to form a glial syncytium. In this context, the supportive role of glial cells was stressed, particularly the regulation of the extracellular milieu through such processes as transport of nutrients from the blood, buffering of potassium and uptake and processing of neurotransmitters (see Orkand 1995 for review). More recently, the development of the patch-clamp technique has allowed the demonstration that glial cells express a broad array of voltage-gated ion channels, including those permeable to sodium, calcium, and potassium, thus conferring upon them some of the excitable properties of neurons (see Duffy et al. 1995; Sontheimer and Ritchie 1995 for review).

Somewhat more problematic has been the characterization of glial membrane responses to neurotransmitter release. Responses of glial cells in situ to application of exogenous neurotransmitters were first recorded in the cerebral cortex (Krnjevic and Schwartz 1967). Initially, these responses were thought to represent an indirect effect upon glial membranes of potassium release from adjacent neurons (Hosli et al. 1981a,b). However, subsequent experiments using immunocytochemically defined glial cultures showed direct membrane voltage responses to application of glutamate (Bowman and Kimelberg 1984; Kettenmann et al. 1984). The demonstration that application of glutamate to retinal glial cells resulted in depolarization mediated by electrogenic glutamate uptake suggested this process as the sole basis for the depolarizing effect (Brew and Attwell 1987). Further work using patch-clamp recording in conjunction with the appropriate receptor agonists and antagonists would show that inward currents evoked by glutamate application in cerebellar and cortical astrocytes were mediated by both electrogenic glutamate uptake and activation of an 2-(aminomethyl)phenylacetic acid (AMPA)–kainate glutamate receptor (Sontheimer et al. 1988; Usowicz et al.

1989; Wyllie et al. 1991; see Steinhauser and Gallo 1996 for review). In cerebellar astrocytes, this AMPA-kainate receptor activation was shown to gate an ion channel permeable to calcium as well as sodium and potassium (Burnashev et al. 1992; Muller et al. 1992; Tempia et al. 1996). These electrophysiological findings were complemented by the glial localization of the cloned ionotropic glutamate receptor subunits (Blackstone et al. 1992; Petralia and Wenthold 1992; Baude et al. 1994; Burnashev et al. 1992; Patneau et al. 1994) and excitatory amino acid transporters (Rothstein et al. 1994; Chaudry et al. 1995) by immunocytochemistry and in situ hybridization.

Activation of brain astrocytes by exogenous glutamate may also be detected by measuring changes in glial cytosolic calcium using microfluorimetric techniques (see Verkhratsky and Kettenmann 1996 for review). Glutamate-evoked calcium increases in brain glia seem to represent at least three different modes of calcium signaling: direct influx via calcium-permeable AMPA-kainate receptors (Muller et al. 1992), calcium influx via voltage-gated calcium channels as triggered by AMPA-kainate receptor–mediated depolarization (Glaum et al. 1990), and activation of phosphoinositide-linked metabotropic glutamate receptors and the consequent mobilization of calcium from inositol 1,4,5-triphosphate (InsP$_3$)–gated internal stores (Glaum et al. 1990; Jensen and Chiu 1990, Cornell-Bell et al. 1990; Cornell-Bell and Finkbeiner 1991, Porter and McCarthy 1995). These calcium responses can take the form of brief spikes, prolonged oscillations, or slow (6 to 30 mm/second) traveling waves. In a glial syncytium, these waves readily travel between cells, allowing for a form of long-range glial signaling (Cornell-Bell et al. 1990; Charles et al. 1991; Cornell-Bell and Finkbeiner 1991).

These results clearly show that membrane currents and cytosolic calcium responses may be evoked in glia by application of exogenous neurotransmitter, but they do not address the question of whether glial cells can respond to neurotransmitter released from synaptic terminals. The details of this question are of great computational importance. Do glia only have the ability to respond slowly to relatively small changes in neurotransmitter concentration which occur in the bulk extracellular fluid or do they have the ability to respond rapidly to localized release of neurotransmitter in the manner of neurons? Repetitive neuronal stimulation has been shown to produce a slow depolarization of the glial membrane mediated by an increase in the concentration of extracellular potassium in several preparations (Orkand et al. 1966; Ransom and Goldring 1973; Futamachi and Pedley 1976; Schwartzkroin and Prince 1979; Roitbak and Fanardjian 1981). A similar stimulation protocol (sustained 8-Hz stimulation applied to hippocampal mossy fibers in an organotypic slice culture) was found to evoke slow calcium waves in astrocyte networks of the CA$_3$ region (Dani et al. 1992). This result has recently been confirmed and extended by Porter and McCarthy (1996) who showed that tetanic stimulation (50-Hz, two seconds) of Schaffer collateral fibers in an acutely prepared hippocampal slice resulted in slow calcium waves in an astrocyte network of area CA1, and that these calcium responses were antagonized by blockers of ionotropic glutamate receptors, metabotropic glutamate receptors, and voltage-gated calcium channels. A related approach was taken by Murphy et al. (1993) who recorded membrane currents from individual, immunocytochemically identified cortical astrocytes simultaneous with microfluorimetric calcium signals from adjacent neurons. They found that spontaneous calcium transients in neurons, which corresponded to neuronal action potentials, were often very closely associated with inward currents in an adjacent glial cell (latencies less than 10 ms).

While the aforementioned experiments suggest that brain glia respond to synaptically released neurotransmitter (presumably glutamate), they are not definitive. Mennerick and Zorumski (1994) used the microisland culture technique to record simultaneously from an adjacent neuron and a glial cell derived from dispersed hippocampus. As neurons on microislands form extensive self-synapses (autapses), autaptic and glial currents may be recorded following a brief depolarizing voltage step applied to the neuronal somata. When an action potential was evoked, both autaptic and glial inward currents were recorded within 5 ms. The autaptic current was sensitive to antagonists of ionotropic glutamate receptors (AP5, CNQX, GYKI). Conversely, the glial current was largely insensitive to glutamate receptor antagonists. Furthermore, the glial current was very sensitive to replacement of external sodium with lithium as well as the reuptake inhibitor hydroxyaspartate, and did not reverse at a command potential of $+50$ mV, all characteristics of a glutamate reuptake mechanism. Manipulations which attenuated the glial current resulted in a prolongation of the autaptic current consistent with a role for this current in extracellular glutamate clearance.

In the intermediate lobe of the pituitary, unusual synaptoid contacts exist between the fibers of the pituitary stalk, and stellate glial cells (Van Leeuwen et al. 1983; see Theodosis and MacVicar 1996 for review). These axonal contacts are immunopositive for γ-aminobotyric acid (GABA) and contain vesicles and a presynaptic density. Activation of the pituitary stalk with a single brief pulse gives rise to a biphasic response in stellate glia, a small, rapid depolarization, mediated by activation of GABA$_A$ receptors and consequent chloride efflux, followed by a large, rapid hyperpolarization mediated by D$_2$ dopamine receptors and consequent potassium influx (Mudrick-Donnon et al. 1993). It is suggested, but not proved, that these synaptic currents are mediated by the aforementioned synaptoid contacts.

GLIAL SYNAPTIC CURRENTS IN CEREBELLAR CULTURE

The cerebellar cortex is a particularly good location to investigate neuron-to-glia signaling as Bergmann glial cells ensheath the parallel fiber–Purkinje neuron synapse unusually tightly and completely (Spacek 1985). Furthermore, the Bergmann glia express a high density of ionotropic glutamate receptors (Blackstone et al. 1992; Hampson et al. 1992; Petralia and Wenthold 1992; Martin et al. 1993; Petralia et al. 1994) on the plasma membrane adjacent to these synapses (Baude et al. 1994). This striking localization led Baude et al. (1994) to conclude, "It is reasonable to assume that glutamate released from parallel fiber terminals acts on AMPA receptors in the glial membrane" (p. 2839). As elaborated in the following section, I have confirmed this assumption using cell pair recording in cultures of embryonic mouse cerebellum.

Glial cells were identified in culture as large cells with nontapering processes and a stellate or fusiform shape. When recordings were made in current clamp mode with a potassium-based saline, granule and Purkinje neurons but not glial cells generated action potentials upon injection of positive current. In some cases, this identification was confirmed with immunocytochemistry for glial fibrillary acidic protein which was positive for glial cells and negative in adjacent neurons. Conversely, glial cells were negative for calbindin-D$_{28K}$, a specific marker for Purkinje neurons. Whole-cell patch-clamp recordings of glial cells were initially made using a standard KCl-based internal saline and a standard NaCl-based external saline supplemented with picrotoxin to block GABA$_A$ receptors. With this recording configuration the glial resting potential was -82.7 ± 9.5 mV (n = 19) and the input resistance was 2.1 ± 1.0 MΩ (n = 19). The low input resistance was due, in part, to a high degree of gap junctional coupling between astrocytes. When octanol (200 µM), a blocker of gap junctions (Bernardini et al. 1984), was applied, input resistance increased in 5 of 11 cells to 6.3 ± 2.8 MΩ (n = 5; the other six, which were unaffected, had input resistance of 2.0 ± 0.8 MΩ). However, a more important determinant of input resistance was a large passive potassium conductance. When recordings were made using a cesium-tetraethylammonium (TEA)–based internal saline to block potassium conductances, the recorded input resistance was higher yet (15.9 ± 4.4 MΩ, n = 20). This increase in input resistance was accompanied by the improved resolution of small spontaneous inward currents measured in voltage-clamp mode at a holding potential of -80 mV (figure 6.1A). These spontaneous currents had a mean amplitude of 132 ± 41 pA and a mean interval of 198 ± 45 ms (n = 100 events in a single cell). Cs-TEA–based internal salines were used in all subsequent glial recordings.

Following establishment of a whole-cell recording from a glial cell, a loose patch electrode was attached to the soma of a nearby granule neuron. In an attempt to evoke glial synaptic currents, a brief voltage step (0.1 to -0.25 ms, 50 to -200 V) was applied to the loose patch electrode to produce an action potential in the granule neuron. This resulted in an evoked glial synaptic current in approximately 30% of granule neuron-glial cell pairs. When a glial synaptic current could not be evoked after repeated stimulation, the loose patch electrode was detached with brief positive pressure and moved to another granule neuron for a subsequent attempt. Figure 6.1B shows a glial synaptic current evoke by granule neuron stimulation, superimposed upon a subsequent trace in which granule neuron stimulation failed to evoke a glial synaptic current. This particular cell pair had 36 of 100 failures in successive stimuli delivered at 0.05 Hz.

A

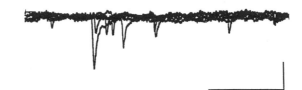

B

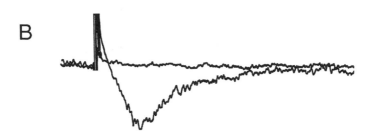

Figure 6.1 Synaptic currents in cultured cerebellar glial cells. (A) Spontaneous synaptic currents recorded in a glial cell. Five sequential traces are superimposed. Scale bar = 80 ms, 50 pA. (B) Glial synaptic current and a failure evoked by stimulation of a single granule neuron. Scale bar: 25 ms, 50 pA. The stimulus artifact has been truncated. (From Linden 1997.)

When glial membrane potential was systematically changed, a current-voltage relation of the evoked currents emerged that displayed slight double rectification. This form of current-voltage relation is typically found in cells which express AMPA-kainate receptor subunits, but which lack the particular glutamate receptor subunit GluR2 and are thereby rendered highly calcium-permeable (Hollman et al. 1991). This has previously been reported for currents evoked by application of exogenous kainate in Bergmann glial cells (Burnashev et al. 1992; Muller et al. 1992; Tempia et al. 1996). In contrast, cerebellar Purkinje neurons, which strongly express GluR2, have linear I-V relations and AMPA-kainate receptors which are very weakly calcium-permeable as assessed using either the present cell culture protocol (Linden et al. 1993) or the cerebellar slice preparation (Tempia et al. 1996). To further characterize the evoked glial synaptic current, a series of drugs were added to the external saline. Neither octanol (200 μM), a blocker of gap junctions, nor L-trans-pyrrolidine-2,4,-dicarboxylate (PDC, 300 μM), which blocks electrogenic glutamate reuptake (Bridges et al. 1991), produced a significant alteration in the amplitude of the evoked glial synaptic current (107.5 ± 9.3 and 94.0 ± 8.3% of baseline, respectively, n = 5 per group). Similarly, neither D-AP5 (50 μM), an antagonist of the N-methyl-D-aspartate (NMDA) receptor, nor this compound applied together with (+)-MCPG (300 μM), an antagonist of metabotropic glutamate receptors, altered the glial synaptic current (92.5 ± 8.9 and 96.4 ± 7.5% of baseline, respectively, n = 5 per group).

However, the AMPA-kainate receptor antagonist CNQX (30 μM) was effective, reducing the glial synaptic current to $11.5 \pm 5.8\%$ of its initial amplitude ($n = 5$). The remaining current is likely to be mediated by electrogenic glutamate reuptake as it failed to reverse when the glial membrane potential was set at $+50$ mV and was reduced to approximately 30% of its original amplitude by PDC. These results suggest that the glial synaptic current is predominantly mediated by AMPA-kainate receptors. For comparison, when 30 μM CNQX was applied to granule neuron–Purkinje neuron excitatory postsynaptic currents (EPSCs), the currents that resulted were $3.4 \pm 1.9\%$ of their initial amplitude ($n = 5$ cells), a similar degree of attenuation to that seen with Purkinje neuron responses to exogenous quisqualate (Linden et al. 1991).

As previous work has shown that responses to exogenous AMPA-kainate receptor agonists in cerebellar Bergmann glia are mediated by opening of an ion channel with high calcium permeability (Burnashev et al. 1992; Muller et al. 1992; Tempia et al. 1996), it became necessary to address this issue for the glial synaptic current. To assess the effects of synaptic AMPA-kainate receptor activation in cultured cerebellar glial cells, I measured glial calcium responses to granule neuron stimulation using fura-2 microfluorimetry. When the glial membrane potential was set to -80 mV, peak internal calcium was 82 ± 26 nM ($n = 4$). Spontaneous synaptic currents were associated with calcium transients, usually limited to a small portion of the glial cell. Stimulation of a granule neuron to evoke a single synaptic current was associated with a calcium transient (peak amplitude 308 ± 41 nM, $n = 4$) which typically decayed to baseline values within approximately 2 seconds (figure 6.2). When this experiment was repeated with the glial cell held in current clamp mode, the peak amplitude of the evoked calcium transient was not significantly different, suggesting that voltage-sensitive calcium channels do not significantly contribute to this measure (data not shown). While the calcium signal contributing to this rise is likely to be dominated by calcium influx through the AMPA-kainate receptor–associated ion channel, it is possible that calcium-induced calcium release is also a factor (Lev-Ram and Ellisman 1995). No evidence of a glial traveling calcium wave was seen.

These experiments suggest that activation of a cerebellar granule neuron can give rise to a rapid inward current in an adjacent glial cell in culture conditions. This current is predominantly mediated by activation of calcium-permeable AMPA-kainate receptors and is largely independent of glutamate reuptake or gap junctional coupling. There are some caveats that should be mentioned in interpreting these results. First, the present recordings were made using a cesium-based, rather than a potassium-based internal saline to improve input resistance and the resolution of small currents. Unfortunately, this will tend to attenuate electrogenic glutamate reuptake, leading to an underestimation of this component by about 30% (Barbour et al. 1988; Szatkowski et al. 1991). Second, it should be emphasized that it is not known

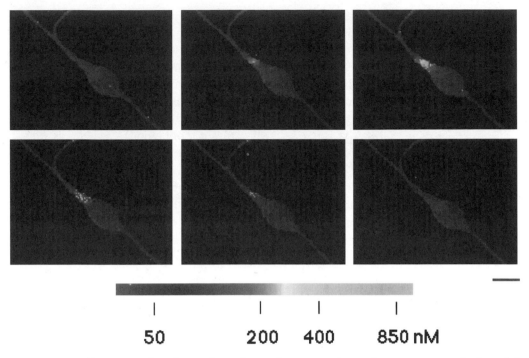

Figure 6.2 Stimulation of a single granule neuron evokes a calcium transient in a fusiform glial cell in cerebellar culture. Fura-2 ratiometric imaging reveals a delimited calcium transient associated with the glial synaptic current. Consecutive frames were acquired at 200-ms intervals (read from the upper left to the lower right). The granule neuron was stimulated to fire a single action potential coincident with the end of the acquisition period for the first frame. Scale bar: 15 μm. (From Linden 1997.)

whether glial cells in this preparation are exclusively detecting glutamate "spillover" from synapses with postsynaptic neuronal elements, or if direct granule neuron-to-glial cell contacts are sometimes formed. Electron microscopic reconstruction of granule cell–glial cell contacts will be required to resolve this issue. Third, it cannot be determined if it is Bergmann glia or some other cerebellar glial cell which detects synaptically released glutamate in culture, as, to my knowledge, there are no unique immunocytochemical or physiological markers for Bergmann glia,. This is particularly important as it has been claimed that astrocytes in culture develop phenotypes that do not correspond to those in vivo (Franklin and Blakemore 1995). While a number of previous recordings from either cultured cerebellar glial cells (Wyllie et al. 1991; Burnashev et al. 1992) or Bergmann glia in cerebellar slice (Muller et al. 1992; Tempia et al. 1996) have not mentioned either spontaneous or evoked synaptic currents, a recent report by Clark and Barbour (1997) has demonstrated synaptic currents evoked in Bergmann glial cells by parallel fiber stimulation in a slice preparation. These synaptic currents were mediated by both electrogenic glutamate uptake and activation of AMPA-kainate receptors with the former predominating.

The present finding of AMPA-kainate receptor–mediated glial synaptic currents differs from that of Mennerick and Zorumski (1994) who found that similar currents in hippocampal microisland culture were mediated by electrogenic glutamate reuptake. A more recent report from this group (Mennerick et al. 1996) finds that while the response of microisland glia to *exogenous* glutamate is dominated by a current mediated by AMPA receptors, the synaptically driven glial current is approximately 20% mediated by these receptors in that it is sensitive to AMPA receptor antagonists and is potentiated by the AMPA receptor desensitization blocker cyclothiazide. These authors suggest that the concentration of glutamate achieved at glial membranes by synaptic release is considerably smaller than that achieved by exogenous application (2 mM glutamate applied with a flow tube), thus allowing the transporter, which has an affinity for glutamate that is approximately 100-fold higher than the AMPA receptor (Arriza et al. 1994; Fairman et al. 1995), to dominate the glial synaptic response.

LONG-TERM POTENTIATION OF NEURONAL AND GLIAL SYNAPTIC CURRENTS IN CEREBELLUM

The cerebellar cortex has been suggested to include an essential circuit for certain forms of motor learning, including associative eye-blink conditioning and adaptation of the vestibulo-ocular reflex (Thompson 1986; Ito 1989; Raymond et al. 1996). One cellular model system thought to contribute to learning in this structure is cerebellar long-term depression (LTD), in which coactivation of climbing fiber and parallel fiber inputs to a Purkinje neuron induces a persistent, input-specific depression of the parallel fiber–Purkinje neuron synapse (Ito et al. 1982; see Linden and Connor 1995 for review). The converse phenomenon, cerebellar LTP, has also been described, in which the parallel fiber–Purkinje neuron synapse is strengthened by repetitive parallel fiber stimulation at low (2 to 8 Hz) frequencies (Sakurai 1987, 1990; Hirano 1990, 1991; Crepel and Jaillard 1991; Shibuki and Okada 1992; Salin et al. 1996) thus endowing this synapse with the capacity for use-dependent bidirectional modification, a computationally important property (Houk and Barto 1991).

Recently, a mechanistic description of cerebellar long-term potentiation (LTP) has been proposed (Salin et al. 1996). It was shown that LTP at this synapse was induced by 8-Hz × 15-seconds stimulation and was not blocked by application of a postsynaptic calcium chelator or blockade of ionotropic glutamate receptors (with bath-applied kynurenate). Cerebellar LTP induction was blocked by removal of external calcium, inhibition of cyclic adenosiae monophosphate (cAMP)–dependent protein kinase, or occlusion via activation of adenylate cyclase. These findings are suggestive of a model previously proposed for LTP induction at the mossy fiber–CA3 synapse in hippocampus (Weisskopf et al. 1994) in which presynaptic calcium entry during axon stimulation resulted in activation of a calcium-sensitive adenylate cyclase, such as the type I isoform of adenylate cyclase, which is enriched in both hippocampal mossy fibers and cerebellar parallel fibers (Xia et al. 1991; Glatt and Snyder 1993), and the consequent activation of cAMP-dependent protein kinase. It has also been suggested that LTP of the parallel fiber–Purkinje neuron synapse is expressed presynaptically, as it is associated with a sustained decrease in paired-pulse facilitation (Salin et al. 1996).

Attributing the locus of expression of long-term use-dependent synaptic change to pre- or postsynaptic structures in the central nervous system (CNS) has been a surprisingly difficult endeavor. Several methods have been suggested to resolve this issue, including analysis of synaptic failure rate, coefficient of variation of EPSCs, paired-pulse facilitation, and minimal stimulation of "silent synapses," but, over time, the applicability of all of these methods has been called into question (Jack et al. 1994; Isaac et al. 1995; Liao et al. 1995; Kullman and Siegelbaum 1995; Kullman et al. 1996; Wang and Kelly 1996). If a non-neuronal detector of synaptically released neurotransmitter could be used to measure use-dependent changes in neurotransmitter release, then this could provide a novel form of evidence for determining locus of expression. In cultures of embryonic mouse cerebellum, glial cells can serve as such a detector and thereby used to examine the expression of cerebellar LTP.

As cerebellar glia in culture can respond to synaptically released glutamate from granule neuron axons (the cell culture analog of parallel fibers), I wanted to determine if cerebellar LTP could be detected using granule neuron–glial cell synaptic currents, and if so, if it had properties similar to those determined for granule neuron–Purkinje neuron EPSCs in the slice preparation. As a control, it was first necessary to determine whether cerebellar LTP could be induced in granule neuron–Purkinje neuron pairs in the present culture system. Activation of a synaptically connected granule neuron–Purkinje neuron pair at 0.1 Hz resulted in a mixture of evoked currents and failures (figure 6.3). LTP was induced by applying 100 pulses at 4 Hz at the test pulse stimulation strength. Induction of LTP was accompanied by a significant decrease in the failure rate ($33 \pm 7\%$ at $t = -2.5$ minutes prior to LTP induction, compared with $17 \pm 10\%$ at $t = 20$ minutes after LTP induction, $n = 6$) and a significant increase in the mean amplitude of evoked EPSCs ($99 \pm 13\%$ of baseline at $t = -2.5$ minutes prior to LTP induction, compared with $193 \pm 24\%$ at $t = 20$ minutes after LTP induction). To determine if cerebellar LTP in culture has similar properties to that described in the slice preparation, 4-Hz stimulation of a granule neuron–Purkinje neuron pair was conducted in the presence of kynurenate plus MCPG to determine whether activation of glutamate receptors was required for cerebellar LTP induction. Upon washout of these drugs and the consequent restoration of synaptic transmission, LTP was revealed (mean EPSC amplitude = $172 \pm 15\%$ of baseline at $t = 22.5$ minutes, $n = 5$), indicating that they are not required. In addition, 4-Hz stimulation of a granule neuron–Purkinje neuron pair was

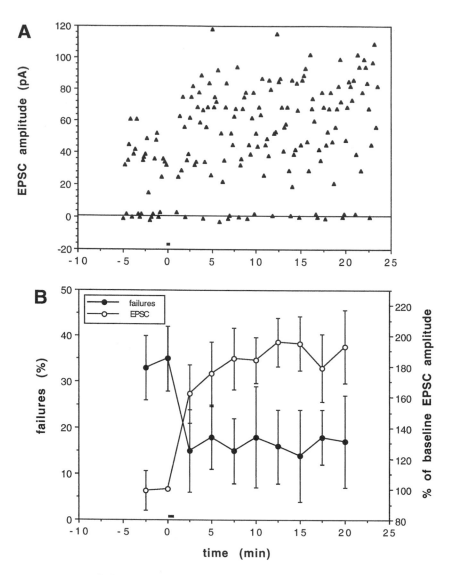

Figure 6.3 Cerebellar long-term potentiation (LTP) in granule neuron–Purkinje neuron pairs. (A) Amplitudes of evoked excitatory postsynaptic currents (EPSCs) following induction of LTP in a granule neuron–Purkinje neuron pair. Each data point represents a single evoked EPSC. LTP was induced by 4-Hz × 100-pulse stimulation (indicated by heavy horizontal bar at t = 0). (B) Cerebellar LTP induction is associated with a decrease in the rate of synaptic failures and an increase in the mean evoked EPSC. Each point represents the mean ± SEM of six cell pairs. The datum for each cell pair was derived from the 2.5-minute recording period prior to the time point indicated. The EPSC amplitude measure was normalized relative to the t = 0 minute time point. C, Representative current traces evoked by four consecutive stimuli two minutes before (left) and ten minutes after (right) induction of LTP in a single granule neuron–Purkinje neuron pair. Scale bars = 10 pA, 10 ms. Stimulus artifacts have been truncated. D, Application of glutamate receptor antagonists (kynurenate 2 mM, (+)-MCPG 500 μM, indicated by the light horizontal bar, t = −7 minutes to 5 minutes) reversibly attenuated synaptic transmission, but failed to block induction of LTP. N = five cell pairs. Removal of external calcium (also indicated by the light horizontal bar) also reversibly attenuated synaptic transmission and did block induction of LTP. N = five cell pairs. (From Linden 1997.)

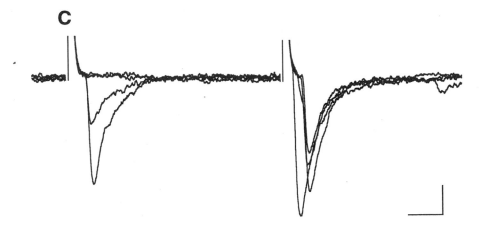

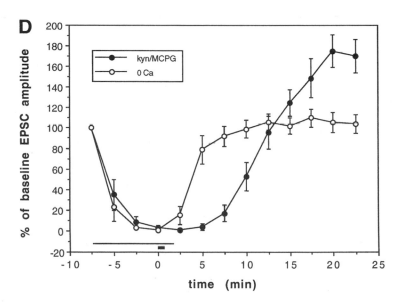

Figure 6.3 (continued)

conducted in the absence of external calcium. When calcium was reintroduced, allowing for the resumption of synchronous transmitter release, no potentiation was evident (mean EPSC amplitude = 108 ± 14% of baseline at t = 22.5 minutes, n = 5). Since all of these experiments were conducted in conditions in which the postsynaptic cell was loaded with calcium chelator and voltage clamped at −80 mV, this suggests that it is calcium influx into the *presynaptic* compartment which is required for cerebellar LTP induction.

When this same set of experiments was repeated using granule neuron–glial cell pairs, equivalent results were obtained (figure 6.4). Activation of a

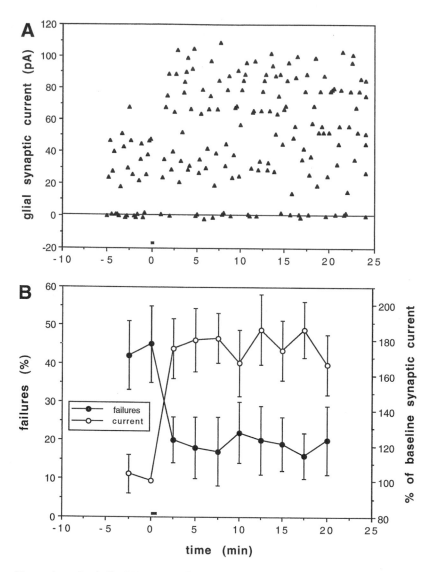

Figure 6.4 Cerebellar LTP in granule neuron–glial cell pairs. (A) Amplitudes of evoked synaptic currents following induction of LTP in a granule neuron–glial cell pair. Each data point represents the amplitude of a single evoked glial synaptic current. LTP was induced by 4-Hz × 100-pulse stimulation (indicated by horizontal bar at t = 0). (B) Cerebellar LTP induction in granule neuron–glial cell pairs is associated with a decrease in the rate of synaptic failures and an increase in the mean glial synaptic current. Each point represents the mean ± SEM of seven cell pairs. (C) Representative current traces evoked by four consecutive stimuli three minutes before (left) and eight minutes after (right) induction of LTP in a single granule neuron–glial cell pair. Scale bars = 10 pA, 10 ms. Stimulus artifacts have been truncated. D, Application of glutamate receptor antagonists (kynurenate 2 mM, (+)-MCPG 500 μM, indicated by the light horizontal bar) during 4-Hz stimulation failed to block induction of LTP. N = five cell pairs. Removal of external calcium (also indicated by the light horizontal bar) blocked induction of LTP. N = five cell pairs. (From Linden 1997.)

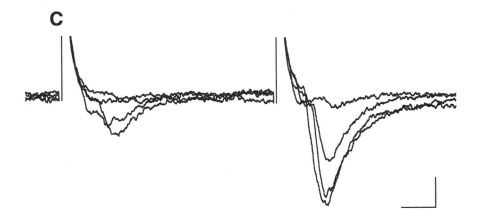

C

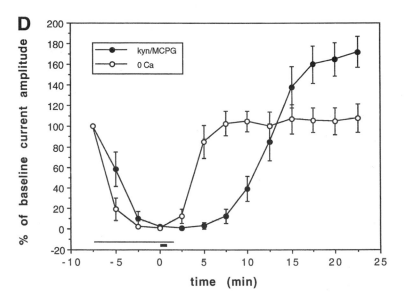

D

Figure 6.4 (continued)

synaptically connected granule neuron–glial cell pair at 0.1 Hz resulted in a mixture of evoked currents and failures, with a slightly higher proportion of failures than granule neuron–Purkinje neuron pairs (42 ± 9% at $t = -2.5$ minutes). Induction of LTP was accompanied by a significant decrease in the failure rate (20 ± 9% at $t = 20$ minutes after LTP induction, $n = 7$) and a significant increase in the mean amplitude of evoked EPSCs (104 ± 11% of baseline at $t = -2.5$ minutes prior to LTP induction, compared with 186 ± 16% at $t = 17.5$ minutes after LTP induction). When 4-Hz stimulation of a granule neuron–glial cell pair was conducted in the presence of kynurenate plus MCPG, LTP was revealed after drug washout (mean EPSC amplitude =

$170 \pm 17\%$ of baseline at $t = 22.5$ minutes, $n = 5$). When this experiment was repeated with external calcium removal during 4-Hz stimulation, no potentiation was seen (mean EPSC amplitude $= 104 \pm 10\%$ of baseline at $t = 22.5$ minutes, $n = 5$).

While the most parsimonious explanation for these results is that cerebellar LTP is expressed as an increase in glutamate release which is detected by AMPA-kainate receptors on either glial cells or Purkinje neurons, it is formally possible that the potentiated response represents the addition of a novel component of synaptic transmission, not mediated by AMPA-kainate receptors. This could potentially result from either the release of a novel cotransmitter after LTP induction, or the postsynaptic alteration of other electrogenic proteins such as NMDA receptors or glutamate transporters. To address this possibility, a saturating dose of an AMPA-kainate receptor antagonist (CNQX, 30 µM) was applied ten minutes after the induction of LTP. In granule neuron–Purkinje neuron pairs, the amplitude of LTP at $t = 10$ minutes was $170.7 \pm 17.7\%$ of baseline, and the current remaining after CNQX application was $5.0 \pm 3.2\%$ of baseline ($t = 25$ minutes). In granule neuron–glial cell pairs, the amplitude of LTP at $t = 10$ minutes was $185.5 \pm 21.0\%$ of baseline, and the current remaining after CNQX application was $13.8 \pm 6.1\%$ of baseline ($t = 25$ minutes). By comparison, unpotentiated synaptic currents were reduced to $3.4 \pm 1.9\%$ and $11.5 \pm 5.8\%$ of baseline for Purkinje neurons and glial cells, respectively. In addition, potentiated glial synaptic currents measured at $t = 8$ minutes reversed at approximately 0 mV and showed slight double rectification similar to that seen for baseline currents. Thus, cerebellar LTP in culture does appear to be *expressed* as an increase in glutamate release which is detected by AMPA-kainate receptors on either glial or Purkinje cells. However, these experiments do not rule out the possible role of a coreleased modulator or MCPG-insensitive metabotropic glotamate receptors (mGluRs) in the cerebellar LTP *induction* process.

The experiments examining cerebellar LTP in granule neuron–Purkinje neuron pairs are entirely consistent with a model in which LTP is triggered by calcium influx and accumulation in the granule neuron axon terminal. Of more interest, the demonstration herein that LTP with similar properties could be induced in either granule neuron–glial neuron or granule neuron–Purkinje neuron cell pairs has important implications for the locus of expression.

One model to explain this finding is that cerebellar LTP is expressed postsynaptically via mechanisms that are common to Purkinje neurons and cerebellar glia. This model would require that these two cell types respond similarly to a common anterograde signal from the granule neuron terminal. Do glial cells have the molecular machinery to express postsynaptic forms of plasticity? Since it has previously been shown that cerebellar long-term depression (LTD) may be induced in the cultured Purkinje neuron when glutamate pulses (to mimic parallel fiber activity) and depolarizing steps (to

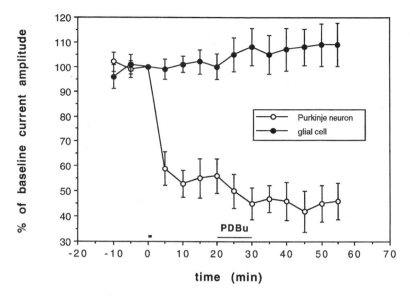

Figure 6.5 Cerebellar long-term depression (LTD) is not induced in glial cells. Glutamate test pulses were applied at 0.05 Hz to Purkinje neurons and glial cells voltage clamped at −80 mV. Neither glutamate nor depolarization conjunctive stimulation (six three-second long depolarizing pulses to 0 mV coincident with glutamate test pulses, indicated by heavy horizontal bar at t = 0 minute) nor bath application of the protein kinase C activator phorbol-12,13-dibutyrate (PDBu) (200 nM, indicated by light bar at t = 20 to 30 minutes) induced a depression of glial responses to glutamate test pulses.

mimic climbing fiber activity) are coapplied (Linden et al. 1991), this protocol was applied to glial cells in an attempt to induce LTD (figure 6.5). This manipulation failed to induce LTD, as did bath application of the protein kinase C activator phorbol-12,13-dibutyrate, another treatment which has been shown to induce a depression of glutamate or AMPA test pulses in Purkinje neurons (Linden and Connor 1991). Thus, cerebellar glial cells in culture do not appear to have the capacity to express LTD.

A second, more parsimonious explanation is that cerebellar LTP is expressed presynaptically and therefore may be detected using either glial or neuronal postsynaptic cells. If this last contention is true, then it makes for a very difficult computational model of the granule neuron–Purkinje neuron synapse, as cerebellar LTD has been shown to be postsynaptically expressed. In such a scheme, cerebellar LTP and LTD would not truly reverse each other (as has been demonstrated for hippocampal LTP and LTD) but rather would be additive, independent phenomena.

NEURON-GLIA SIGNALING IN OTHER MODEL SYSTEMS OF INFORMATION STORAGE

Assessment of the potential roles of glial cells in model systems of information storage has been hampered by a lack of tools to manipulate glial processes specifically. Since glial cells are intimately involved with the development and ongoing basal function of synapses (Pfrieger and Barres 1996), gross interference with glial function produces drastic impairments which preclude the analysis of use-dependent synaptic modification. For example, metabolic poisoning of glial cells with fluoroacetate results in a large, rapid attenuation of glutamatergic synaptic transmission at the Schaffer collateral–CA1 synapse of the hippocampus which results from an inhibition of transmitter release (Keyser and Alger 1994). Conditional ablation of astrocytes in postnatal transgenic mice (through activation of glial fibrillary acidic protein (GFAP) promoter–driven toxin synthesis) results in a disruption of cerebellar cell layering patterns and an excitotoxic depletion of granule neurons within several days (Delaney et al. 1996). While not assessed in this report, it is very likely that basal synaptic properties would be severely disrupted as well.

More subtle perturbations of glial cells that do not appear to affect basal synaptic function have been found to affect LTP and LTD. Application of antiserum directed against the glial protein S-100 has been demonstrated to attenuate the amplitude of hippocampal LTP at the Schaffer collateral–CA1 synapse (Lewis and Teyler 1986). Analysis of hippocampal LTP in transgenic mice in which the intermediate filament GFAP has been rendered null also showed a reduced amplitude of hippocampal LTP (McCall et al. 1996). Similarly, cerebellar LTD was completely blocked in GFAP mutant mice and this was associated with an impairment in associative eye-blink conditioning (Shibuki et al. 1996). Unfortunately, an understanding of the mechanisms by which S-100 or GFAP influence LTP and LTD has yet to emerge.

WHAT ARE THE POTENTIAL CONSEQUENCES OF SYNAPTICALLY DRIVEN GLIAL CURRENTS?

It has been shown that a large number of amino acids and neurotransmitters are released from astrocytes in culture following exposure to glutamate (or glutamate receptor agonists such as kainate). These include glutamate, GABA, aspartate, glycine, and D-serine (Gallo et al. 1991; Levi and Patrizio 1992; Schell et al. 1995). Once released, these substances could act on neuronal receptors either directly, or in the case of glycine and D-serine, as coagonists at the NMDA receptor (Cull-Candy 1995). Indeed, it has been reported that stimuli that evoke calcium increases in cultured astrocytes (such as bradykinin, which triggers phosphoinositide turnover) result in both glutamate release and calcium increase in adjacent neurons (Parpura et al. 1994, 1995c). The neuronal calcium increase could be blocked by NMDA receptor antagonists of removal of external calcium, suggesting that glutamate release acting upon NMDA receptors results in the increase in neuronal calcium. A similar finding was reported by Hassinger et al. (1995) who triggered a calcium wave in a syncytium of cultured cortical glia by mechanical stimulation of a single glia cell. This calcium wave also resulted in calcium elevations in neighboring neurons in a manner that was completely blocked by a combination of NMDA and AMPA receptor antagonists. However, it has been suggested that these results may be an artifact of unusually high concentrations of glutamate in cultured glial cells (Pfrieger and Barres 1996). Nedergaard (1994), using a similar preparation, reported that the rise in neuronal calcium that was evoked by a rise in glial calcium was unaffected by these manipulations, but was inhibited by compounds which block gap junctions. This last result is controversial as other investigators have failed to find evidence of gap junctional coupling between neurons and astrocytes (Murphy et al. 1993; Linden 1997).

The evidence summarized above paints a picture of brain glia, not as passive supportive elements, but as cells which are sometimes capable of responding to and modulating neuronal signals on a millisecond time scale. However, there are still many parts of this story that are unclear. For example, the most definitive evidence for synaptically evoked glial excitatory currents has found these currents to be predominantly mediated by electrogenic glutamate reuptake (Mennerick and Zorumski 1994; Mennerick et al. 1996). It is not straightforward to envision how such a process could, in turn, trigger increases in glial calcium or release of neuroactive amino acids or both (Gallo et al. 1991; Levi and Patrizio 1992; Parpura et al. 1994; Schell et al. 1995). If, in some cases, glial synaptic currents were predominantly mediated by AMPA-kainate receptors, this could evoke glial amino acid release in several ways. First, sodium influx through these receptors could result in *reverse* operation of sodium-coupled glial amino acid transporters (Szatkowski et al. 1990), as has been suggested for glutamate-evoked GABA release from astrocytes (Gallo et al. 1991). Second, an increase in glial calcium produced by direct calcium permeation of the AMPA-kainate receptor (Burnashev et al. 1992; Muller et al. 1992; Tempia et al. 1996), or by indirect activation of voltage-sensitive calcium channels (Glaum et al. 1990), could activate a novel form of glial vesicular release. This is a more problematic proposal. While glia appear to have some of the protein machinery for vesicular release, they are notably lacking some key proteins (Parpura et al. 1995a,b). Finally, glial calcium increases could potentially activate calcium-sensitive enzymes such as phospholipase A_2 and nitric oxide synthase to produce the diffusible messengers arachidonic acid and nitric oxide, respectively. Indeed, glutamate-evoked release of arachidonic acid from cultured astrocytes has been reported (Stella et al. 1994). In conclusion, while glial cells have the potential when activated to signal neurons in turn, whether this signaling comprises "computation" remains to be determined.

ACKNOWLEDGMENTS

Thanks to D. Gurfel who provided skillful technical assistance and to C. Aizenman, K. Narasimhan, A. Parent, and K. Takahashi for helpful suggestions and to A. Ghosh and B. Barres, who provided comments upon an earlier version of the manuscript. Figures 6.1–6.4 are from Linden (1997), reprinted by permission of the copyright holder, Cell Press. This work was supported by PHS MH51106 and NS36842, the McKnight Foundation, the Develbiss Fund, and the National Alliance for Research on Schizophrenia and Depression.

Note added in proof: This chapter represents the state of the field in September, 1997, the time of its last revision. For more recent publications, I suggest searching the recent work of C. E. Jahr, R. A. Nicoll, H. Ohmori and B. Barbour.

REFERENCES

Arriza, J. L., Fairman, W. A., Wadiche, J. A., Murdoch, G. H., Kavanaugh, M. P., and Amara, S. G. (1994). Functional comparisons of three glutamate transporter subtypes cloned from human motor cortex. *J. Neurosci.* 14: 5559–5569.

Barbour, B., Brew, H., and Attwell, D. (1988). Electrogenic glutamate uptake in glial cells is activated by intracellular potassium. *Nature* 335: 433–435.

Baude, A., Molnar, E., Latawiec, D., McIlhinney, R. A. J., and Somogyi, P. (1994). Synaptic and nonsynaptic localization of the GluR1 subunit of the AMPA-type excitatory amino acid receptor in the rat cerebellum. *J. Neurosci.* 14: 2830–2843.

Bernardini, G., Peracchia, C., and Peracchia, L. L. (1984). Reversible effects of octanol on gap junction structure and cell-to-cell electrical coupling. *Eur. J. Cell. Biol.* 34: 307–312.

Blackstone, C. D., Moss, S. J., Martin, L. J., Levey, A. I., Price, D. L., and Huganir, R. L. (1992). Biochemical characterization and localization of a non–N-methyl-D-aspartate glutamate receptor in rat brain. *J. Neurochem.* 58: 1118–1126.

Bowman, C. L., and Kimelberg, H. K. (1984). Excitatory amino acids directly depolarize rat brain astrocytes in primary culture. *Nature* 311: 656–659.

Brew, H., and Attwell, D. (1987). Electrogenic glutamate uptake is a major current carrier in the membrane of axolotl retinal glial cells. *Nature* 327: 707–709.

Bridges, R. J., Stanley, M. S., Anderson, M. W., Cotman, C. W., and Chamberlin, A. R. (1991). Conformationally defined neurotransmitter analogues. Selective inhibition of glutamate uptake by one pyrrolidine-2,4–dicarboxylate diastereomer. *J. Med. Chem.* 34: 717–725.

Burnashev, N., Khodorova, A., Jonas, P., Helm, P. J., Wisden, W., Monyer, H., Seeburg, P. H., and Sakmann, B. (1992). Calcium-permeable AMPA-kainate receptors in fusiform cerebellar glial cells. *Science* 256: 1566–1570.

Charles, A. C., Merrill, J. E., Dirksen, E. R., and Sanderson, M. J. (1991). Intercellular signaling in glial cells: calcium waves and oscillations in response to mechanical stimulation and glutamate. *Neuron* 6: 983–992.

Chaudhry, F. A., Lehre, K. P., van Lookern Campagne, M., Ottersen, O. P., Danbolt, N. C., and Storm-Mathisen, J. (1995). Glutamate transporters in glial plasma membranes: highly differentiated localizations revealed by quantitative ultrastructural immunocytochemistry. *Neuron* 15: 711–720.

Cornell-Bell, A. H., and Finkbeiner, S. M. (1991). Ca^{2+} waves in astrocytes. *Cell Calcium* 12: 185–204.

Cornell-Bell, A. H., Finkbeiner, S. M., Cooper, M. S., and Smith, S. J. (1990). Glutamate induces calcium waves in cultured astrocytes: long-range glial signaling. *Science* 246: 470–473.

Clark, B. A., and Barbour, B. (1997). Currents evoked in Bergmann glial cells by parallel fibre stimulation in rat cerebellar slices. *J. Physiol.* 502: 3335–350.

Crepel, F., and Jaillard, D. (1991). Pairing of pre- and postsynaptic activities in cerebellar Purkinje cells induces long-term changes in synaptic efficacy in vitro. *J. Physiol.* 432: 123–141.

Cull-Candy, S. (1995). NMDA receptors: do glia hold the key? *Curr. Biol.* 5: 841–843.

Dani, J. W., Chernjavsky, A., and Smith S. J. (1992). Neuronal activity triggers calcium waves in hippocampal astrocyte networks. *Neuron* 8: 429–440.

Delaney, C. L., Brenner, M., and Messing, A. (1996). Conditional ablation of cerebellar astrocytes in postnatal transgenic mice. *J. Neurosci.* 16: 6908–6918.

Duffy, S., Fraser, D. D., and MacVicar, B. A. (1995). Potassium channels. In *Neuroglia*, H. Kettenmenn and B. R. Ransom, eds, pp. 185–201. New York, Oxford University Press.

Fairman, W. A., Vandenberg, R. J., Arriza, J. L., Kavanaugh, M. P., and Amara, S. G. (1995). An excitatory amino-acid transporter with properties of a ligand-gated chloride channel. *Nature* 375: 599–603.

Franklin, R. J. M., and Blakemore, W. F. (1995). Glial cell transplantation and plasticity in the O-2A lineage—implications for CNS repair. *Trends Neurosci.* 18: 151–156.

Futamachi, K., and Pedley, T. A. (1976). Glial cells and extracellular potassium: their relationship in mammalian cortex. *Brain Res.* 109: 311–322.

Gallo, V., Patrizio, M., and Levi, G. (1991). GABA release triggered by the activation of neuron-like non-NMDA receptors in cultured type-2 astrocytes is carrier mediated. *Glia* 4: 245–255.

Glatt, C. E., and Snyder, S. H. (1993). Cloning and expression of an adenylyl cyclase localized to the corpus striatum. *Nature* 361: 536–538.

Glaum, S. R., Holzwarth, J. A., and Miller, R. J. (1990). Glutamate receptors activate Ca^{2+} mobilization and Ca^{2+} influx into astrocytes. *Proc. Natl. Acad. Sci. USA* 87: 3454–3458.

Hampson, D. R., Huang, X. P., Oberdorfer, M. D., Goh, J. W., Auyeung, A., and Wenthold, R. J. (1992). Localization of AMPA receptors in the hippocampus and cerebellum of the rat using an anti-receptor monoclonal antibody. *Neuroscience* 50: 11–22.

Hassinger, T. D., Atkinson, P. B., Strecker, G. J., Whalen, L. R., Dudek, F. E., Kossel, A. H., and Kater, S. B. (1995). Evidence for glutamate-mediated activation of hippocampal neurons by glial calcium waves. *J. Neurobiol.* 28: 159–170.

Hirano, T. (1990). Depression and potentiation of the synaptic transmission between a granule cell and a Purkinje cell in rat cerebellar culture. *Neurosic. Lett.* 119: 141–144.

Hirano, T. (1991). Differential pre- and postsynaptic mechanisms for synaptic potentiation and depression between a granule cell and a Purkinje cell in rat cerebellar culture. *Synapse* 7: 321–323.

Hollman, M., Hartley, M., and Heinemann, S. (1991). Calcium permeability of KA-AMPA-gated glutamate receptor channels: dependence on subunit composition. *Science* 252: 851–853.

Hosli, L., Hosli, E., Andres, P. F., and Landolt, H. (1981a). Evidence that the depolarization of glial cells by inhibitory amino acids is caused by an efflux of K^+ from neurones. *Exp. Brain Res.* 42: 43–48.

Hosli, L., Hosli, E., Landolt, H., and Zehtner, C. (1981b). Efflux of potassium from neurones excited by glutamate and aspartate causes a depolarization of cultured glial cells. *Neurosci. Lett.* 21: 83–86.

Houk, J. C., and Barto, A. G. (1991). Distributed sensorimotor learning. In *Tutorials in Motor Behavior II*, G. E. Stelmach and J. Requin, (eds.) Amsterdam, Elsevier.

Isaac, J. T. R., Nicoll, R. A., and Malenka, R. C. (1995). Evidence for silent synapses: implications for the expression of LTP. *Neuron* 15: 427–434.

Ito, M. (1984). *The Cerebellum and Neural Control*. New York, Raven Press.

Ito, M., Sakurai, M., and Tongroach, P. (1982). Climbing fibre induced depression of both mossy fiber responsiveness and glutamate sensitivity of cerebellar Purkinje cells. *J. Physiol.* 324: 113–134.

Jack, J. J., Larkman, A. U., Major, G., and Stratford, K. J. (1994). Quantal analysis of the synaptic excitation of CA1 hippocampal pyramidal cells. *Adv. Second Messenger Phosphoprote in Res.* 29: 275–299.

Jensen, A. M., and Chiu, S. Y. (1990). Fluorescence measurement of changes in intracellular calcium induced by excitatory amino acids in cultured cortical astrocytes. *J. Neurosci.* 10: 1165–1175.

Kettenmann, H., Backus, K. H., and Schachner, M. (1984). Aspartate, glutamate, and γ-aminobutyric acid depolarize cultured astrocytes. *Neurosci. Lett.* 52: 25–29.

Keyser, D. O., and Pellmar, T. C. (1994). Synaptic transmission in the hippocampus: critical role for glial cells. *Glia* 10: 237–243.

Krnjevic, K., and Schwartz S. (1967). Some properties of unresponsive cells in the cerebral cortex. *Exp. Brain Res.* 3: 306–319.

Kullman, D. M., and Siegelbaum, S. A. (1995). The site of expression of NMDA receptor–dependent LTP: new fuel for an old fire. *Neuron* 15: 997–1002.

Kullman, D. M., Erdemli, G., and Asztely, F. (1996). LTP of AMPA and NMDA receptor-mediated signals: evidence for presynaptic expression and extrasynaptic glutamate spill-over. *Neuron* 17: 461.

Levi, G., and Patrizio, M. (1992). Astrocyte heterogeneity: endogenous amino acid levels and release evoked by non-*N*-methyl-D-aspartate receptor agonists and by potassium induced swelling in type-1 and type-2 astrocytes. *J. Neurochem* 58: 1943–1952.

Lev-Ram, V., and Ellisman, M. H. (1995). Axonal activation-induced calcium transients in myelinating Schwann cells, sources, and mechanisms. *J. Neurosci.* 15: 2628–2637.

Lewis, D., and Teyler, T. J. (1986). Anti-S-100 serum blocks long-term potentiation in the hippocampal slice. *Brain Res.* 383: 159–164.

Liao, D., Hessler, N. A., and Malinow, R. (1995). Activation of postsynaptically silent synapses during pairing-induced LTP in CA1 region of hippocampal slice. *Nature* 375: 400–404.

Linden, D. J. (1997). Long-term potentiation of glial synaptic currents in cerebellar culture. *Neuron* 18: 983–994.

Linden, D. J., and Connor, J. A. (1991). Participation of postsynaptic PKC in cerebellar long-term depression in culture. *Science* 254: 1656–1659.

Linden, D. J., and Connor, J. A. (1995). Long-term synaptic depression. *Annu. Rev. Neurosci.* 18: 319–357.

Linden, D. J., Dickinson, M. H., Smeyne, M., and Connor, J. A. (1991). A long-term depression of AMPA currents in cultured cerebellar Purkinje neurons. *Neuron* 7: 81–89.

Linden, D. J., Smeyne, M., and Connor, J. A. (1993). Induction of cerebellar long-term depression in culture requires postsynaptic action of sodium ions. *Neuron* 11: 1093–1100.

Martin, L. J., Blackstone, C. D., Levey, A. I., Huganir, R. L., and Price, D. L. (1993). AMPA glutamate receptor subunits are differentially distributed in brain. *Neuroscience* 53: 327–358.

McCall, M. A., Gregg, R. G., Behringer, R. R., Brenner, M., Delaney, C. L., Galbreath, E. J., Zhang, C. L., Pearce, R. A., Chiu, S. Y., and Messing, A. (1996). Targeted delection in astrocyte intermedaite filament (GFAP) alters neuronal physiology. *Proc. Natl. Acad. Sci. USA* 93: 6361–6366.

Mennerick, S., and Zorumski, C. F. (1994). Glial contributions to excitatory neurotransmission in cultured hippocampal cells. *Nature* 368: 59–62.

Mennerick, S., Benz, A., and Zorumski, C. F. (1996). Components of glial responses to exogenous and synaptic glutamate in rat hippocampal microcultures. *J. Neurosci.* 16: 55–64.

Mudrick-Donnan, L. A., Williams, P. J., Pittman, Q. J., and MacVican, B. A., Postsynaptic potentials mediated by GABA and dopamine evoked in stellate glial cells of the pituitary pass intermedia. *J. Neurosci.* 13: 4660–4668.

Muller, T., Moller, T., Berger, T., Schnitzer, J., and Kettenmann, H. (1992). Calcium entry through kainate receptors and resulting potassium-channel blockade in Bergmann glial cells. *Science* 256: 1563–1566.

Murphy, T. H., Blatter, L. A., Wier, W. G., and Baraban, J. M. (1993). Rapid communication between neurons and astrocytes in primary cortical culture. *J. Neurosci.* 13: 2672–2679.

Nedergaard, M. (1994). Direct signalling from astrocytes to neurons in cultures of mammalian brain cells. *Science* 263: 1768–1771.

Orkand, R. K. (1995). Effects of nerve impulses on glial membranes. In *Neuroglia*, H. Kettenmenn and B. R. Ransom, eds, pp. 460–470. New York, Oxford University Press.

Orkand, R. K., Nicholls, J. G., and Kuffler, S. W. (1966). Effect of nerve impulses on the membrane potential of glial cells in the central nervous system of amphibia. *J. Neurophysiol.* 29: 788–806.

Parpura, V., Basarsky, T. A., Liu, F., Jeftinija, K., Jeftinija, S., and Haydon, P. G. (1994). Glutamate-mediated astrocyte-neuron signaling. *Nature* 369: 744–747.

Parpura, V., Fang, Y., Basarsky, T., Jahn, R., and Haydon, P. G. (1995a). Expression of synaptobrevin II, cellubrevin and syntaxin but not SNAP-25 in cultured astrocytes. *FEBS Lett.* 377: 489–492.

Parpura, V., Liu, F., Brethorst, S., Jeftinija, K., Jeftinija, S., and Haydon, P. G. (1995b). α-Latrotoxin stimulates glutamate release from cortical astrocytes in cell culture. *FEBS Lett.* 360: 266–270.

Parpura, V., Liu, F., Jeftinija, K. V., Haydon, P. G., and Jeftinija, S. D. (1995c). Neuroligand-evoked calcium-dependent release of excitatory amino acids from Schwann cells. *J. Neurosci.* 15: 5831–5839.

Patneau, D. K., Wright, P. W., Winters, C., Mayer, M. L., and Gallo, V. (1994). Glial cells of the oligodendrocytes lineage express both kainate- and AMPA-preferring subtypes of glutamate receptor. *Neuron* 12: 357–371.

Petralia, R. S., and Wenthold, R. J. (1992). Light and electron immunocytochemical localization of AMPA-selective glutamate receptors in the rat brain. *J. Comp. Neurol.* 318: 329–354.

Petralia, R. S., Wang, Y.-X., and Wenthold (1994). Histological and ultrastructural localization of the kainate receptor subunits, KA2 and GluR6/7, in the rat nervous system using selective anti-peptide antibodies. *J. Comp. Neurol.* 349: 85–110.

Pfrieger, F. W., and Barres, B. A. (1996). New views on synapse-glia interactions. *Curr. Opin. Neurobiol.* 6: 615–621.

Porter, J. T., and McCarthy, K. D. (1995). GFAP-positive astrocytes in situ respond to glutamatergic neuroligands with increases in $[Ca^{2+}]_i$. *Glia* 13: 101–112.

Porter, J. T., and McCarthy, K. D. (1996). Hippocampal astrocytes in situ respond to glutamate released from synaptic terminals. *J. Neurosci.* 16: 5073–5081.

Ransom, B. R., and Goldring, S. (1973). Slow depolarizations in cells presumed to be glia in the cerebral cortex of the cat. *J. Neurophysiol.* 36: 869–878.

Raymond, J. L., Lisberger, S. G., and Mauk, M. D. (1996). The cerebellum: a neuronal learning machine? *Science* 272: 1126–1131.

Roitbak, A. I., and Fanardjian, V. V. (1981). Depolarization of cortical glial cells in response to electrical stimulation of the cortical surface. *Neuroscience* 6: 2529–2537.

Rothstein, J. D., Martin, L., Levey, A. I., Dykes-Hoberg, M., Jin, L., Wu, D., Nash, N., and Kuncl, R. W. (1994). Localization of neuronal and glial glutamate transporters. *Neuron* 13: 713–725.

Sakurai, M. (1987). Synaptic modification of parallel fiber-Purkinje cell transmission in *in vitro* guinea-pig cerebellar slices. *J. Physiol.* 394: 463–480.

Sakurai, M. (1990). Calcium is an intracellular mediator of the climbing fiber in induction of cerebellar long-term depression. *Proc. Natl. Acad. Sci. USA* 87: 3383–3385.

Salin, P. A., Malenka, R. C., and Nicoll, R. A. (1996). Cyclic AMP mediates a presynaptic form of LTP at cerebellar parallel fiber synapses. *Neuron* 16: 797–806.

Schell, M. J., Molliver, M. E., and Snyder, S. H. (1995). D-serine, an endogenous synaptic modulator: localization to astrocytes and glutamate stimulated release. *Proc. Natl. Acad. Sci. USA* 92: 3948–3952.

Schwartzkroin, P. A., and Prince D. A. (1979). Recordings from presumed glial cells in the hippocampal slice. *Brain Res.* 161: 533–538.

Shibuki, K., and Okada, D. (1992). Cerebellar long-term potentiation under suppressed postsynaptic Ca^{2+} activity. *NeuroReport* 3: 231–234.

Shibuki, K., Gomi, H., Chen, L., Bao, S., Kim, J. J., Wakatsuki, H., Fujisaki, T., Fujimoto, K., Katoh, A., Ikeda, T., Chen. C., Thompson, R. F., and Itohara, S. (1996). Deficient cerebellar long-term depression impaired eyeblink conditioning and normal motor coordination in GFAP mutant mice. *Neuron* 16: 587–599.

Somogyi, P., Halasy, K., Somogyi, J., Storm-Mathisen, J., and Ottersen, O. P. (1986). Quantification of immunogold labelling reveals enrichment of glutamate in mossy and parallel fiber terminals in cat cerebellum. *Neuroscience* 19: 1045–1050.

Sontheimer, H., and Ritchie, J. M. (1995). Voltage gated sodium and calcium channels. In *Neuroglia*, H. Kettenmenn and B. R. Ransome, eds. pp. 202–220. New York, Oxford University Press.

Sontheimer, H., Kettenmann, H., Backus, K. H., and Schachner, M. (1988). Glutamate opens Na/K channels in cultured astrocytes. *Glia* 1: 328–336.

Spacek, J. (1985). Three-dimensional analysis of dendritic spines. III. Glial sheath. *Anat. Embryol.* 171: 245–252.

Staub, C., Vranesic, I., and Knopfel, T. (1992). Responses to metabotropic glutamate receptor activation in cerebellar Purkinje cells: induction of an inward current. *Eur. J. Neurosci.* 4: 832–839.

Steinhauser, C., and Gallo, V. (1996). News on glutamate receptors in glial cells. *Trends Neurosci.* 19: 339–345.

Stella, M., Tencé, M., Glowinski, J., and Prémont, J. (1994). Glutamate-evoked release of arachidonic acid from mouse brain astrocytes. *J. Neurosci.* 14: 568–575.

Szatkowski, M., Barbour, B., and Attwell, D. (1990). Non-vesicular release of glutamate from glial cells by reversed electrogenic glutamate uptake. *Nature* 348: 443–446.

Tempia, F., Kano, M., Schneggenburger, R., Schirra, C., Garaschuk, O., Plant, T., and Konnerth, A. (1996). Fractional calcium current through neuronal AMPA-receptor channels with a low calcium permeability. *J. Neurosci.* 16: 456–466.

Theodosis, D. T., and MacVicar, B. (1996). Neurone-glia interactions in the hypothalamus and pituitary. *Trends Neurosci.* 19: 363–367.

Thompson, R. F. (1986). The neurobiology of learning and memory, *Science* 233: 941–947.

Usowicz, M. M., Gallo, V., and Cull-Candy, S. G. (1989). Multiple conductance channels in type-2 cerebellar astrocytes activated by excitatory amino acids. *Nature* 339: 380–383.

Van Leeuwen, F. W., Pool, C. W., and Sluiter, A. A. (1983). Enkephalin immunoreactivity in synaptoid elements on glial cells in the rat neural lobe. *Neuroscience* 8: 229–241.

Verkhratsky, A., and Kettenmann, H. (1996). Calcium signalling in glial cells. *Trends Neurosci.* 19: 346–352.

Wang, J. -H., and Kelly, P. T. (1996). Regulation of synaptic facilitation by postsynaptic Ca^{2+}/CaM pathways in hippocampal CA1 neurons. *J. Neurophysiol.* 76: 276–286.

Weisskopf, M. G., Castillo, P. E., Zalutsky, R. A., and Nicoll, R. A. (1994). Mediation of hippocampal mossy fiber long-term potentiation by cyclic AMP, *Science* 265: 1878–1882.

Wyllie, D. J. A., Mathie, A., Symonds, C. J., and Cull-Candy S. G. (1991). Activation of glutamate receptors and glutamate uptake in identified macroglial cells in rat cerebellar cultures. *J. Physiol.* 432: 235–258.

Xia, Z., Refsdal, C. D., Merchant, K. M., Dorsa, D. M., and Storm, D. R. (1991). Distribution of mRNA for the calmociulin-sensitive adenylate cyclase in rat brain: expression in areas associated with learning and memory. *Neuron* 6: 431–443.

7 Anatomical Plasticity in the Striatum during Development and after Lesions in the Adult Rat

Marie-Françoise Chesselet, A. K. Butler, J. A. Napieralski, W. V. Morehouse, F. G. Szele, and K. Uryu

The striatum, a large subcortical nucleus, is an integral part of the basal ganglia, a group of interconnected structures involved in various aspects of the control of movement (Calabresi et al. 1997; Chesselet and Delfs 1996; Marsden and Obeso 1994). For many years, much of the work devoted to the striatum has focused on the input it receives from the substantia nigra pars compacta, the dopaminergic nigrostriatal pathway (Bjorklund and Lindvall 1984). This interest has been sustained by the realization, in the early 1960s, that loss of dopaminergic neurons in the pars compacta is the hallmark of Parkinson's disease, a neurodegenerative disease characterized by severe motor and cognitive dysfunction (Bernheimer et al. 1973). As a result, many studies have focused on the development and plasticity of the nigrostriatal pathway (Murrin and Ferrer 1984; Voorn et al. 1988; Weihmuller and Bruno 1989; Zigmond and Striker 1989).

Little, if any, evidence of axonal sprouting and reactive synaptogenesis has been found in the striatum following the loss of dopaminergic inputs in adult rats or primates, either after experimental lesion or in Parkinson's disease (Zigmond and Striker 1989). This has led to the idea that the adult striatum may lack molecular mechanisms that promote or sustain anatomical plasticity. Supporting this hypothesis, molecules thought to play a critical role in axonal plasticity, such as the growth-associated protein-43 (GAP-43) and the polysialylated form of the neural cell adhesion molecule (PSA-NCAM) are expressed at high levels during development, but are undetectable in a majority of the striatum in adult rats (Aaron and Chesselet 1989; Benowitz et al. 1988; Bonfanti et al. 1992; Szele et al. 1994). In this respect, the striatum seemed markedly different from other brain regions, such as the hippocampus and the hypothalamus, which retain a high degree of anatomical plasticity in adult rats, and continue to express these molecules into adulthood (Cotman et al. 1981; Mathews et al. 1976; Theodosis et al. 1991).

In this review, we summarize recent evidence from our laboratory suggesting that robust axonal plasticity and reactive synaptogenesis do occur in the striatum, not only during late postnatal development but also in adult rats. Our work has focused on the corticostriatal input, a massive glutamatergic projection which forms asymmetrical synapses with the dendritic spines of medium-sized spiny neurons of the striatum (Bolam and Bennett 1995). This class of neurons comprises approximately 95% of striatal neurons and forms the main output pathway of the striatum (Bolam and Bennett 1995; Parent and Hazrati 1995). In the first part of the review, we describe our recent work on the development of the corticostriatal pathway and evidence for corticostriatal plasticity in rat pups. In the second part, we review our work on corticostriatal plasticity in adults. Unless otherwise specified, all data concern the dorsolateral part of the striatum in rats. This region is the target of most inputs from the sensorimotor cortex (Donoghue and Herkenham 1986; McGeorge and Faull 1989) and its developmental time course and adult characteristics differ from those of the medial striatum, which receives inputs from medial regions of the prefrontal cortex, matures later in development, and retains immature characteristics in adults (Sesack et al. 1989; Szele et al. 1994; Uryu and Chesselet, unpublished observations).

DEVELOPMENT OF THE CORTICOSTRIATAL PATHWAY IN RATS

Ipsilateral and Contralateral Corticostriatal Inputs

Previous studies in rats have revealed that striatal neurons are born embryonically, migrate from the ganglionic eminence, and undergo developmentally regulated cell death during the first postnatal week (Bayer 1984; Fentress et al. 1981; Fishell and van der Kooy 1991; Halliday and Cepko 1992; Liu and Graybiel 1992; Phelps et al. 1989; Semba et al. 1988; Song and Harlan 1994). Efferent neurons, which form the very large majority of striatal neurons, have reached their target regions by postnatal day 7 (Fishell and Van der Kooy 1987, 1989; Iniguez et al. 1990; Tepper et al. 1990). Earlier evidence from Golgi studies indicate that the axons of corticostriatal neurons have reached the striatum at birth (Wise et al. 1979). Studies with retrograde tracers also detected corticostriatal inputs early in development (Iniguez et al. 1990); however, these results can be confounded by uptake of the dye by en passage fibers. This is particularly difficult to avoid for injections into the striatum because the injection needle must go through the corpus callosum which is located between the cerebral cortex and the striatum (figure 7.1). Furthermore, in the rat, corticofugal fibers cross the striatum on their way to other subcortical regions (Paxinos and Watson 1986). Therefore, retrograde labeling of neuronal cell bodies in the cerebral cortex could result from the uptake of the tracer by axon terminals innervating the striatum, or by axons destined to other regions.

We have examined (Butler et al. 1997; Morehouse et al., unpublished observations) the developmental time course of the projection from the sensorimotor cortex to the striatum in rat pups with the anterograde tracer Di I (1,1-dioctadecyl-3,3,3,3,-tetra-methylindocarbocyanine perchlorate, Molecular Probes, Eugene, OR), which is particularly suitable for tracing studies prior to axonal myelination and the development of spontaneous neuronal

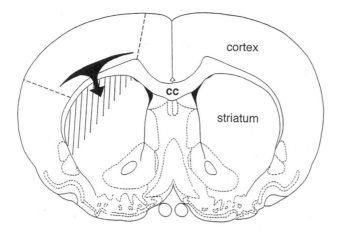

Figure 7.1 Schematic diagram of a frontal section from a rat brain at the level of the rostral striatum. The hatched area represents the region of the striatum innervated by the corticostriatal inputs which were removed by the cortical lesions (dotted lines) performed in the experiments from our laboratory, both in rat pups and in adults. CC, corpus callosum.

activity (Godment et al. 1987). Indeed, in our hands, several other tracers such as neurobiotin and Fluoro-Ruby were ineffective in labeling the corticostriatal pathway prior to postnatal day 21. In contrast, postmortem deposits of Di I into the sensorimotor cortex of 2-day-old rat pups labeled a dense network of axons in the ipsilateral dorsolateral striatum (figure 7.2). Even at this age, the labeled axons showed extensive branching, suggestive of terminal fields. Although preliminary data suggest that a significant contralateral corticostriatal pathway may exist transiently during the first postnatal week, corticostriatal inputs were already primarily ipsilateral on postnatal day 7 (P7), as they are in adults (Ebrahimi et al. 1992; McGeorge and Faull 1989). The intensity of labeling in the ipsilateral striatum increased progressively between P2 and P14 (see figure 7.2; Butler et al. 1997).

Synaptogenesis in the Developing Striatum

Both the number of growth cones (Uryu et al. 1999, in preparation) and immunolabeling for GAP-43 (Dani et al. 1991; Butler and Chesselet, unpublished observations) decreased markedly in the dorsolateral striatum of rat pups after P7, suggesting that this period marks the end of massive axonal growth within the dorsolateral striatum. At this time, however, the striatum remained very immature, and asymmetrical synapses, the type of synapses formed by corticostriatal inputs (Bolam and Bennett, 1995), were extremely rare. Notably, the dendritic spines, which are the normal targets of most asymmetrical synapses, were still absent at this age, and did not form until the third postnatal week (also see Lu and Brown 1977; Misgeld et al. 1986; Tepper and Trent, 1993). It has been known since the 1970s that the third postnatal week is also the period of massive synaptogenesis in the striatum

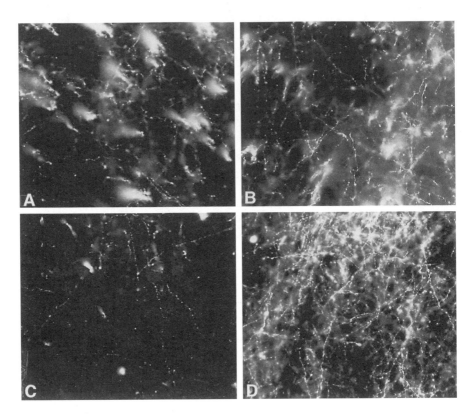

Figure 7.2 Photomicrographs of striatal sections of pups sacrificed at postnatal day 2 (A), 4 (B and C), and 7 (D). A postmortem deposit of Di I was made in the sensorimotor cortex and sections examined 6 to 8 weeks later. Axons were labeled with Di I in the dorsolateral striatum ipsilateral to the lesion at all ages examined (A, B, and D), and the density of labeled axons increased with age. At postnatal day 4, a few labeled fibers were detected in the contralateral dosrolateral striatum (B), but this labeling was no longer observed at postnatal days 7 (not shown) and 14. (From Butler et al. 1997.)

(Hattori and McGeer 1973; Lu and Brown 1977). However, information on the time course of synaptic formation in rat striatum was not very detailed.

We have reexamined the temporal and topographical aspects of synaptogenesis in the developing rat striatum in a recent study (Uryu et al., 1999). All analyses were performed in Sprague-Dawley rats. Litters were culled to ten pups at birth, and both males and females were included in the study. The development of both asymmetrical synapses, which are formed primarily by excitatory (glutamatergic) inputs from the cerebral cortex and the thalamus, and symmetrical synapses, which are formed primarily by dopaminergic and serotonergic inputs, as well as by intrinsic GABAergic terminals (Bolam and Bennett 1995), were examined. Quantitative analysis of synapse numbers was performed with the physical dissector method (Coggeshall and Lekan 1996), which is required for reliable synaptic quantification, especially during development when synapse size may change significantly (Brand and Rakic 1984; DiFiglia et al. 1980). It should be noted, however, that stereological techniques were not used for the present studies because these measurements can only be performed in regions with anatomically defined boundaries. Our studies clearly indicate marked regional differences in the time course of synaptogenesis in the lateral vs. the medial part of the striatum (see below). In addition, it is likely that marked caudorostral differences accompany caudorostral developmental gradients (Bayer 1984; Phelps et al. 1989; Szele et al. 1994). Therefore, measuring the numbers of synapses in the entire striatum, as prescribed for the use of stereological methods, would be of little interest.

Our analysis has confirmed a threefold increase in the number of asymmetrical synapses in the dorsolateral striatum between P14 and P18, as previously reported (Hattori and McGeer 1973; Lu and Brown 1977). However, several significant new observations were made in this study. Surprisingly, a 40% decrease in asymmetrical synapse density was seen between P18 and P25. Because there was little change in striatal size between P18 and P25 in the rat, the decrease in synaptic density is likely to represent a substantial decrease in synapse number. The density of asymmetrical synapses was similar at P25 and in adult rats in this region. The data suggest that a previously unreported synaptic pruning occurs in the dorsolateral striatum during, or just before, the fourth postnatal week. Pruning of asymmetrical synapses was unrecognized in previous studies, probably because these studies examined different subregions of the striatum. Indeed, there were marked differences in both the density and the time course of development of asymmetrical synapses in the dorsolateral vs. the dorsomedial striatum. The number of asymmetrical synapses was much lower in the dorsomedial, as compared to the dorsolateral, striatum at all time points examined. Furthermore, although the number of asymmetrical synapses also increased in the dorsomedial striatum between P14 and P18, it was not significantly different at P18, P25, and in the adult in this region (see Butler et al. 1998).

Major differences were also found between the developmental patterns of symmetrical vs. asymmetrical synapses. The number of symmetrical synapses was much lower than the number of asymmetrical synapses at all time points examined, in both the dorsomedial and the dorsolateral striatum. The density of symmetrical synapses did not change at any of the time points examined in the dorsomedial striatum. However, in the dorsolateral striatum, symmetrical synaptic density was higher than in the adult, not only at P18, but already at P14, suggesting that symmetrical synapses develop earlier than asymmetrical synapses (see Butler et al. 1998). This is further supported by the observation that, at P14, some symmetrical synapses already have mature characteristics, whereas the presynaptic elements of all asymmetrical synapses still retain growth cone—like characteristics at this age.

PSA-NCAM Expression in the Developing Striatum

In the same study, we examined the ultrastructural location of immunolabeling for PSA-NCAM with an antibody that specifically recognizes the long

Normal striatal development

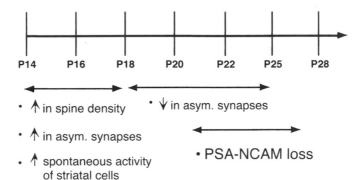

Figure 7.3 Schematic illustration of the time course of critical events in striatal development in rats. P14 to P28: postnatal days 14 to 28; asym., asymmetrical; PSA-NCAM, polysiated form of the neural cell adhesion molecule.

chains of polysialic acids which are characteristic of the immature form of NCAM in vertebrates (Rougon and Marshak 1986). PSA-NCAM is the predominant form of NCAM during development, and only persists in the adult brain in regions exhibiting high levels of neuronal plasticity (Aaron and Chesselet 1989; Bonfanti et al. 1992; Goldowitz et al. 1990; Le Gall La Salle et al. 1992; Seki and Arai 1991; Szele and Chesselet 1996; Szele et al. 1994). During development, PSA-NCAM has been shown to play a critical role in cell migration, axonal growth and fasciculation, and synaptic plasticity (reviewed by Kiss and Rougon 1997).

In rat striatum, intense immunoreactivity for PSA-NCAM was observed until P14. PSA-NCAM immunolabeling then decreased between P14 and P18, and progressively disappeared from the dorsolateral striatum between P22 and P25 (Aaron and Chesselet 1989; Szele et al. 1994) (figure 7.3). At the light microscopic level, PSA-NCAM immunoreactivity remained detectable only in the medial striatum in adult rats (Bonfanti et al. 1992; Szele et al. 1994; Szele and Chesselet 1996). Confirming results from these light microscopic studies, ultrastructural examination (Uryu et al., 1999) showed that intense immunoreactivity for PSA-NCAM was associated with neuronal membranes during early postnatal development in the striatum. After P14, PSA-NCAM immunoreactivity took on a progressively more punctate appearance. At the ultrastructural level, this corresponded to a loss of immunoreactivity along the cytoplasmic membrane of neuronal cell bodies, and the preservation of PSA-NCAM expression in pre- and postsynaptic elements. At the peak of asymmetrical synapse formation (P18), most asymmetrical synapses (88%) expressed PSA-NCAM. At this age, 50% of asymmetrical synapses expressed PSA-NCAM immunoreactivity in both the pre- and the postsynaptic elements, and 38% expressed PSA-NCAM on the postsynaptic side only. Although the density of asymmetrical synapses only

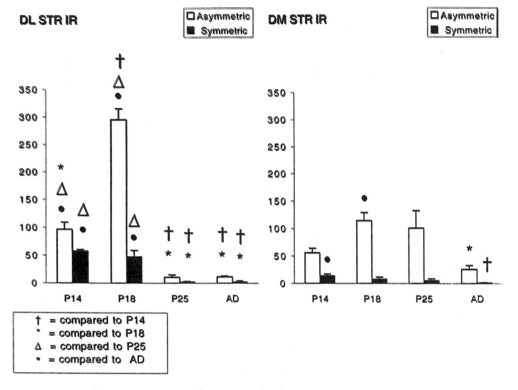

Figure 7.4 Density of asymmetrical and symmetrical synapses expressing polysialylated form of neural cell adhesion molecule (PSA-NCAM) immunoreactivity (IR) in the dorsolateral (DL) and dorsomedial (DM) striatum (STR). X-axes indicate the number of synapses per 2000 μ^2 measured with the physical dissector method. Y-axes indicate postnatal ages. Statistical analysis was done with ANOVA (analysis of variance) followed by the Fisher post hoc test. n = 3.

decreased by 40% between P18 and P25, PSA-NCAM immunoreactivity became practically undetectable at this age, indicating that the loss of PSA-NCAM immunoreactivity was not solely due to the loss of synapses, but also to a downregulation of PSA-NCAM expression at remaining synapses (figure 7.4). A very similar pattern of expression was observed in the symmetrical synapses of the dorsolateral striatum.

In contrast to the dorsolateral striatum, the density of asymmetrical synapses expressing PSA-NCAM immunoreactivity did not change significantly between P14 and P25 in the dorsomedial striatum, and about half of the asymmetrical synapses remained labeled at P25 in this region. There were very few symmetrical synapses in the dorsomedial striatum, and the number of labeled symmetrical synapses decreased progressively in the dorsomedial striatum between P14 and P25.

These data provide several important observations. First, during the period of synaptogenesis, PSA-NCAM was present not only in the axons of striatal inputs but also in striatal neurons. This indicates that the late expression of PSA-NCAM during striatal development was not solely due to the immaturity of striatal inputs (van den Pol et al. 1986). Second, although PSA-NCAM was no longer continuously expressed along the somatic, axonal, and dendritic membranes of striatal neurons and their inputs late in development, it remained localized at synapses for a longer period of time. PSA-NCAM has been shown to play a role in early, activity-independent developmental events, such as axonal growth and fasciculation, and synapse formation (Kiss and Rougon 1997). The expression of PSA-NCAM during a protracted period of striatal development, which encompasses not only the period of axonal growth but also the later period of synaptogenesis, is compatible with similar roles for PSA-NCAM in the developing striatum. Third, synapses expressing PSA-NCAM in only the presynaptic element were extremely rare at all time points examined, suggesting that PSA-NCAM expression decreased in the presynaptic elements prior to its loss from the postsynaptic side of the synapses. Finally, PSA-NCAM remained expressed in the dorsolateral striatum during a period of synaptic pruning. Recent results have suggested that PSA-NCAM may also be involved in activity-dependent developmental processes such as synapse stabilization (Tang and Landmesser 1993). This is compatible with the recently described role of PSA-NCAM in long-term potentiation (LTP) in the hippocampus (Muller et al. 1996). Our data suggest that PSA-NCAM could serve a similar role in the late phases of striatal synaptogenesis.

To further examine the mechanisms involved in the regulation of PSA-NCAM expression and synapse numbers in the developing striatum, we examined the effects of cortical ablation and of treatments with antagonists of the N-methyl-D-aspartate (NMDA) subtype of glutamate receptors in rat pups.

LESIONS OF THE CEREBRAL CORTEX IN DEVELOPING RATS

Previous studies have shown that large ablations of the cerebral cortex in the immediate postnatal period result in a marked compensatory innervation of the denervated striatum by the contralateral cortex (Kolb et al. 1992). It was unclear, however, whether this effect was due to sprouting of axons which would not normally innervate the contralateral striatum, or to a lack of pruning of a transient contralateral input. It was also unclear how late in development lesion-induced axonal sprouting could occur in the rat striatum.

Effects of Postnatal Cortical Lesions on Axonal Plasticity in the Striatum

Thermocoagulation of pial blood vessels overlying the sensorimotor cortex was performed on P14 (Butler et al. 1997) (see figure 7.1). This procedure has been used extensively to perform cortical lesions in adult rats (Errami and Nieoullon 1986; Napieralski et al. 1996; Salin and Chesselet 1992, 1993; Szele et al. 1995) and is particularly effective for performing extensive lesions of the cerebral cortex in pups. Indeed, the size of the cortex and the absence of myelination of the corpus callosum make it difficult to control the depth of the lesion at this age when lesions are performed by aspriation or other similar procedures. In contrast, when thermocoagulation of pial blood vessels is performed with a hot probe, without piercing the dura mater, the cerebral cortex degenerates in a few days, leaving the corpus callosum and the striatum intact (Butler et al. 1997).

Supporting the occurrence of axonal sprouting in response to the lesion, a marked increase in axonal growth cones was observed in the denervated striatum ten days after the lesion (Butler et al. 1997). Furthermore, the synaptic density was similar to controls in the dorsolateral striatum on the side of the lesion, despite removal of the ipsilateral sensorimotor cortex, which normally provides the cortical input to this region of the striatum (McGeorge and Faull 1987). Although the origin of the axons forming these synapses was not identified, it is likely that sprouting axons from the contralateral cortex participated in the reactive synaptogenesis which led to the restoration of a normal density of asymmetrical synapses. Indeed, evidence for the sprouting of axons from contralateral cortical neurons was obtained in experiments with the anterograde tracer Fluoro-Ruby.

Fluoro-Ruby (Schmued et al. 1990) was used for these tracing studies because Di I injections resulted in an extremely diffuse labeling pattern, confirming that this dye is not suitable for tracing studies of myelinated fibers (Balice-Gordon et al. 1993). When injected on P25 into the sensorimotor cortex contralateral to a thermocoagulatory lesion performed on P14, Fluoro-Ruby labeled a dense network of axons in the contralateral striatum. In contrast, very few axonal fibers were labeled in the striatum contralateral to a similar injection in control rats. This strongly suggests that cortical neurons contralateral to the lesion were the source of at least some of the axonal sprouting in the denervated striatum. Since our tracing studies in rat pups (Butler et al. 1997; see above) indicated that the corticostriatal pathway was already primarily ipsilateral at P7, the presence of labeled axons in the contralateral striatum was not due to a lack of axonal pruning of an early contralateral projection. These data demonstrate that axonal and synaptic plasticity in rat striatum is not limited to the immediate postnatal period (Kolb et al. 1992), when increased contralateral projections could be the result of a maintenance of transient projections.

Effects of Postnatal Cortical Lesions on PSA-NCAM Expression in the Striatum

Previous studies have shown that developmental alterations, such as the delay in synaptogenesis occurring in mice with the staggerer mutation, cause a delay in PSA-NCAM maturation in developing brain (Edelman and Chuong 1982). To determine whether cortical lesions produced a similar effect, groups of rats with and without cortical lesions performed on P14 were sacrificed on P25 and their striatum examined for PSA-NCAM immunoreactivity (Butler et al. 1997). Although immunolabeling for PSA-NCAM was very low or undetectable in the dorsolateral striatum of control animals at this age, it was much stronger in lesioned rats, indicating a delay in the loss of PSA-NCAM immunoreactivity compared to normal development. A similar result was obtained in rats sacrificed on P28.

These data suggest that alterations in the development of the corticostriatal pathway affect the timing of PSA-NCAM loss. Considering that cortical lesions induced robust axonal sprouting from the contralateral homotypic cortex and reactive synaptogenesis in the striatum on the side of the lesion, it was unclear from these data whether the delay in the loss of PSA-NCAM observed after cortical lesions during development was due to the loss of glutamatergic inputs per se, or rather to the anatomical reorganization of the corticostriatal input triggered by the lesion. To further examine the role of glutamatergic inputs during this late phase of striatal development, we have examined the effects of glutamate antagonists on PSA-NCAM expression and synaptic density in the developing striatum.

N-METHYL-D-ASPARTATE ANTAGONISTS AND STRIATAL DEVELOPMENT

The NMDA subtype of glutamate receptors has been shown to play a critical role in brain development (Constantine-Paton 1994; Scheetz and Constantine-Paton 1994; Bear 1996). However, its specific role remains unclear (Kasamatsu et al. 1997), and other factors are likely to contribute to the effects originally attributed to glutamate (Shi et al. 1997). In contrast to the visual system, there is surprisingly little information on the role of NMDA receptors in the developing striatum, despite extensive evidence that NMDA receptors are present in the striatum as early as the first postnatal week (Chaudieu et al. 1991; Colwell et al. 1998; Enomoto et al. 1996; Insel et al. 1990; Laurie and Seeburg 1994; Monyer et al. 1994; Portera-Caillau 1996; Riva et al. 1994; Snyder-Keller and Constantini 1996). It is impractical to perform repeated intracerebral drug injections in pups, and therefore an initial set of studies was performed with MK-801 ((5R,10S)-(+)-5-methyl-10,11-dihydro-5H-dibenzo[a,d]cyclo-hepten-5,10-imine hydrogen maleate), the only readily available NMDA antagonist that crosses the blood-brain barrier. Pups were treated for various periods of time with peripherally administered MK-801, sacrificed twenty-four hours after the last injection, and their brains processed for PSA-NCAM immunohistochemistry (Butler et al., 1999).

Injections of MK-801 (0.25 mg/kg intraperitoneally) from P14 to P16, P14 to P18, or P18 P19 did not induce noticeable changes in immunolabeling for PSA-NCAM in the dorsolateral striatum (figure 7.5). In contrast, MK-801 administered from P14 to P24 and from P18 to P20 markedly reduced PSA-

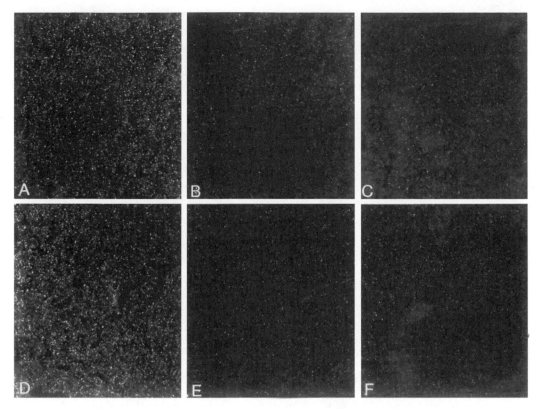

Figure 7.5 Photomicrographs of the gradient of punctate immunolabeling for PSA-NCAM in the medial (A and D), central (B and E) and lateral (C and F) dorsal striatum of 19-day-old rat pups. There was no significant difference in the intensity of labeling for PSA-NCAM in the striatum of control rats (A, B, and C), and of rats treated with the antagonist of N-methyl-D-aspartate receptors MK-801 (0.25 mg/kg introperitoneally) from day 16 to day 18 (D, E, and F).

NCAM immunoreactivity in this region, and in most of the cerebral cortex (figure 7.6). Immunolabeling in the medial striatum, the subventricular zone, and the hippocampus, all regions that still express PSA-NCAM immunoreactivity in the adult (Aaron and Chesselet 1989; Bonfanti et al. 1992; Szele et al. 1994), was not significantly affected by the treatment, indicating that the effect of the NMDA antagonist was regionally specific.

A comparison of the regimens which did, and did not, affect PSA-NCAM expression in the dorsolateral striatum suggested that P20 was critical for the effect observed. To further test this hypothesis, we injected MK-801 into the striatum on day 20. This single injection reproduced the effect of peripheral injections, although the effect was limited to the striatum. This confirmed that the effect of the peripheral injections was mediated by the blockade of striatal receptors. In addition, the loss of PSA-NCAM in dorsolateral striatum was reproduced by a single intrastriatal injection of ketamine and of APV (DL-2-amino-5-phosphonovaleric acid), a competitive glutamate antagonist, on P20.

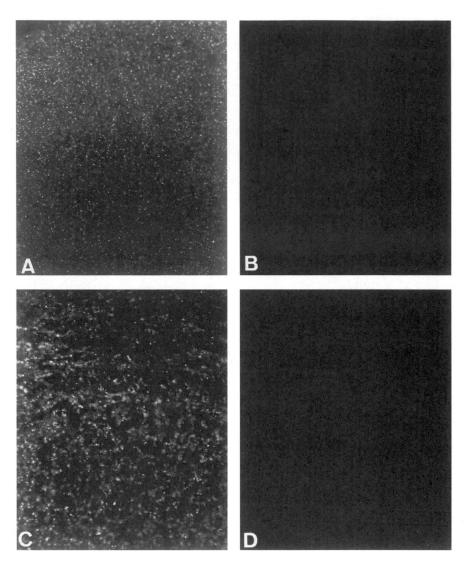

Figure 7.6 Photomicrographs of sections of the sensorimotor cortex (A and B) and dorso-lateral striatum (C and D) in 25-day-old rats injected with vehicle (A and C) or MK-801 (0.25 mk/kg) from postnatal day 14 to 24 (B and D).

Although some of the MK-801 regimens slowed weight gain in the injected pups, the loss of PSA-NCAM immunoreactivity was not related to this effect because MK-801 administration from P18 to P20 did not affect weight gain but markedly decreased PSA-NCAM immunoreactivity in the dorsolateral striatum. The same treatment regimen was chosen to test the hypothesis that the loss of PSA-NCAM, which was selectively expressed at synapses during the period of treatment examined (see above), was due to a loss of synapses. Administration of MK-801 (P18 to P20) induced a 30% decrease in the density of asymmetrical synapses in the dorsolateral striatum, without affecting the density of symmetrical synapses, which do not use the neurotransmitter glutamate (Bolam and Bennett 1995).

MK-801 did not affect PSA-NCAM expression early in development, despite the fact that functional postsynaptic NMDA receptors are present in the striatum as early as the first postnatal week (Colwell et al. 1998). Instead, the effect of MK-801 on PSA-NCAM expression was detected after the development of functional corticostriatal synapses (Tepper and Trent 1993), suggesting that MK-801 acted by blocking the effects of synaptically released glutamate. It is unlikely that MK-801 exerted its effect by inducing a general decrease in neuronal activity. Indeed, most corticostriatal responses at this age are mediated by 2-(aminomethyl)phenylacetic acid (AMPA)– kainate receptors (Hurst and Levine, personal communication, 1998).

There is a clear difference between the moderate effect of MK-801 on the density of asymmetrical synapses (-30% compared to same-age controls), and its effect on PSA-NCAM, which became undetectable in the treated rats. During normal development, PSA-NCAM was expressed by virtually all asymmetrical synapses at the onset of treatment (P18), but progressively decreased in parallel with synaptic pruning between P18 and P25 (see above). Considering that PSA-NCAM expression was restricted to synapses at this time in development, it is likely that the loss of PSA-NCAM after MK-801 treatment was due to the loss of those synapses which expressed the adhesion molecule. The sensitivity of these synapses to MK-801 treatment suggests that they depend on glutamate for their maintenance during this period of development. A preferential expression of PSA-NCAM at these synapses is compatible with a role in synaptic plasticity, and in particular in LTP (Muller et al. 1996).

SIGNIFICANCE OF THE DEVELOPMENTAL DATA

Much of our work on the developing rat striatum has focused on the pattern of expression and regulation of PSA-NCAM. This was made possible by the availability of a specific antibody (Rougon and Marshack 1986) permitting a detailed topographical analysis with immunohistochemical approaches, and was motivated by the growing body of evidence suggesting that PSA-NCAM is involved both in activity-independent and in activity-dependent developmental events (Kiss and Rougon 1997). The data provide the most detailed analysis of PSA-NCAM expression during development in any brain region so far. They demonstrate that PSA-NCAM expression is tightly regulated in both a topographical and a temporal manner during postnatal development (Szele et al. 1994). Furthermore, disruption of normal striatal development following lesions of its cortical inputs delays the loss of PSA-NCAM in striatal neurons postsynaptic to the lesion (Butler et al. 1997). This effect is likely due to the synaptic plasticity induced by the lesion because blockade of receptors to glutamate, the neurotransmitter of corticostriatal neurons, precipitates rather than delays PSA-NCAM loss.

Our data, which show the robust axonal and synaptic plasticity of corticostriatal inputs several weeks after birth in rats, are compatible with clinical observations that children with large cortical ablations for intractable epilepsy fare very well as long as the surgery is performed before age five years (Peacock et al. 1996). However, the sensitivity of a subset of synapses to NMDA antagonists during a narrow period of development raises concerns about the use of this type of drug in children. It is clear that we need to know much more about the long-term consequences of perturbation of striatal development, and the correspondence between developmental landmarks in experimental animals and in humans.

In summary, we are only beginning to understand the various steps leading to the formation of a mature striatum (see figure 7.3). Elucidating the molecular mechanisms of striatal development first requires a better grasp of the detailed time course of inputs and synapse formation in the striatum. It is likely that many of the events described in other brain regions, such as activity-dependent synaptic remodeling (Goodman and Shatz 1993; Lahof et al. 1996; Katz and Shatz 1996), also take place in the striatum, but, their molecular mechanisms remain largely unknown. These questions are of great clinical importance because abnormal striatal development is likely to play a role in developmental disorders such as early-onset dystonia, Tourette's syndrome, possibly schizophrenia, and some forms of mental retardation, such as Rett's syndrome (Armstrong 1997, Carlsson and Carlsson 1990, Leckman et al. 1997).

CORTICOSTRIATAL PLASTICITY IN ADULTS

In many experimental systems, PSA-NCAM expression has been related to axonal sprouting or fasciculation, both during development and in response to neuronal injury in adults (Doherty et al. 1990; Landmesser et al. 1990; Le Gal la Salle et al. 1992; Miller et al. 1994; Muller et al. 1994; Zhang et al. 1992). Therefore, PSA-NCAM could be critical for the robust axonal sprouting observed after cortical lesions during development. The hypothesis that the loss of PSA-NCAM in the dorsolateral striatum of adult rats contributes to decreased axonal plasticity in this region was supported by earlier data indicating that cortical lesions in adult rats induced little, if any, axonal sprouting in the striatum (Chen and Hillman 1990; however, see Cheng et al. 1997). We decided to examine this question in more detail with immunohistochemical, ultrastructural, and tract-tracing approaches (Szele et al. 1995; Napieralski et al. 1996; Uryu and Chesselet, in preparation). Our data confirm previous results showing a paucity of axonal sprouting after aspiration lesions of the cerebral cortex. However, we found that robust sprouting of corticostriatal axons does occur in adult striata after ischemic lesions of the cerebral cortex, and that reexpression of PSA-NCAM is not necessary for this effect to occur.

Effects of Aspiration and Thermocoagulatory Lesions of the Sensorimotor Cortex: Light Microscopic Studies

Extensive lesions of the sensorimotor cortex were performed in adult rats, either by the classic method of aspiration or by thermocoagulation of pial blood vessels (Errami and Nieoullon 1986; Salin and Chesselet 1992) (see figure 7.1). In contrast to the aspiration lesions, which instantly sever cortical neurons and their axons, the thermocoagulatory lesions cause a progressive ischemic lesion, resulting in cortical degeneration in five to seven days (Szele et al. 1995). Neither lesion induced neuronal loss, nor the expression of the immediate early gene *c-fos* or of the microtubule-associated protein MAP-2 in the dorsolateral striatum, and both respected the corpus callosum (Szele et al. 1995).

Previous work has shown that thermocoagulatory lesions of the sensorimotor cortex in adult rats induced long-lasting changes in the level of expression of neuropeptide transmitters in the striatum (Salin and Chesselet 1992; Salin et al. 1990). Similar effects were not observed after aspiration lesions, suggesting that the two types of lesion had different consequences on striatal function (Napieralski et al. 1996; Somers and Beckstead 1990; Uhl et al. 1988). Similarly, thermocoagulatory lesions increased the expression of glutamic acid decarboxylase and of its messenger RNA (mRNA), whereas aspiration lesions had no effect (Salin and Chesselet 1993, Napieralski and Chesselet, unpublished observations). These observations prompted us to compare the effects of these two lesions on the expression of molecules known to play a role in axonal plasticity in brain (Szele et al. 1995). Immunohistochemical methods were used so that regional differences could be readily determined. Indeed, the region of the cerebral cortex removed by the lesion projects primarily to the dorsolateral striatum in rats (McGeorge and Faull 1987). Therefore, changes induced by the loss of corticostriatal inputs would be expected to be restricted to this region of the striatum.

Groups of rats with either type of lesion were sacrificed six hours, and 3, 5, 7, 12, 16, 21, and 42 days after surgery and data were compared with results in unlesioned rats. The patterns of expression of a number of molecules believed to play either a facilitating (basic fibroblast growth factor [bFGF], PSA-NCAM, laminin) or an inhibiting (tenascin, chondroitin sulfate proteoglycans [CSPGs]) role in axonal sprouting were examined. In addition, the effects of the two lesions on glial acidic fibrillary protein (GFAP, a marker of activated astrocytes); OX42, a marker of microglia; synaptophysin, a marker of synaptic vesicles; and on GAP-43, were also examined.

Both lesions induced a marked decrease in labeling for bFGF, which is normally expressed by astrocytes in the dorsolateral striatum. Following either type of lesion, immunostaining for bFGF markedly decreased as early as day 1, became virtually undetectable at day 7, and slowly recovered to control levels by day 21. These changes in bFGF immunostaining differ markedly from observations in the hippocampus. Indeed lesions of the ento-rhinal cortex, which are followed by robust axonal plasticity of remaining inputs to the hippocampus, induced an increase in bFGF expression (Gomez-Pinilla et al. 1992). Also in contrast to observations in the hippocampus (Le Gal La Salle 1992; Miller et al. 1994), lesions of the corticostriatal pathway did not induce expression of PSA-NCAM in the areas denervated by the lesion. Laminin, another molecule believed to favor axonal sprouting (Rivas et al. 1992), was not affected after either lesion in the neuropil of the dorso-lateral striatum. On the other hand, tenascin and CSPG, two adhesion mole-cules which are believed to impair axonal sprouting by contributing to the formation of a glial scar (McKeon et al. 1991; Pindzola et al. 1993), were not increased in the dorsolateral striatum after either type of lesion.

These data suggested that although no molecular obstacle to axonal sprouting was formed in response to the cortical lesion, a lack of stimulatory molecules could contribute to the reported lack of sprouting. Further analy-sis, however, led us to reconsider this hypothesis. Indeed, although all the other molecules examined did not differ in the two experimental models, levels of GAP-43 were markedly different after thermocoagulation vs. aspi-ration lesions (Szele et al. 1995). GAP-43 is enriched in growth cones and has been shown to be necessary for axonal sprouting (Chong et al. 1994; Curtis et al. 1993; Strittmatter et al. 1995). Expression of GAP-43 is increased in the hippocampus after entorhinal lesions, and the time course and topography of this effect corresponds to axonal sprouting in the dener-vated hippocampus (Benowitz et al. 1990; Masliah et al. 1991).

In the adult striatum, levels of GAP-43 are low (Benowitz et al. 1988; Szele et al. 1994), but the molecule remains expressed in unmyelinated fibers, and in some dendritic spines (DiFiglia et al. 1990). Lesions by aspiration induced a marked decrease in the expression of GAP-43, which becomes sig-nificant 12 days post lesion. This probably corresponds to the degeneration of corticostriatal axons, and is compatible with the lack of axonal sprouting reported in utrastructural studies after this type of lesion (Chen and Hilman 1990). In contrast to aspiration lesions, thermocoagulatory lesions were not followed by a decrease in GAP-43 immunostaining in the denervated stria-tum. Considering that both lesions removed a similar area of cortex, the data suggested either that GAP-43 expression was increased in unlesioned neu-rons after the thermocoagulatory lesion, or that the lesion induced axonal sprouting. The latter was confirmed by ultrastructural and tracing studies.

Ultrastructural Analysis of the Dorsolateral Striatum after Cortical Lesions

Tissue from rats with either type of lesion sacrificed 16 days after surgery, and from the corresponding controls, was processed for GAP-43 immunos-taining and examined with electronmicroscopy (Uryu and Chesselet, in preparation). The data confirmed the absence of neuronal degeneration in the striatum after both lesions, and showed a marked increase in the number of growth cones and filopodia labeled with GAP-43 after thermocoagulatory lesions. After aspiration lesions, a slight increase was also noted compared to controls, but, this was very modest compared to the effects of the thermocoagulatory lesions. These results indicate the presence of significant axonal sprouting after thermocoagulatory, but not aspiration, lesions. Furthermore, analysis of synaptic density showed a quasi-recovery in the number of asymmetrical synapses, the type of synapses made by corticostriatal inputs, in the dorsolateral striatum of rats with thermocoagulatory lesions. In contrast, the number of asymmetrical synapses was markedly reduced in the same region in rats with an aspiration lesion of the sensorimotor cortex. The analysis was performed with a physical dissector method adapted from Coggeshal and Lekan (1996) to prevent errors resulting from changes in synaptic sizes after the lesion. Because the lesions did not affect the size of the striatum, the recovery of synaptic density after the lesion is likely to reflect reactive synaptogenesis.

It is interesting to note that immunolabeling for synaptophysin, a molecule associated with synaptic vesicles (Jahn et al. 1985), was not significantly changed at the light microscopic level after aspiration lesion, and was only slightly decreased at 16 days after thermocoagulatory lesions. The dissociation between synaptophysin immunoreactivity and synapse number commands caution in the use of this antigen as a marker of synaptic density. The absence of a significant decrease in immunolabeling after aspiration lesions, despite a marked decrease in the density of asymmetrical synapses, may be due to a compensatory synaptic enlargement as reported by Chen and Hillman (1990). This may also explain the lack of a decrease in synaptophysin labeling at earlier time points after thermocoagulatory lesions, despite the fact that the reactive synaptogenesis detected 16 days after surgery is unlikely to be immediate.

The results of ultrastructural studies suggest that thermocoagulatory lesions induced robust axonal plasticity in the adult striatum. However, the origin of the sprouting axons was not identified in these experiments. To address this question, we performed tracing studies after both types of lesion.

Sprouting of Contralateral Corticostriatal Neurons after Thermocoagulatory Lesions of the Sensorimotor Cortex

We hypothesized that the homotypic contralateral cortex was a likely source of sprouting axons in the denervated striatum after thermocoagulatory lesions. To test this hypothesis, the anterograde tracer Fluoro-Ruby was injected into the sensorimotor cortex contralateral to the lesion (one month after surgery) in rats with either aspiration or thermocoagulatory cortical lesions, as well as in control rats (Napieralski et al. 1996). Rats were sacrificed one week after injection, and the tissue was examined with fluorescence microscopy for the presence of labeled axons. The pattern of axonal labeling was identical in rats with aspiration lesions and in control rats. In both cases, a dense network of labeled axons was seen in the dorsolateral striatum on the side of the lesion, but hardly any labeled fibers could be detected in the contralateral striatum (figure 7.7). In contrast, in rats with thermocoagulatory lesions, axonal labeling was as dense in the contralateral striatum as on the side of the injection (see figure 7.7). This indicated a marked increase in the projection from the homotypic cortex contralateral to the lesion to the denervated striatum. Therefore, crossed corticostriatal neurons are likely to contribute significantly to the increase in growth cones and the reactive synaptogenesis observed in the striatum on the side of the cortical lesion.

The data indicate that, in contrast to conclusions based on the results of aspiration lesions only (Chen and Hilman 1990), the striatum of adult rats can support robust axonal sprouting and reactive synaptogenesis. Therefore, there are no fundamental differences between the striatum and brain areas traditionally considered as the locus of axonal plasticity in adults, such as the hippocampus (Cotman and Nieto-Sampedro, 1984). However, the mechanisms of sprouting may be lesion- /or region-specific, or both. In particular, sprouting in the striatum occurred in the absence of increases in bFGF (Szele et al. 1995) and brain-derived growth factor (Napieralski, Butler and Chesselet, unpublished observations), which are believed to play a critical role in hippocampal sprouting (Beck et al. 1993; Gomez-Pinilla et al. 1992). Furthermore, axonal sprouting in the adult striatum occurred in the absence of reexpression of PSA-NCAM, either in neurons or in glial cells. This result was unexpected because it has been proposed that expression of PSA-NCAM in many regions of the adult brain, such as the hippocampus, the hypothalamus, and the interpeduncular nucleus, was critical for the high level of axonal plasticity occurring in these regions (Aaron and Chesselet 1989; Le Gal La Salle et al. 1992; Muller et al. 1994; Theodosis et al. 1991). Furthermore, in both the adult hippocampus and spinal cord, lesions that resulted in axonal sprouting also triggered the reexpression of PSA-NCAM by glial cells or neurons, or both (Bonfanti et al. 1996; Gimenez y Ribotta et al. 1995; Miller et al. 1994; Styren et al. 1994). In contrast, our results indicate that, although PSA-NCAM may be necessary for sprouting after lesion in other regions, it is not required for the occurrence of robust axonal sprouting in the dorsolateral striatum.

The mechanism underlying the differences in sprouting after aspiration and thermocoagulatory lesions of the sensorimotor cortex remains unclear. It is unlikely that differences in the striatum itself explain the differences in responses. Indeed, the same region of the striatum was denervated after both lesions, and the pattern and time course of expression of GFAP, a marker of reactive astrocytes (Szele et al. 1995), and of OX42, a marker of activated microglia (Zhang and Chesselet, in preparation), did not differ significantly after the two lesions. After thermocoagulatory lesions, the cortex degenerates slowly, and during degeneration is invaded by glial cells which presum-

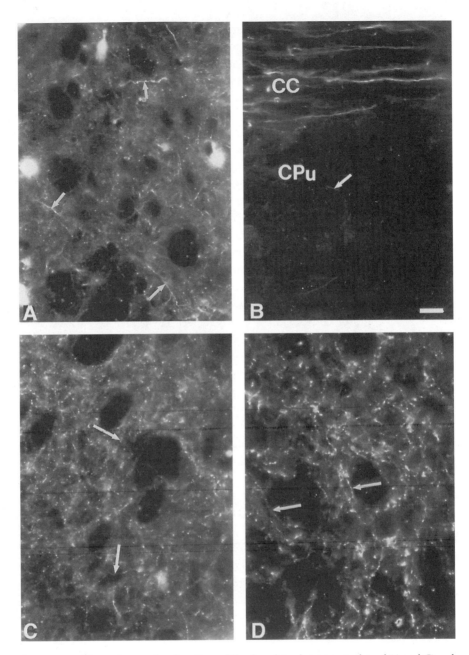

Figure 7.7 Photomicrographs of sections of the dorsolateral striatum ipsilateral (A and C) and contralateral (B and D) to an injection of the anterograde tracer Fluoro-Ruby in the sensorimotor cortex. Arrows indicate labeled axons. The rat illustrated in A and B had an intact cortex contralateral to the dye injection; note that the corticostriatal projection is primarily ipsilateral, despite the fact that labeled axons were seen traveling in the contralateral corpus callosum (CC) above the striatum (CPu). The rat illustrated in C and D had a thermocoagulatory lesion of the sensorimotor cortex contralateral to the dye injection: note the marked increase in axonal labeling in the doroslateral striatum on the side of the lesion (D). Scale bar (shown in B): 25 µm for all panels.

Anatomical Plasticity in Rat Striatum

ably express a large number of cytokines or growth factors. These diffusible factors could act upon axons traveling in the corpus callosum, just adjacent to the lesion site. The corpus callosum contains the axons of crossed cortico-cortical projections, as well as a small number of crossed corticostriatal projections (Ebrahimi et al. 1992; McGeorge and Faull 1987; Wilson 1987). Axons traveling in the corpus callosum are clearly critical since no sprouting was observed when the corpus callosum was accidentally damaged by the lesion (Napieralski et al. 1996). It is possible that factors secreted by cells in the degenerating cortex stimulated sprouting from these axons, in particular those from the corticocortical axons which were deprived of their target by the lesion or the few crossed corticostriatal axons which normally innervate the striatum (Ebrahimi et al. 1992; Wilson 1987). Alternatively, the thermo-coagulatory lesions may result in changes in neuronal activity which alter the firing of the contralateral spared cortex, as observed in other models of cortical ischemia (Luhmann 1996). Finally, limb use may be critical for the axonal plasticity observed, as previously reported for the dendritic plasticity induced in the contralateral cortex by a kainic acid–induced lesion of the motor cortex (Jones and Schallert 1994). These various, and nonexclusive, possibilities are presently being investigated in our laboratory.

Effects of Cortical Lesions on the Medial Striatum and Subventricular Zone

Although the cortical lesions performed in these experiments removed the region of the cortex projecting to the dorsolateral striatum, the effects of the lesion were not restricted to this area of the striatum. The most dramatic effect of the lesions was observed in the subventricular zone (SVZ), an area immediately adjacent to the layer of ependymal cells bordering the ventricle. This region is known to contain dividing precursor cells in adults (Smart 1961; Lois and Alvarez-Buylla 1993). Some of the cells originating in the SVZ migrate to the olfactory bulb, where they can differentiate into neurons (Lois and Alvarez-Buylla 1994; Luskin 1993). In addition, after infusion of growth factors in the ventricle, cells of the SVZ can migrate into the adjacent striatum and differentiate into neurons or glia (Goldman and Luskin 1998). Little is known, however, about the regulation of these dividing cells by endogenous factors in adults.

By seven days after cortical lesions, the number of cells in the SVZ at the level of the rostral striatum had doubled (figure 7.8). This increase was observed after both thermocoagulatory and aspiration lesions, and was further characterized after aspiration lesions (Szele and Chesselet 1996). The increase in cell number in the SVZ was paralleled by a marked increased in immunostaining for PSA-NCAM, which labels cells having accomplished their last division (Bonfanti and Theodosis 1994). Increases in the number of cells labeled by a single administration of bromodeoxyuridine were only observed in some of the rats after cortical lesions, suggesting that cell divi-

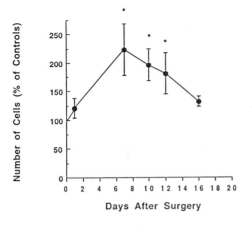

Dorsolateral Subventricular Zone

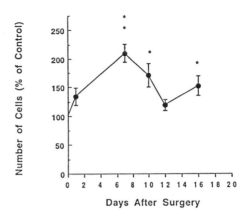

Striatal Subventricular Zone

Figure 7.8 Increase in cell number in the dorsolateral (left) and striatal (right) regions of the subventricular zone ipsilateral to an aspiration lesion of the sensorimotor cortex. Data are mean ± SEM of number of cells in lesioned rats expressed in percent of number of cells in controls. *$P < .05$ when absolute values in lesioned rats are compared with the unlesioned controls with an ANOVA and post hoc Dunnett test (n = 3–6).

sions increased, but only transiently. No increase in labeling for markers of mature neurons (neuron-specific enolase) or glial cells (GFAP, carbonic anhydrase) was observed in the SVZ of lesioned rats. Expression of bFGF decreased in the SVZ, as it did in the dorsolateral striatum, but no immunolabeling for epidermal growth factor was detected, either before or after lesion.

In addition to dramatic changes in cell numbers in the SVZ, the lesions also induced changes in immunolabeling in the medial striatum. Immunoreactivity to tenascin, a glial cell adhesion molecule believed to oppose neuronal migration in some conditions (Laywell et al. 1992, Lochter et al. 1991), decreased, whereas immunoreactivity for PSA-NCAM, believed to facilitate cell migration (Doetsch and Alvarez-Buylla 1996; Hu et al. 1996; Ono et al. 1994; Wang et al. 1994), increased in the medial striatum immediately adjacent to the SVZ. In addition, a conspicuous change in the morphology of GFAP-positive astrocytes was noted in this region (Szele et al. 1995). In the medial striatum of unlesioned rats, astrocytes displayed a typical stellar morphology, whereas after lesions, GFAP-positive processes extended from the SVZ into the medial striatum, similar to the radial processes seen during the first few postnatal weeks (Butler and Chesselet, upublished observations). These changes in immunoreactivity are reminiscent of patterns observed during development, and suggest that the medial striatum presents a milieu favorable to cell migration after cortical lesions. However, we were unable to detect a significant migration of bromodeoxyuridine-labeled cells into the striatum after cortical lesions. It is possible, however, that other markers would permit the detection of migrating cells. Alternatively, the cortical lesions may induce limited increases in cytokines and growth factors which incompletely mimic the effects of exogenous factors (Goldman and Luskin 1998).

CONCLUSIONS

In conclusion, much work over the last twenty years has been focused on the hippocampus as one of the few loci of axonal plasticity in response to brain injury in adults. Our data indicate that these properties are far from being limited to the hippocampus. It was particularly surprising to find such a high level of axonal plasticity in the dorsolateral striatum because many of the molecules that are thought to be associated with anatomical plasticity are absent or expressed at a much lower level in the dorsolateral striatum than in other brain regions believed to have a high degree of plasticity. Therefore, although axonal plasticity may rely on similar molecular mechanisms in a subset of brain regions, it is likely that regional differences exist in these mechanisms. It is of particular interest that shortly after our finding of a robust axonal plasticity in the adult striatum, Charpier and Denial (1997) demonstrated significant LTP in the dorsolateral striatum of adult rats. The existence of LTP has also been thought to be restricted to specialized highly "plastic" brain regions. Furthermore, PSA-NCAM has been shown to play a role in LTP in the hippocampus (Muller et al. 1996). Therefore, both functional and anatomical plasticity may be much more widespread in adult brain than previously believed, but their underlying mechanisms may be regionally specific. Understanding the regional differences in the molecular mechanisms of neuronal plasticity is important to improve recovery of function after brain injury or in neurodegenerative disease.

ACKNOWLEDGMENTS

Work in our laboratory has been supported by PHS grants NS-29230 and MH-10794. We thank Dr. G. Rougon, Marseille, France for the gift of antibodies against PSA-NCAM and many stimulating discussions in the course of these studies, Dr. P. Zhang and Mr. C. Alexander for help with some of the experiments, and Mr. John Sharpe for help with the manuscript and illustrations.

REFERENCES

Aaron, L. I., and Chesselet, M-F. (1989). Heterogeneous distribution of polysialylated neuronal-cell adhesion molecule during post-natal development and in the adult: an immunohistochemical study. *Neuroscience* 28: 701–710.

Armstrong, D. D. (1997). Review of Rett syndrome. *J. Neuropathol. Exp. Neurol.* 56: 843–849.

Balice-Gordon, R. J., Chua, C. K., Nelson, C. C., and Lichtman, J. W. (1993). Gradual loss of synaptic cartels precedes axon withdrawal at developing neuromuscular junctions. *Neuron* 11: 801–815.

Bayer, S. A. (1984). Neurogenesis in the rat neostriatum. *Int. J. Dev. Neurosci.* 2: 163–175.

Bear, M. F. (1996). NMDA-receptor–dependent synaptic plasticity in the visual cortex. *Prog. Brain Res.* 108: 205–208.

Beck, K. D., Lamballe, F., Klein, R., Barbacid, M., Schauwecker, E., McNeil, T. H., Finch, C. E., Hefti, F., and Day, J. R. (1993). Induction of noncatalytic TrkB neurotrophin receptors during axonal sprouting in the adult hippocampus. *J. Neurosci.* 13: 4001–4014.

Benowitz, L. I., Apostolides, P. J., Perrone-Bizzorero, N., Finklestein, S. P., and Zwiers, H. (1988). Anatomical distribution of the growth associated protein GAP-43/B-50 in the adult rat brain. *J. Neurosci.* 8: 339–352.

Benowitz, L. I., Rodriguez, W. R., and Neve, R. L. (1990). The pattern of GAP-43 immunostaining changes in the rat hippocampal formation during reactive synaptogenesis. *Mol. Brain Res.* 8: 17–23.

Bernheimer, H., Birkmayer, W., Honykiewicz, O., Jellinger, K., and Seitelberger, F. (1973). Brain dopamine and the syndromes of Parkinson and Huntington. *J. Neurol. Sci.* 20: 415–455.

Bjorklund, A., and Lindvall, O. (1984). Dopamine-containing systems in the CNS. *Handbook of Chemical Neuroanatomy*, Vol. 2: *Classical Transmitters in the CNS*, Part I, A. Bjorklund, and T. Hokfelt, eds., pp. 55–122. Amsterdam, Elsevier.

Bolam, J., and Bennett, D. (1995). Microcircuitry of the neostriatum: molecular and Cellular Mechanisms of Neostriatal Function. In *Molecular and Cellular Mechanisms of Neostriatal Function*, M. A. Ariano, D. J. Surmeier, eds., pp. 1–20. Austin, TX, R. G. Landes.

Bonfanti, L., and Theodosis, D. T. (1994). Expression of polysialylated neural cell adhesion molecule by proliferating cells in the subependymal layer of the adult rat, in its rostral extension and in the olfactory bulb. *Neuroscience* 62: 291–305.

Bonfanti, L., Olive, S., Poulain, D. A., and Theodosis, D. T. (1992). Mapping of the distribution of polysialylated neural cell adhesion molecule throughout the central nervous system of the adult rat: an immunohistochemical study. *Neuroscience* 49: 419–436.

Bonfanti, L., Merighi, A., and Theodosis, D. T. (1996). Dorsal rhizotomy induces transient expression of the highly sialylated isoform of the neural cell adhesion molecule in neurons and astrocytes of the adult rat spinal cord. *Neuroscience* 74: 619–623.

Brand, S., and Rakic, P. (1984). Cytodifferentiation and synaptogenesis in the neostriatum of fetal and neonatal rhesus monkeys. *Anat. Embryol.* 169: 21–34.

Butler, A. K., Uryu, K., Morehouse, V., Rougon, G., and Chesselet, M-F. (1997). Regulation of the polysialylated form of the neural cell adhesion molecule in the developing striatum: effects of cortical lesions. *J. Comp. Neurol.* 389: 289–308.

Butler, A. K., Uryu, K., and Chesselet, M-F. (1998). A role for NMDA receptors in the regulation of synaptogenesis and PSA-NCAM expression in the developing striatum. *Dev. Neurosci.*

Butler, A. K., Uryu, K., Rougon, G., and Chesselet, M-F. NMDA receptor blockade affects PSA-NCAM expression and synapse number during striatal development. *Neuroscience*, in press.

Calabresi, P., De Murtas, M., and Bernardi, G. (1997). The neostriatum beyond the motor function: experimental and clinical evidence. *Neuroscience* 78: 39–60.

Carlsson, M., and Carlsson, A. (1990). Schizophrenia: a subcortical neurotransmitter imbalance syndrome? *Schizophr. Bull.* 16: 425–432.

Charpier, S., and Deniau, J. M. (1997). In vivo activity-dependent plasticity at cortico-striatal connections: evidence for physiological long-term potentiation. *Proc. Natl. Acad. Sci. USA* 94: 7036–7040.

Chaudieu, I., Mount, I., Quirion, R., and Boksa, P. (1991). Transient postnatal increases in excitatory amino acid binding sites in rat ventral mesencephalon. *Neurosci. Lett.* 133: 267–270.

Chen, S., and Hillman, D. E. (1990). Robust synaptic plasticity of striatal cells following partial deafferentation. *Brain Res.* 520: 103–114.

Cheng, H. W., Rafols, J. A., Goshgarian, H. G., Anavi, Y., Tong, J., and McNeill, T. H. (1997). Differential spine loss and regrowth of striatal neurons following multiple forms of deafferentation: a Golgi study. *Exp. Neurol.* 147: 287–298.

Chesselet, M.-F., and Delfs, J. M. (1996). Basal ganglia and movement disorders: an update. *Trends Neurosci.* 19: 417–422.

Chong, M. S., Reynolds, M. L., Irwin, N., Coggeshall, R. E., Emson, P. C., Benowitz, L. I., and Woolf, C. J. (1994). GAP-43 expression in primary sensory neurons following central axotomy. *J. Neurosci.* 14: 4375–4384.

Coggeshall, R. E., and Lekan, H. A. (1996). Methods for determining numbers of cells and synapses: a case for more uniform standards of review. *J. Comp. Neurol.* 364: 6–15.

Colwell, C. S., Cepeda, C., Crawford, C., and Levine, M. (1998). Postnatal development of NMDA evoked responses in the neostriatum. *Dev. Neurosci.*, 20: 154–163.

Constantine-Paton, M. (1994). Effects of NMDA receptor antagonists on the developing brain. *Psychopharmacol. Bull.* 30: 561–565.

Cotman, C., Nieto-Sampedro, M., and Harris, E. (1981). Synapse replacement in the nervous system of adult vertebrates. *Physiol. Rev.* 61: 684–784.

Cotman, C. W., and Nieto-Sampedro, M. (1984). Cell biology of synaptic plasticity. *Science* 255: 1287–1294.

Curtis, R., Green, D., Lindsay, R. M., and Wilkin, G. P. (1993). Up-regulation of GAP-43 and growth of axons in rat spinal cord after compression injury. *J. Neurocytol.* 22: 51–64.

Dani, J. W., Armstrong, D. M., and Benowitz, L. I. (1991). Mapping the development of the rat brain by GAP-43 immunocytochemistry. *Neuroscience.* 40: 277–287.

DiFiglia, M., Pasik, P., and Pasik, T. (1980). Early postnatal development of the monkey neostriatum: a Golgi and ultrastructural study. *J. Comp. Neurol.* 190: 303–331.

DiFiglia, M., Roberts, R., and Benowitz, L. I. (1990). Immunoreactive GAP-43 in the neuropil of the adult rat neostriatum: localization in unmyelinated fibers, axon terminals, and dendritic spines. *J. Comp. Neurol.* 302: 992–1001.

Doetsch, F., and Alvarez-Buylla, A. (1996). Network of tangential pathways for neuronal migration in adult mammalian brain. *Proc. Natl. Acad. Sci. USA* 93: 14895–14900.

Doherty, P., Cohen, J., and Walsh, F. (1990). Neurite outgrowth in response to transfected N-CAM changes during development and is modulated by polysialic acid. *Neuron* 5: 209–219.

Donoghue, J. P., and Herkenham, M. (1986). Neostriatal projections from individual cortical fields conform to histochemically distinct striatal compartments in the rat. *Brain Res.* 365: 397–403.

Ebrahimi, A., Pochet, R., and Roger, M. (1992). Topographical organization of the projections from physiologically identified areas of the motor cortex to the striatum in the rat. *Neurosci. Res.* 14: 39–60.

Edelman, G. M., and Chuong, C.-M. (1982). Embryonic to adult conversion of neural cell adhesion molecules in normal and staggerer mice. *Proc. Natl. Acad. Sci. USA* 79: 7036–7040.

Enomoto, R., Ogita, K., Kawanami, K., Azuma, Y., and Yoneda, Y. (1996). Simultaneous determination of binding of a variety of radioligands related to ionotropic excitatory amino acid receptors in fetal and neonatal rat brains. *Brain Res.* 723: 100–109.

Errami, M., and Nieoullon, A. (1986). Development of a micromethod to study the Na^+-independent L-(^{3}H)glutamic acid binding to rat striatal membranes. II. Effects of selective striatal lesions and deafferentations. *Brain Res.* 366: 178–186.

Fentress, J. C., Stanfield, B. B., and Cowan, W. M. (1981). Observation on the development of the striatum in mice and rats. *Anat. Embryol.* 163: 275–298.

Fishell, G., and van der Kooy, D. (1987). Pattern formation in the striatum: developmental changes in the distribution of striatonigral neurons. *J. Neurosci.* 7: 1969–1978.

Fishell, G., and van der Kooy, D. (1989). Pattern formation in the striatum: developmental changes in the distribution of striatonigral projections. *Dev. Brain Res.* 45: 239–255.

Fishell, G., and van der Kooy, D. (1991). Pattern formation in the striatum: neurons with early projections to the substantia nigra survive the cell death period. *J. Comp. Neurol.* 312: 33–42.

Gimenez y Ribotta, M., Rajaofetra, N., Morin-Richaud, C., Alonso, G., Bochelen, D., Sandillon, F., Legrand, A., Mersel, M., and Privat, A. (1995). Oxysterol (7 beta-hydroxycholesteryl-3–oleate) promotes serotonergic reinnervation in the lesioned rat spinal cord by reducing glial reaction. *J. Neurosci. Res.* 41: 79–95.

Godment, P., Vanselow, J., Thanes, S., and Bonhoeffer, F. (1987). A study in developing visual systems of a new method of staining neurons and their processes in fixed tissue. *Development* 101: 697–713.

Goldman, S. A., and Luskin, M. B. (1998). Strategies utilized by migrating neurons of the postnatal vertebrate forebrain. *Trends Neurosci.* 21: 107–113.

Goldowitz, D., Barthels, D., Lorenzon, N., Junblut, A., and Wille, W. (1990). NCAM gene expression during the development of the cerebellum and dentate gyrus in the mouse. *Dev. Brain Res.* 52: 151–160.

Gomez-Pinilla, F., Lee, J. W., and Cotman, C. W. (1992). Basic FGF in adult rat brain: cellular distribution and response to entorhinal lesion and fimbria-fornix transection. *J. Neurosci.* 12: 345–355.

Goodman, C. S., and Shatz, C. J. (1993). Developmental mechanisms that generate precise patterns of neuronal connectivity. *Neuron 10 (suppl.):* 77–98.

Halliday, A. L., and Cepko, C. L. (1992). Generation and migration of cells in the developing striatum. *Neuron* 9: 15–26.

Hattori, T., and McGeer, P. L. (1973). Synaptogenesis in the corpus striatum of infant rat. *Exp. Neurol.* 38: 70–79.

Hu, H., Tomaseiwicz, H., Magnuson, T., and Rutishauser, U. (1996). The role of polysialic acid in migration of olfactory bulb interneuron precursors in the subventricular zone. *Neuron* 16: 735–743.

Iniguez, C., De Juan, J., Al-Majdalawi, A., and Gayoso, M. J. (1990). Postnatal development of striatal connections in the rat: a transport study with wheat germ agglutinin–horseradish peroxidase. *Dev. Brain Res.* 57: 43–53.

Insel, T. R., Miller, L. P., and Gelhard, R. E. (1990). The ontogeny of excitatory amino acid receptors in rat forebrain-I. N-methyl-D-aspartate and quisqualate receptors. *Neuroscience* 35: 31–43.

Jahn, R., Schiebler, W., Ouimet, C., and Greengard, P. (1985). A 38,000—dalton membrane protein (p38) present in synaptic vesicles. *Proc. Natl. Acad. Sci. USA* 12: 4137—4141.

Kasamatsu, T., Imamura, K., Mataga, N., Hartveit, E., Heggelund, U., and Heggelund, P. (1997). Roles of *N*-methyl-D-aspartate receptors in ocular dominance plasticity in developing visual cortex: a re-evaluation. *Neuroscience* 82: 687—700.

Katz, L. C., and Shatz, C. J. (1996). Synaptic activity and the construction of cortical circuits. *Science* 274: 1133—1138.

Kiss, J. Z., and Rougon, G. (1997). Cell biology of polysialic acid. *Curr. Opin. Neurobiol.* 7: 640—646.

Kolb, B., Gibb, R., and van der Kooy, D. (1992). Cortical and striatal structure and connectivity are altered by neonatal hemidecortication in rats. *J. Comp. Neurol.* 322: 311—324.

Lahof, A. M., N. D.-B. and J. M. (1996). Synapse elimination in the central nervous system: functional significance and cellular mechanisms. *Rev. Neurosci.* 7: 85—101.

Landmesser, L., Dahm, L., Tang, J., and Rutishauser, U. (1990). Polysialic acid as a regulator of intramuscular nerve branching during embryonic development. *Neuron* 4: 655—667.

Laurie, D. J., and Seeburg, P. H. (1994). Regional and developmental heterogeneity in splicing of the rat brain NMDAR1 mRNA. *J. Neurosci.* 14: 3180—3194.

Laywell, E. D., Dorries, U., Bartsch, U., Faissner, A., Schachner, M., and Steindler, D. A. (1992). Enhanced expression of the developmentally regulated extracellular matrix molecule tenascin following adult brain injury. *Proc. Natl. Acad. Sci. USA* 89: 2634—2638.

Leckman, J. F., Peterson, B. S., Anderson, G. M., Arnsten, A. F., Pauls, D. L., and Cohen, D. J. (1997). Pathogenesis of Tourette's syndrome. *J. Child Psychol. Psychiatry* 38: 119—142.

Le Gal La Salle, G., Rougon, G., and Valin, G. (1992). The embryonic form of the neural cell adhesion molecule (E-NCAM) in the rat hippocampus and its reexpression on glial cells following kainic acid—induced status epilepticus. *J. Neurosci.* 12: 872—882.

Liu, F-C., and Graybiel, A. M. (1992). Transient calbindin-D28K—positive systems in the telencephelon: ganglionic eminence, developing striatum and cerebral cortex. *J. Neurosci.* 12: 674—690.

Lochter, A., Vaughan, L., Kaplony, A., Prochiantz, A., Schachner, M., and Faissner, A. (1991). J1/tenascin in substrate-bound and soluble form displays contrary effects on neurite outgrowth. *J. Cell Biol.* 113: 1159—1171.

Lois, C., and Alvarez-Buylla, A. (1993). Proliferating subventricular zone cells in the adult mammalian forebrain can differentiate into neurons and glia. *Proc. Natl. Acad. Sci. USA* 90: 2074—2077.

Lois, C., and Alvarez-Buylla, A. (1994). Long-distance neuronal migration in the adult mammalian brain. *Science* 264: 1145—1148.

Lu, E. J., and Brown, W. J. (1977). An electron microscopic study of the developing caudate nucleus in euthyroid and hypothyroid. *Anat. Embryol.* 150: 335—364.

Luhmann, H. J. (1996). Ischemia and lesion-induced imbalances in cortical function. *Prog. Neurobiol.* 48: 131—166.

Luskin, M. B. (1993). Restricted proliferation and migration of postnatally generated neurons derived from the forebrain subventricular zone. *Neuron.* 11: 173—189.

Marsden, C. D., and Obeso, J. A. (1994). The functions of the basal ganglia and the paradox of stereotaxic surgery in Parkinson's disease. *Brain* 117: 877—897.

Chesselet et al.

Masliah, E., Fagan, A. M., Terry, R. D., DeTeresa, R., Mallory, M., and Gage, F. H. (1991). Reactive synaptogenesis assessed by snaptophysin immunoreactivity is associated with GAP-43 in the dentate gyrus of the adult rat. *Exp. Neurol.* 113: 131–142.

Matthews, D. A., Cotman, C., and Lynch, G. (1976). An electron microscopic study of lesion-induced synaptogenesis in the dentate gyrus of the adult rat. II. Reappearance of morphologically normal synaptic contacts. *Brain Res.* 115: 23–41.

McGeorge, A. J., and Faull, R. L. M. (1987). The organization and collateralization of corticostriate neurons in the motor and sensory cortex of the rat brain. *Brain Res.* 423: 318–324.

McGeorge, A. J., and Faull, R. L. M. (1989). The organization of the projection from the cerebral cortex to the striatum in the rat. *Neuroscience* 29: 503–537.

McKeon, P., Schoureiber, R. C., Rudge, J. S., and Silver, J. (1991). Reduction of neurite outgrowth in a model of glial scarring following CNS injury is correlated with the expression of inhibitory molecules on reactive astrocytes. *J. Neurosci.* 11: 3398–3411.

Miller, P. D., Styren, S. D., Lagenaur, C. F., and DeKosky, S. T. (1994). Embryonic neural cell adhesion molecule (NCAM) is elevated in the denervated dentate gyrus. *J. Neurosci.* 14: 4217–4225.

Misgeld, U., Dodt, H. U., and Frotscher, M. (1986). Late development of intrinsic excitation in the rat neostriatum: an in vitro study. *Dev. Brain Res.* 27: 59–67.

Monyer, H., Burnashev, N., Laurie, D. J., Sakmann, B., and Seeburg, P. H. (1994). Development and regional expression in the rat brain and functional properties of four NMDA receptors. *Neuron* 12: 529–540.

Muller, D., Stoppini, L., Wang, C., and Kiss, J. Z. (1994). A role for poylsialylated neural cell adhesion molecule in lesion induced sprouting in hippocampal organotypic cultures. *Neuroscience* 61: 441–445.

Muller, D., Wang, C., Skibo, G., Toni, N., Cremer, H., Calaora, V., Rougon, G., and Kiss, J. Z. (1996). PSA-NCAM is required for activity-induced synaptic plasticity. *Neuron* 17: 413–422.

Murrin, C., and Ferrer, J. R. (1984). Ontogeny of the rat striatum: correspondence of dopamine terminals, opiate receptors and acetylcholinesterase. *Neurosci. Lett.* 47: 155–160.

Napieralski, J. A., Butler, A. K., and Chesselet, M-F. (1996). Anatomical and functional evidence for lesion specific sprouting of corticostriatal input in the adult rat. *J. Comp. Neurol.* 373: 484–497.

Ono, K., Tomasiewicz, H., Magnuson, T., and Rutishauser, U. (1994). N-CAM mutation inhibits tangential neuronal migration and is phenocopied by enzymatic removal of polysialic acid. *Neuron* 13: 595–609.

Parent, A., and Hazrati, L.-N. (1995). Functional anatomy of the basal ganglia. I. The cortico-basal ganglia-thalamo-cortical loop. *Brain Res. Rev.* 20: 91–127.

Paxinos, G., and Watson, C. (1986). *The Rat Brain in Stereotaxic Coordinates.* New York, Academic Press.

Peacock, W. J., Wehby-Grant, M. C., Shields, W. D., Shewmon, D. A., Chugani, H. T., Sankar, R., and Vinters, H. V. (1996). Hemispherectomy for intractable seizures in children: a report of 58 cases. *Childs Nerv. Syst.* 12: 376–384.

Phelps, P. E., Brady, D. R., and Vaughn, J. E. (1989). The generation and differentiation of cholinergic neurons in rat caudate-putamen. *Dev. Brain Res.* 46: 47–60.

Pindzola, R. R., Doller, C., and Silver, J. (1993). Putative inhibitory extracellular matrix molecules at the dorsal root entry zone of the spinal cord during development and after root and sciatic nerve lesions. *Dev. Biol.* 156: 34–48.

Portera-Cailliau, C., Price, D. L., and Martin, L. J. (1996). N-methyl-D-aspartate receptor proteins NR2A and NR2B are differentially distributed in the developing rat central nervous system as revealed by subunit-specific antibodies. *J. Neurochem.* 66: 692–700.

Riva, M. A., Tascedda, F., Molteni, R., and Racagni, G. (1994). Regulation of NMDA receptor subunit mRNA expression in the rat brain during postnatal development. *Mol. Brain Res.* 25: 209–216.

Rivas, R. J., Burmeister, D. W., and Goldberg, D. J. (1992). Rapid effects of laminin on the growth cone. *Neuron* 8: 107–115.

Rougon, G., and Marshak, D. (1986). Structural and immunological characterization of the amino-terminal domain of mammalian neural cell adhesion molecules. *J. Biol. Chem.* 261: 3396–3408.

Salin, P., and Chesselet, M-F. (1992). Paradoxical increase in striatal neuropeptide gene expression following ischemic lesions of the cerebral cortex. *Proc. Natl. Acad. Sci. USA* 89: 9954–9958.

Salin, P., and Chesselet, M-F. (1993). Expression of GAD (Mr 67,000) and its messenger RNA in basal ganglia and cerebral cortex after ischemic cortical lesions in rats. *Exp. Neurol.* 119: 291–301.

Salin, P., Kerkerian-Le Goff, L., Heidet, V., Epelbaum, J., and Nieoullon, A. (1990). Somatostatin-immunoreactive neurons in the rat striatum: effects of corticostriatal and nigrostriatal dopaminergic lesions. *Brain Res.* 521: 23–32.

Scheetz, A. J., and Constantine-Paton, M. (1994). Modulation of NMDA receptor function: implications for vertebrate neural development. *FASEB J.* 8: 745–752.

Schmued, L., Kyriakidis, K., and Heimer, L. (1990). In vivo anterograde and retrograde axonal transport of the fluorescent rhodamine-dextran amine, Fluoro-Ruby, within CNS. *Brain Res.* 526: 127–134.

Seki, T., and Arai, Y. (1991). Expression of highly polysialylated NCAM in the neocortex and piriform cortex of the developing and adult rat. *Anat. Embryol.* 184: 395–401.

Semba, K., Vincent, S. R., and Fibiger, H. C. (1988). Different times of origin of choline acetyltransferase and somatostatin-immunoreactive neurons in the rat striatum. *J. Neurosci.* 8: 3937–3944.

Sesack, S. R., Deutch, A. Y., Roth, R. H., and Bunney, B. S. (1989). The topographical organization of the efferent projections of the medial prefrontal cortex in the rat: an anterograde tract-tracing study with *Phaseolus vulgaris* Leucoagglutinin. *J. Comp. Neurol.* 290: 213–242.

Shi, J., Aamodt, S. M., and Constantine-Paton, M. (1997). Temporal correlations between functional and molecular changes in NMDA receptors and GABA neurotransmission in the superior colliculus. *J. Neurosci.* 17: 6264–6276.

Smart I. (1961). The subventricular zone of the mouse brain and its cell production as shown by radioautography after thymidine-H3 injection. *J. Comp. Neurol.* 116: 325–338.

Snyder-Keller, A., and Costantini, L. C. (1996). Glutamate receptor subtypes localize to patches in the developing striatum. *Dev. Brain Res.* 94: 246–250.

Somers, D. L., and Beckstead, R. M. (1990). Striatal preprotachykinin and preproenkephalin mRNA levels and the levels of nigral substance P and pallidal met[5−] enkephalin depend on coricostriatal axons that use the excitatory amino acid neurotransmitters aspartate and glutamate: quantitative radioimmunocytochemical and in situ hybridization evidence. *Mol. Brain Res.* 8: 143–158.

Song, D. D., and Harlan, R. E. (1994). Genesis and migration patterns of neurons forming the patch and matrix compartments of the rat striatum. *Dev. Brain Res.* 83: 233–245.

Strittmatter, S. M., Frankhauser, C., Huang, P. L. Mashimo, H., and Fishman, M. C. (1995). Neuronal pathfinding is abnormal in mice lacking the neuronal growth cone protein GAP-43. *Cell* 80: 445–452.

Styren, S. D., Lagenaur, C. F., Miller, P. D., and DeKosky, S. T. (1994). Rapid expression and transport of embryonic N-CAM in dentate gyrus following entorhinal cortex lesion: ultrastructural analysis. *J. Comp. Neurol.* 349: 486–492.

Szele, F. G., and Chesselet, M-F. (1996). Cortical lesions induce an increase in cell number and PSA-NCAM expression in the subventricular zone of adult rats. *J. Comp. Neurol.* 368: 439–454.

Szele, F. G., Dowling, J. J., Gonzales, C., Theveniau, M., Rougon, G., and Chesselet, M-F. (1994). Pattern of expression of highly polysialylated neural cell adhesion molecule in the developing and adult rat striatum. *Neuroscience* 60: 133–144.

Szele, F: G., Alexander, C., and Chesselet, M-F. (1995). Expression of molecules associated with neuronal plasticity in the striatum after aspiration and thermocoagulatory lesions of the cerebral cortex in adult rats. *J. Neurosci.* 15: 4429–4448.

Tang, J., and Landmesser, L. (1993). Reduction of intramuscular nerve branching and synaptogenesis is correlated with decreased motoneuron survival. *J. Neurosci.* 13: 3095–3103.

Tepper, J. M., and Trent, F. (1993). In vivo studies of the postnatal development of rat neostriatal neurons. *Prog. Brain Res.* 99: 35–50.

Tepper, J. M., Trent, F., and Nakamura, S. (1990). Postnatal development of the electrical activity of rat nigrostriatal dopaminergic neurons. *Dev. Brain Res.* 54: 21–33.

Theodosis, D. T., Rougon, G., and Poulain, D. (1991). Retention of embryonic features by an adult neuronal system capable of plasticity: polysialylated neural cell adhesion molecule in the hypothalamo-neurohypophysial system. *Proc. Natl. Acad. Sci. USA* 88: 5494–5498.

Uhl, G. R., Navia, B., and Douglas, J. (1988). Differential expression of preproenkephalin and preprodynorphin mRNAs in striatal neurons: high levels of preproenkephalin expression depend on cerebral cortical afferents. *J. Neurosci.* 8: 4755–4764.

Uryu, K., Butler, A. K., and Chesselet, M-F.: Synaptogenesis and ultrastructural localization of the polysialylated neural cell adhesion molecule in the developing striatum. *J. Comp. Neurol.*, in press.

van den Pol, A. N., diPorzio, U., and Rutishauser, U. (1986). Growth cone localization of neural cell adhesion molecule on central nervous system neurons in vitro. *J. Cell Biol.* 102: 2281–2294.

Voorn, P., Kalsbeek, A., Jorritsma-Byham, B., and Groenewegen, H. J. (1988). The pre- and postnatal development of the dopaminergic cell groups in the ventral mesencephalon and the dopaminergic innervation of the striatum of the rat. *Neuroscience* 25: 857–887.

Wang, C., Rougon, G., and Kiss, J. Z. (1994). Requirement of polysialic acid for the migration of the O-2A glial progenitor cell from neurohypophyseal explants. *J. Neurosci.* 14: 4446–4457.

Weihmuller, F. B., and Bruno, J. P. (1989). Age-dependent plasticity in the dopaminergic control of sensorimotor development. *Behav. Brain Res.* 35: 95–109.

Wilson, C. J. (1987). Morphology and synaptic connections of crossed corticostriatal neurons in the rat. *J. Comp. Neurol.* 263: 567–580.

Wise, S. P., Fleshman, J. W., and Jones, E. G. (1979). Maturation of pyramidal cell form in relation to developing afferent and efferent connections of rat somatic sensory cortex. *Neuroscience* 4: 1275–1297.

Zhang, H., Miller, R. H., and Rutishauser, U. (1992). Poysialic acid is required for optimal growth of axons on a neuronal substrate. *J. Neurosci.* 12: 3107–3114.

Zigmond, M. J., and Striker, E. M. (1989). Animal models of parkinsoninsm using selective neurotoxins: clinical and basic implications. *Int. Rev. Neurobiol.* 31: 1–79.

8 Pathway-Specific Regulation of Synapses in the Thalamocortical System

Barry W. Connors, Ziv Gil, Carole E. Landisman,
Jay R. Gibson, and Yael Amitai

The functions of the thalamus and neocortex are inextricable. Neural information from sensory organs is relayed to first-order central nuclei (in the brainstem and spinal cord, or retina), then to the thalamus, then to a primary sensory area of the cortex, and on to other higher sensory areas. Intracortical axons synaptically interconnect cortical neurons. The cortex sends dense connections back to the thalamus. This arrangement allows a remarkable orchestration of simultaneous operations: new information continually streams upward to the cortex, the cortex processes information through parallel and hierarchical networks, the cortex influences thalamic function and regulates the upward information stream, the thalamus reroutes information descending from one region of the cortex upward to other regions, and the cortex and thalamus sustain a variety of synchronous oscillatory patterns (Sherman and Guillery 1996; Steriade 1997).

The interactions between thalamus and cortex rely on three types of excitatory glutamatergic contacts: thalamocortical (TC), intracortical (IC), and corticothalamic (CT) synapses (figure 8.1). These are general categories; anatomically, there are multiple subclasses of each pathway, but whether there are differences of synaptic function in these subclasses remains to be tested. In this chapter we review recent research comparing TC, IC, and CT synapses and the neural networks they interconnect. Our general conclusion is that each type of synaptic pathway has its own rules of dynamic behavior and regulation. These diverse properties may help to determine the flow of information through the thalamocortical axis, the modification of this flow during changes in behavioral state, and the long-term synaptic alterations that mediate learning and memory. We begin by describing in vitro analyses of specific synapses which suggest that each pathway in the thalamocortical system may be differentially regulated by neural activity and chemical modulators (Gil et al. 1997a; Landisman et al. 1997). Then we describe how two parallel thalamocortical pathways tested in vivo display very different dynamic properties (Castro-Alamancos and Connors 1996b–d). The dynamics of these pathways depends not only on intrinsic synaptic properties but also on the particular cortical subcircuit engaged, and the behavioral state of the animal (Castro-Alamancos and Connors 1996c,e).

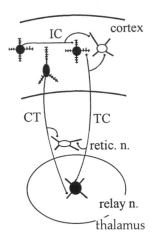

Figure 8.1 Schematic circuit diagram of the thalamocorticothalamic loop. Neurons in relay nuclei project thalamocortical (TC) axons into neocortex; cortical cells are interconnected by intracortical (IC) axons; corticothalamic (CT) axons in turn project back to the thalamus. Closed cells symbolize spiny, excitatory neurons; open cells symbolize inhibitory neurons. Retic. n., reticular nucleus.

DIFFERENTIAL DYNAMICS OF THALAMOCORTICAL AND INTRACORTICAL SYNAPSES

The Variability of Synapse Properties in Cerebral Cortex

The basic molecular mechanisms of chemical synapses are highly conserved (Ferro-Novick and Jahn 1994; Bennett and Scheller 1994). Synapses have nevertheless evolved a wide range of functional characteristics. Not only do transmitter type and postsynaptic receptors vary among synapses but release probability, quantal content, plasticity, and presynaptic modulation are also highly diverse, yet can be specific for different synapse types (Malenka and Nicoll 1993; Davis and Murphey 1994). A further complication is that the efficacy of a chemical synapse is not static, but changes with use and time (Magleby 1987; Zucker 1989). The complexity of these processes is reflected in the abstruse nomenclature of the field. Some synaptic changes are "long-term," lasting for tens of minutes to hours and days, and may either potentiate or depress efficacy ("long-term potentiation, LTP" or "long-term depression, LTD"). Long-term changes may be limited to only certain synapse types, but all synapses display "short-term" (milliseconds to minutes) changes in efficacy—termed "facilitation," "depression," "augmentation," and "potentiation."

Mechanisms of synaptic plasticity are being actively investigated. Most short-term forms seem to involve presynaptic mechanisms (e.g., see Zucker 1989), although postsynaptic processes may sometimes contribute. For example, facilitation apparently depends on a small, residual increase in presynaptic internal $[Ca^{2+}]$ following activation (Katz 1962; Kamiya and Zucker

1994; Regehr et al. 1994). Synapses with an inherently low probability of release tend to display large facilitation, because when release fails on the first of a stimulus pair the increased internal $[Ca^{2+}]$ makes it more likely that the second stimulus will evoke release. In contrast, synapses with an inherently high probability of release tend to display stronger depression, presumably because the pool of available vesicles for release becomes more rapidly depleted (Stevens and Wang 1995; Debanne et al. 1996; Murthy et al. 1997). So far these aspects of synaptic function cannot be predicted from structure alone. However, it has been proposed that the strength of a synapse (Pierce and Lewin 1994), or more specifically its probability of transmitter release (Schikorski and Stevens 1997), is related to the size of the presynaptic terminal or its active zones.

Thalamocortical and Intracortical Synapses Have Similar Quantal Properties

According to classic theory, synaptic neurotransmitter is quantized (Katz 1962). When comparing different types of excitatory synapses, the first question we might ask is: do they have the same size quanta? Differences in quantal size, everything else being equal, could imply interesting differences in the microphysiology of synapse types. Quantal size could also be an important determinant of synaptic efficacy. In recent experiments we compared quantal sizes in TC and IC synapses that converge onto single neurons (Gil et al. in press). Whole-cell recording was used in slices of rat somatosensory cortex in vitro. Slices were cut in a plane that preserved some of the pathways between thalamus and cortex (Agmon and Connors 1991), and stimulation was applied separately to a horizontal intracortical pathway or to the ventrobasal thalamus to activate thalamocortical fibers, while spiny cells were recorded in deep layer 3 or layer 4 (Gil and Amitai 1996b). GABAergic inhibition, voltage-dependent postsynaptic currents, and N-methyl-D-aspartate (NMDA) receptor—mediated reponses were suppressed pharmacologically.

Measuring quantal size from defined pathways in the brain is complicated by the small size of the quanta, by the large variety of synaptic inputs to each neuron, and by the difficulty of distinguishing single from multiple quantal events. Quantal excitatory postsynaptic potentials (EPSPs) or excitatory postsynaptic currents (EPSCs) were isolated from either the thalamocortical or intracortical pathway with two different methods (Gil et al. in press). First, the Ca^{2+} in the bathing medium was replaced with Sr^{2+}, which causes a large number of long-latency, asynchronously released quanta (Oliet et al. 1996). With quantal events so spread out in time, it becomes possible to measure the size and shape of single quantal EPSPs reliably. Second, the probability of transmitter release was reduced to low levels by adding 10 to 20 $\mu M\ Cd^{2+}$ to the bath. Cd^{2+} blocks the entry of Ca^{2+} into the presynaptic terminals, and leads to frequent failures of transmission. The results from experiments using the Sr^{2+} and Cd^{2+} strategies yielded very

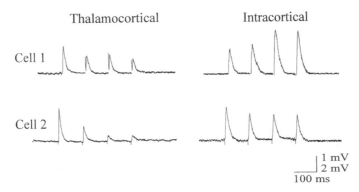

Figure 8.2 Thalamocortical synapses (left) are more strongly depressed by 10-Hz activation than are intracortical synapses (right). Examples of each type of synaptic input are shown for two different neurons. (From Gil et al. 1997a.)

similar results. The quantal EPSP size distributions implied for both TC and IC synapses had mean amplitudes of about 0.4 mV, and each synapse generated mean peaks of about 14 pA under voltage clamp conditions (Gil et al. in press). The evoked quantal EPSPs were also indistinguishable from the amplitude distributions of spontaneous EPSPs in the same cells. The results suggest that two classes of glutamatergic synapses, which arise from very different presynaptic cells (i.e., thalamic relay cells and cortical pyramidal cells) but converge on the same postsynaptic cortical pyramidal cell, have equal quantal size.

Short-Term Dynamics of Thalamocortical, Intracortical, and Corticothalamic Synapses

Despite the central importance of the thalamocorticothalamic loops, no study has directly assessed the short-term dynamics of the synapses within them. We have examined these in thalamocortical slices by stimulating specific pathways with either paired pulse or short trains of variable frequency. When convergent TC and IC synapses were compared in the paradigm described above (Gil et al. 1997a), clear differences were evident. Whereas the IC synapses generated either weak depression or slight facilitation during stimulus trains, the TC synapses were inevitably strongly depressed (figure 8.2). Paired-pulse stimuli revealed the largest differences between TC and IC synapses at the shorter interstimulus intervals, from 10 to 100 ms; the pathways were less distinctive at intervals greater than 100 ms. The paired-pulse ratio (measured at a 50-ms interval) for IC synapses almost always exceeds that for TC synapses when tested on the same neuron (figure 8.3).

Within the parallel pathways between thalamus and cortex lie enormous feedback connections (the CT fibers of figure 8.1), which may greatly outnumber the feedforward connections. For example, relay nuclei of the thala-

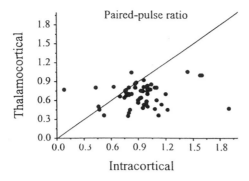

Figure 8.3 Comparison of short-term plasticity for TC and IC synapses. Paired stimuli (50-ms interstimulus interval) were delivered to TC or IC axons, and the paired-pulse ratio was calculated as the size of the second response relative to the first. Each point plots data from one neuron (n = 57), and the line has a unity slope. (From Gil et al. 1997a.)

mus contribute fewer than 20% of the total synapses onto neurons of cortical layer 4, the main input layer for primary sensory areas (LeVay and Gilbert 1976; White and Keller 1989). Feedback connections to thalamus from cortex may outnumber feedforward connections by up to fortyfold, and account for about 50% of the synapses on thalamic relay neurons (Sherman and Koch 1986). There have been few physiological studies of identified CT synapses (cf. Kao and Coulter 1997). We have prepared living thalamocortical slices, demonstrated with rhodamine-dextran axonal tracers that some of the corticothalamic pathways remain intact, and renamed them corticothalamic slices (Bourassa et al. 1995). These slices have been used to study the physiology of CT synapses onto cells of a relay nucleus (ventral posterior, VP) and the posteromedial (Pom) nucleus of the somatosensory thalamus (Landisman et al. 1997; Castro-Alamancos et al. 1997). Intracellular recordings from thalamic neurons reveal fast, glutamatergic EPSPs when stimuli are applied to cortical layer 6. CT synapses usually produce facilitation during paired-pulse or short-train stimulus protocols. This stands in sharp contrast to the ascending TC synapses, which strongly depress under the same conditions, and the IC synapses, which only rarely show a weak facilitation.

The results from TC, IC, and CT synapses (schematized in figure 8.4) emphasize the wide range of synaptic behaviors governing interconnections within the thalamus-neocortex axis. Previous work on cerebral cortex emphasizes that variability is indeed the rule. For example, some hippocampal pathways show strong facilitation, while neocortical synapses more often depress (Thomson and Deuchars 1994; Abbott et al. 1997; Varela et al. 1997). Post-tetanic potentiation has not been described in neocortex, but it is quite potent in hippocampal pathways (Kirkwood et al. 1993; Malenka 1995; Castro-Alamancos et al. 1995). The survey of neocortical synapses is far from complete, but it is clear that different classes of synapses may have very different properties. Excitatory synapses between layer 5 pyramidal cells usually show depression (along with a high probability of release to the

Pathway-Specific Regulation of Synapses

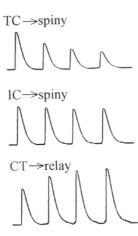

TC→spiny

IC→spiny

CT→relay

Figure 8.4 Schematic summary of the different dynamics of three types of synapses within the thalamocorticothalamic loop. During brief 10-Hz stimulation TC synapses most strongly depress, IC synapses depress less or occasionally facilitate, while CT synapses usually facilitate.

first stimulus; Thomson and Deuchars 1994; Tsodyks and Markram 1997), while layer 5 pyramidal cell synapses ending on some inhibitory interneurons show dramatic facilitation (and low probability of first release; Thomson and Deuchars 1994, 1997). These results imply that presynaptic function might be determined by the postsynaptic neuron. This is not universally true, however, as numerous studies of invertebrate systems imply (e.g., see Davis and Murphey 1994). Data presented here, as well as the results of Stratford et al. (1996) from visual cortex, show that differences of dynamics are correlated with the presynaptic neuron type.

Theory predicts interesting implications for short-term synapse dynamics. Depression may serve to enhance the information capacity of intracortical synapses (Abbott et al. 1997; Tsodyks and Markram 1997). When the rate of depression is relatively fast (as in TC synapses), postsynaptic responses will reflect the temporal coherence of the presynaptic firing. On the other hand, slower rates (as in many IC synapses), while providing some gain control, tend to evoke firing postsynaptically that is related to the intensity of the input. The general implications of facilitating synapses (such as CT synapses) were not considered in previous analyses. In general, however, we can predict that the diverse dynamics of synapses will strongly influence the interactions within thalamocortical loops.

Pathway-Specific Neuromodulation of Thalamocortical and Intracortical Synapses

Neurotransmitters in the neocortex have two general modes of action: (1) rapid excitation and inhibition, mainly via glutamate and γ-aminobutyric acid (GABA) acting on ligand-gated ion channels, and (2) slower modulation of pre- or postsynaptic excitability, mediated mainly by acetylcholine (ACh), norepinephrine (NE), serotonin, histamine, dopamine, various peptides, and glutamate and GABA themselves, virtually all operating via G protein–coupled receptors (McCormick 1992). Each type has distinctly different anatomical systems. Fast glutamate and GABA mechanisms use local intra-cortical axons, as well as specific, spatially discrete inputs from the thalamus. Modulators mainly arise from small sets of subcortical neurons that inner-vate large regions of neocortex. The slower-acting modulators can signifi-cantly alter neural network properties, and they are important regulators of the general functional state of the forebrain.

The membranes of presynaptic terminals express a variety of neuro-modulator receptors (Marder 1996; McGehee and Role 1996; Wu and Saggau 1997). Activation of these may lead to either enhancement or reduc-tion of transmitter release probability (e.g., see Manzoni et al. 1994; Capogna et al. 1995; Chen and Regehr 1997). While the postsynaptic effects of neuro-modulators have been relatively well characterized in neocortex, their pre-synaptic influence has been largely ignored. We have studied the presynaptic effects of two ubiquitous modulators in the cortex: GABA acting via the GABA$_B$ receptor, and ACh acting via either G protein–coupled muscarinic receptors or ionotropic nicotinic receptors. The experimental setup was the same as described above: both TC and IC synaptic inputs were recorded from single layer 3 pyramidal cells in vitro. Possible postsynaptic effects of the neuromodulators were suppressed by pharmacologically blocking K$^+$ currents and GABA$_A$ receptors in the recorded neuron.

The sensitivity of thalamocortical and intracortical terminals to the tested modulators proved to be dramatically different (figure 8.5A; Gil et al. 1997a). Transmitter release from the IC synapses was depressed by application of the GABA$_B$ receptor agonist baclofen, but the response from TC synapses was unaffected. In contrast, nicotinic cholinergic agonists *enhanced* release only from TC synapses, but had no effect on IC synapses. Specific muscarinic receptor activation was not pathway-selective; it depressed release from both synapse types.

The effect of presynaptic modulation was not a simple scaling of efficacy upward or downward. Instead, modulators also affected the dynamic proper-ties of each synapse (figure 8.5B), as assessed by paired-pulse measurements. Activation of GABA$_B$ receptors on IC synapses reduced paired-pulse depres-sion, but TC synapses were insensitive to GABA$_B$ manipulation. Somewhat paradoxically, an antagonist of GABA$_B$ receptors (CGP35348) also reduced depression, presumably by blocking the action of GABA released endge-nously by the first stimulus of the pair. Muscarinic activation reduced de-pression in both TC and IC synapses. However, nicotine, which enhanced low-frequency transmission only in the TC pathway, also increased paired-pulse depression there.

Our results demonstrate that distinct sets of synapses within the neo-cortex are differentially affected by neuromodulators. This suggests a poten-tial mechanism for adjusting the relative strengths and dynamics of input and

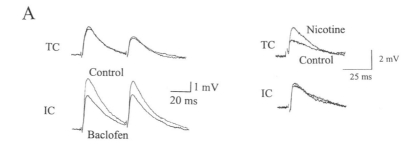

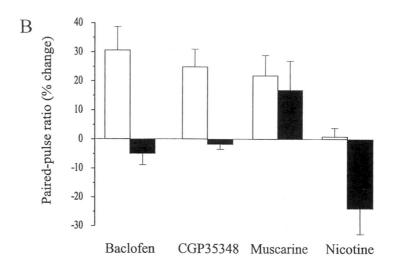

Figure 8.5 Differential regulation of TC and IC synapses by neuromodulators. (A) Application of the GABA$_B$ receptor agonist baclofen to TC and IC synapses on the same cell yields suppression only in the IC synapses; TC synapses are unaffected. On the other hand, activation of nicotinic acetylcholine receptors enhances TC synapses, while IC synapses are unaffected. (B) Modulators differentially affect synapse dynamics as well. The histogram plots changes in paired-pulse ratios (50-ms intervals) during activation (baclofen) or antagonism (CGP35348) of presynaptic GABA$_B$ receptors, or activation of muscarinic or nicotinic presynaptic receptors in TC or IC synapses. Positive values imply that the drug caused an increase in paired-pulse ratio; negative values imply a decrease. (From Gil et al. 1997.)

associational pathways during changes of behavioral state. Neuromodulators can be divided into two basic types: those released from sources intrinsic to a local circuit, and those that arise from extrinsic sources (Katz and Frost 1996). We tested one of each type: GABA is largely intrinsic to the cortex, and its release rate is expected to parallel the level of local activity in cortical circuits, while ACh is derived from control circuits extrinsic to neocortex (Rye et al. 1984; Eckenstein and Baughman 1987). We found that TC (input) synapses and IC (associational) synapses have qualitatively different sensitivities to each modulator. Synapses of piriform cortex and hippocampus may also be differentially modulated by ACh (Kahle and Cotman 1989; Hasselmo and Bower 1992; Gray et al. 1996) and $GABA_B$ receptors (Colbert and Levy 1992; Tang and Hasselmo 1994). Taken together, these results reinforce the suggestion of Hasselmo (1995), that the selective modulation of intrinsic and afferent synapses is a general organizational feature of the cerebral cortex.

PATHWAY-SPECIFIC DYNAMICS OF THALAMOCORTICAL ACTIVITY IN VIVO

Our studies of the forebrain in vitro imply that thalamocortical transmission is very sensitive to repetitive activation. If the properties of first-order synapses alone determine thalamus-to-cortex transformations, then activating the ascending pathways in vivo should lead to strongly depressing responses at frequencies faster than about 1 Hz. But other factors are likely to complicate this prediction. First, are the properties of individual synapses characterized in brain slices in vitro similar to those in vivo? Synaptic function is so easily modified by local conditions, such as the particular cocktail of neuromodulators in the local milieu, that synapses in slices might poorly represent the status of working synapses in situ. Second, how does local circuitry alter the ascending flow of activity from thalamus to cortex? Relevant circuitry might include parallel pathways onto excitatory and inhibitory neurons, lateral connections between these cells, and even recurrent connections from cortex back to thalamus. Third, is there a role for intrinsic postsynaptic membrane properties in temporal dynamics of the pathways? Both cortical and thalamic neurons are notable for their complex and wide-ranging intrinsic properties (Connors and Gutnick 1990), and the possible cell-specificity of thalamic connections could engage neuronal populations with very different dynamic characteristics (Agmon and Connors 1992; Gil and Amitai 1996b). We have begun to sort out some of these issues using a simple test of thalamocortical responses assessed in vivo.

Ventroposterolateral vs. Ventrolateral Pathways to Sensorimotor Cortex

The ventroposterolateral (VPL) nucleus of the thalamus relays somatosensory information to the sensorimotor cortex; adjacent to VPL is the ventrolateral (VL) nucleus, which has motor functions and also sends axons into sensorimotor regions of the cortex. The areas of VPL and VL termination in cortex partly overlap, although they have different laminar selectivities (figure 8.6A; Donoghue et al. 1979). Electrical stimulation of a primary thalamocortical pathway, such as VPL, produces a characteristic response in the cortex of an anesthetized animal. One way to reveal the spatiotemporal response patterns is to measure extracellular voltage at regular intervals through the cortical

A

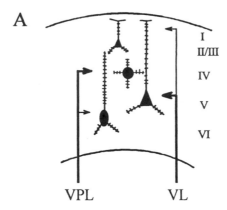

I
II/III
IV
V
VI

VPL   VL

B

Decremental Response   Augmenting Response

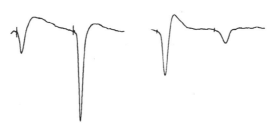

Figure 8.6 A, Schematic diagram of the dominant projection laminae of the ventroposterolateral (VPL) and ventrolateral (VL) nuclei into sensorimotor cortex of the rat. B, Field potential responses of cortex to paired stimuli (100-ms intervals) to either the VPL nucleus (Decremental Response) or the VL nucleus (Augmenting Response). (Data from Castro-Alamancos and Connors 1996b.)

depth, and calculate a map of current source density (CSD). We have tested cortical responses from VPL stimulation in the ketamine-anesthetized rat. Activation of VPL axons generates short-latency current sinks in layers 6 and 4, followed by spread of the upper sink into layer 3 (Castro-Alamancos and Connors 1996b). This spatial pattern of current flow agrees well with the anatomy of primary thalamocortical projections. The VPL-to-cortex response is relatively invariant at low frequencies of activation, but at higher frequencies (i.e., especially above 5 Hz) the response to the second stimulus becomes strongly depressed (figure 8.6B). We have called this depression the *decremental response*, and it is strongly reminiscent of the intrinsic frequency-dependent depression of TC synapses observed in vitro (Gil et al. 1997a) and described above.

In contrast, stimulation delivered to the parallel VL thalamocortical pathway produces a response beginning with a relatively small current sink in layer 5 of the cortex, and in many cases an even smaller sink in layer 1 (Castro-Alamancos and Connors 1996b). This spatial pattern of currents is also consistent with the anatomical projections of VL and similar types of thalamic nuclei (see Castro-Alamancos and Connors 1997b for review). The VL response is relatively stable at low stimulation rates, but activation at frequencies of about 7 to 14 Hz generates, paradoxically, a strong enhancement of the response (see figure 8.6B). A very similar type of thalamocortical enhancement was originally described by Dempsey and Morison (1943), who dubbed it the *augmenting response*. At first glance, we might suspect that augmenting implies that the VL-to-cortex synapses behave quite differently from the VPL-to-cortex synapses, since VPL synapses tend to depress so strongly. However there is no evidence that the two types of TC synapses differ, and close evaluation of the CSD patterns from VPL and VL reveal that the monosynaptic TC components of both depress when activated at frequencies that produce augmenting in the VL pathway. Indeed, augmenting occurs *in spite of* the intrinsic tendency of TC synapses to depress. As we shall see, the mechanisms of augmenting are complex, with critical and interacting contributions from intrinsic synapse and membrane properties, and from local circuitry.

Sources of Short-Term Depression in Primary Thalamocortical Responses

When tested with paired-pulse stimuli, responses of the primary (VPL) thalamocortical pathway in vivo have a biphasic temporal profile. It starts with prominent depression at interstimulus intervals (ISIs) shorter than 200 ms, falls back to baseline after about 300 ms, and ends with a period of weaker depression at longer intervals until recovery is attained at two to five seconds (figure 8.7). Within the cortex VPL axons strongly activate cells in layer 4, and their axons in turn synapse densely upon layer 3 neurons, as implied by the upwardly propagating current sink. Activating this layer 4–to-3 pathway in a slice in vitro yields depression similar to that of the VPL-to-cortex pathway (Castro-Alamancos and Connors 1997a; Abbott et al. 1997). It is important to note that frequency-dependent depression is not a consequence of anesthesia, nor of slicing, since it occurs in awake, intact animals (Castro-Alamancos and Connors 1996b).

What is the source of the frequency-dependent depression of the primary thalamocortical response and the second-order intracortical pathway? We have investigated the issue in neocortical slices and intact animals and identified several potential causes of depression. First, the excitatory synapses along these pathways may have a relatively high baseline probability of transmitter release, leading to depression when initial activity reduces the immediately available pool of releasable neurotransmitter (Gil et al. 1997, in press). Second, a strong and long-lasting disynaptic inhibition is recruited by the thalamocortical pathways, and shunts the monosynaptic excitatory input (Castro-Alamancos and Connors 1996b; Gil and Amitai 1996a,b; Swadlow 1995). Finally, stimulus-induced release of neuromodulatory substances

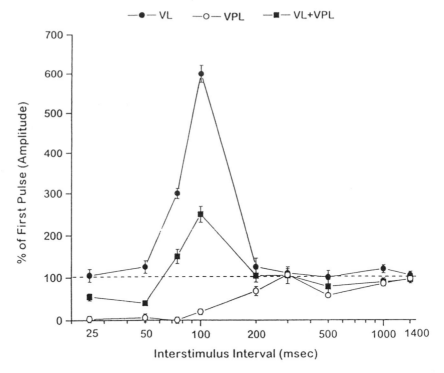

Figure 8.7 Effects of paired-pulse stimuli, of varying intervals, when applied to VL, VPL, or both while recording in sensorimotor cortex of the rat. Data are expressed as the percentage of change in the amplitude of the second response relative to the first. (From Castro-Alamancos and Connors 1996.)

within the cortex can temporarily decrease the efficacy of synapses by acting on presynaptic terminals (Castro-Alamancos and Connors 1996e; Gil et al. 1997a). The relative importance of each of these during normal function remains to be determined.

Mechanisms of Augmenting Responses of Secondary Thalamocortical Responses

Why should the response to one thalamic pathway so strongly depress, while a parallel pathway, activating the same region of cortex, displays such a sharp enhancement? Morison and Dempsey (1943) attributed the augmenting response to a purely thalamic mechanism. More recent work points to the cortex as a primary site for the augmenting response, however. Neither thalamic lesions (Morin and Steriade 1981; Ferster and Lindstrom 1985) nor reversible inactivation of thalamic circuitry with microinjections of GABA or kynurenic acid impair the augmenting response (Castro-Alamancos and Connors 1996b). Thus it is very unlikely that the augmenting response is exclusively due to a polysynaptic intrathalamic process that is relayed to the cortex, although in the decorticate brain the thalamus can generate enhanced responses similar to cortical augmenting (Steriade and Timofeev 1997). How does the cortex generate augmenting? In considering the likely mechanisms of this augmenting response, several characteristics are particularly informative (Castro-Alamancos and Connors 1996b,c,d):

First, the frequency dependence of the augmenting response is peculiar. Augmented responses can be generated only within a narrow time interval following a single conditioning stimulus—the second stimulus must occur between 50 and 200 ms. Intervals longer or shorter than this yield responses near control levels (see figure 8.7).

Second, concurrent with the termination of the opportune augmenting interval, at around 200 ms, is the onset of a long-latency event within the cortex; this event consists of a slow, negative field potential component when measured extracellularly, and a barrage of EPSPs when measured intracellularly (figure 8.8). If a second, augmenting, stimulus is applied before this late-onset event, then the late EPSPs and field potential are occluded.

Third, current-source density analysis and single-cell recordings reveal that the response to the first stimulus, the augmenting response, and the long-latency potentials all occur in layer 5. The layer 5 current sink for the augmenting response is much stronger than the sink for the first response, concurrent with a similar increase in amplitude of a current source located in the upper layers. This dipolar arrangement suggests that the elongated pyramidal cells of layer 5 are the primary generators of the currents of the augmenting response.

Fourth, intracellular recordings in vivo reveal that a correlate of the narrow time interval for generating the augmenting response is a prominent hyperpolarization of layer 5 cells. This hyperpolarization is generated by fast and slow IPSPs (Connors et al. 1988) recruited by thalamocortical activation of inhibitory interneurons, and it is terminated by the long-latency depolarizing (EPSP) event.

Fifth, layer 5 has a subpopulation of pyramidal cells with specific membrane conductances that can be activated or deinactivated by hyperpolarization. These conductances apparently mediate low-threshold calcium currents (I_T) and hyperpolarization-activated cationic currents (I_H). Activation of these currents can generate rebound bursts of spikes in these layer 5 neurons following brief hyperpolarizations (Silva et al. 1991).

These and other observations indicate that augmenting responses arise initially from neural circuitry within cortical layer 5. Anterograde tracers show that the main terminations of the VL projection are within layers 1 and 5 (Yamamoto et al. 1990) or layers 1, 3, and 5 (Herkenham 1986) in the rat motor cortex. CSD analysis of responses to VL stimulation shows two current sinks, with the earliest located in layer 5 and a longer-latency component in layer 1. Thus, unlike the VPL pathway, VL afferents seem to directly excite neurons within layer 5 (see figure 8.6A). We suspect that this distinction is critical.

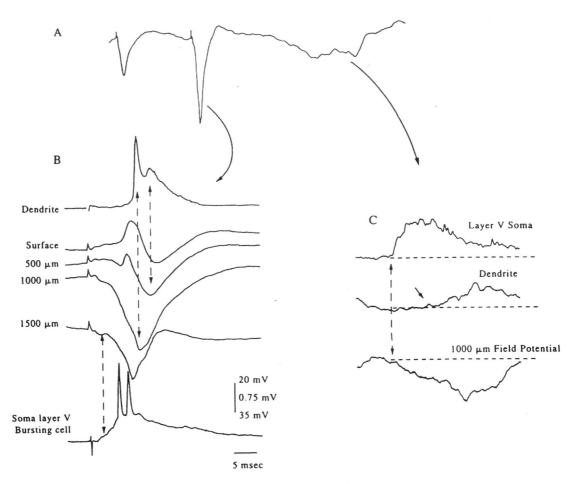

Figure 8.8 Augmenting responses originate in layer 5 and propagate to upper cortical layers. (A) Augmenting field potential in response to paired VL stimuli (100-ms interstimulus interval). (B) Augmented (second) responses recorded as field potentials from various cortical depths (top five traces) or as an intracellular response from the soma of an intrinsically bursting neuron of layer 5 (bottom). (C) Long-latency responses following the second, augmented response, recorded as a field potential or as intracellular recordings from a presumed dendrite or layer 5 soma. (From Castro-Alamancos and Connors 1997.)

Our hypothetical mechanism for the augmenting response (Castro-Alamancos and Connors 1996d) begins with excitatory VL synapses terminating on the large pyramidal cells of layer 5, and briefly depolarizing them. Because the membrane channels mediating I_T and I_H in layer 5 cells are largely inactivated at resting potential, the first postsynaptic response of the thalamocortical synapses is modest. However VL afferents monosynaptically activate inhibitory interneurons, and the fast IPSPs they trigger transiently hyperpolarize the pyramidal cells of layer 5, thus activating I_H and deinactivating I_T. If a subsequent excitatory thalamocortical input occurs after an appropriate interval, it can trigger larger depolarizing responses in postsynaptic neurons because of the activation of I_T-like currents and the addition of I_H. In addition, spike firing by layer 5 pyramidal cells is reinforced because of their tendency to mutually excite one another through local axon collaterals (Chagnac-Amitai et al. 1990; Amitai and Connors 1995; Nicoll and Blakemore 1993; Markram and Tsodyks 1996). If a second VL stimulus is not applied, then the long-latency EPSPs that occur after about 200 ms imply that rebound bursting is occurring nevertheless in a subset of layer 5 cells. As these cells depolarize and burst, they signal the end of the augmenting opportunity because I_T and I_H are once again inactivated.

Once generated, an augmenting response propagates horizontally into adjacent cortical territory (Castro-Alamancos and Connors 1996b,c), and also vertically from layer 5 into the upper layers. In addition to the synaptically mediated spread of the augmenting response through the local neuronal network, an augmented response may also propagate upward (retrogradely) within the apical dendrites of layer 5 pyramidal cells via mechanisms involving active dendritic conductances (Castro-Alamancos and Connors 1996d).

If the proposed model for generation of the augmenting response in vivo is correct, then appropriate stimuli delivered to isolated slices of cortex in vitro should trigger an augmenting response. Indeed, stimulation and recording locally within layer 5 of a slice does generate a nascent augmenting effect, while the network of layer 3 cells displays only depression. Finally, if it is true that postsynaptic membrane properties and network amplification mediate the augmenting response, then we would predict that augmenting (unlike synaptic facilitation) should not be input-specific. In a test of this prediction, stimulation of two independent pathways converging onto layer 5 cells in vitro showed that augmenting can be conditioned by a stimulus to either pathway, and triggered by a subsequent stimulus to the other pathway (see Castro-Alamancos and Connors 1996d).

Augmenting Responses Are Rapidly Modified by Behavior and Neuromodulators

The augmenting response provides an exciting window onto some of the mechanisms that modulate the excitability of the cortex during awake behavior. We found that the response was simple to assess with field potentials, yet is a sensitive and rapid indicator of function in the thalamocortical pathway. Most notably, in unrestrained, spontaneously behaving rats the augmenting response is prominent when animals are immobile and resting (but nevertheless awake), and it promptly inactivates during active exploration of the environment or performance of a skilled motor task (figure 8.9; Castro-Alamancos and Connors 1996c). The behavioral modulation of augmenting is remarkably specific; during exploration the primary (first) thalamocortical response is unaltered, but subsequent responses delivered at optimal intervals are not augmented. This implies that the frequency-selectivity of the VL-to-cortex pathway is modulated moment by moment during behavior.

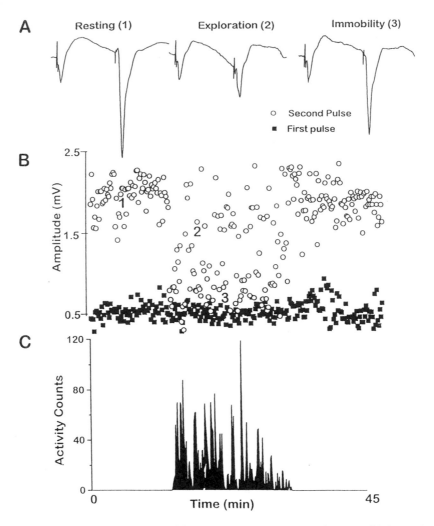

Figure 8.9 Rapid modulation of the augmenting response as a function of behavioral state. Cortical field potential responses were recorded from awake, freely behaving rats over a period of forty-five minutes. (A) Raw responses are illustrated during awake resting, during active exploration, and during a brief period of awake immobility. (B) The amplitudes of the first and second evoked responses are plotted as a function of time; numbered points refer to the times of examples in A. (C) Gross motor activity was recorded by a series of photobeams and detectors, and displayed as activity counts as a function of time. (From Castro-Alamancos and Connors 1996.)

Our analysis of the characteristics and mechanisms for the behavioral modulation of the augmenting response are far from complete. Modulation seems to correlate more with a general state change, rather than with a particular movement or task. This suggests that the effect arises from a change in the activity of some diffuse neuromodulatory system associated with arousal or attention. There are several possible candidates for this putative modulator(s), and a much longer list of the receptor subtypes it might activate. These receptors are widely distributed, with the potential to modify just about every corner of the thalamocortical system, including pre- and postsynaptic elements, excitatory and inhibitory neurons, and even axons and glia (McCormick and Bal 1997). However the cellular distribution of each particular receptor is very selective, as we described for the presynaptic modulation of TC and IC synapses (Gil et al. 1997a).

In preliminary experiments to characterize the modulators of the augmenting response, we used continuous perfusion through cortically implanted microdialysis probes while recording and stimulating in anesthetized animals (Castro-Alamancos and Connors 1996e). The dialysis probes provide a stable, repeatable, and reversible way to deliver (rather than to measure, as they are most often used) pharmacological agents locally, while testing electrophysiological function. We have so far tested only a few cholinergic and adrenergic agonists and antagonists, but the results are most consistent with the hypothesis that behavioral modulation of the augmenting response is mediated by the diffuse noradrenergic system. Perfusion of norepinephrine or certain of its agonists mimicked the specific effect of behavioral modulation on augmenting, without influencing primary thalamocortical responses. Cholinergic agonists had complex and interesting effects, but they did not resemble the behavioral modulation.

IMPLICATIONS

Neurons and synapses are exquisitely sensitive to the timing of impulses, and there is abundant evidence that timing is critical to the coding of information within the brain (Perkel and Bullock 1968; Rieke et al. 1997). The responsiveness of neocortical neurons to sensory stimuli depends on the frequency of those stimuli. Frequency-dependent depression in primary thalamocortical pathways may help to optimize the temporal integration of sensory inputs (Mountcastle et al. 1990; Recanzone et al. 1992). Cortical responses to tactile stimuli in the monkey strongly diminish at higher frequencies (Mountcastle et al. 1969). Similarly, responses of neurons in the barrel cortex rapidly decline during repetitive whisker displacements faster than about 15 Hz (Simons 1978), and frequency-dependent depression is stronger in cortex than in thalamus (Simons and Carvell 1989). This suggests that the connection between thalamus and cortex is one important locus of depression, and our measurements from TC synapses in vitro and in vivo confirm this directly. Our studies in vitro imply that the dynamic properties of synapses within the thalamocortical system vary widely, but with pathway-specificity—TC synapses depress strongly, some IC synapses depress weakly, and CT synapses most often facilitate. Thus synapse dynamics is an important variable in analyzing forebrain circuits, and no single synapse will serve as a general model for the rest. So far most synaptic pathways remain untested.

The dependence of the augmenting response on stimulus timing suggests a sharp and powerful resonance in certain thalamocortical pathways, centered at about 10 Hz. Many neurons and circuits within the isolated and intact cortex have a propensity to oscillate spontaneously in this frequency range (Connors and Amitai 1997). During augmenting responses, neural activity is strongly synchronized over large regions of neocortex. The mechanisms involved in augmenting may be similar or identical to those that underlie several oscillatory phenomena observed in the rat sensorimotor system. Brief whisker deflections will often generate a damped membrane oscillation in cortical cells, with a period of about 75 ms (Simons and Carvell 1989), and sensorimotor cortex of the rat can generate widespread 7 to 12-Hz oscillations during certain awake behavioral states (Semba and Komisaruk 1984; Buzsaki 1991; Nicolelis et al. 1995). The functions of these synchronous oscillations are not at all clear, but speculation includes roles in temporally encoding stimulus or whisker position, and in aspects of motor planning (Nicolelis et al. 1995; Fee et al. 1997; Ahissar et al. 1997).

A remarkable feature of the vertebrate brain is its ability to adapt rapidly to the vacillating and often unpredictable environment. This is accomplished in part by the diffuse ascending modulatory systems, whose activity varies sharply during changes of behavioral state and sleep-wake cycles (Aston-Jones and Bloom 1981; Steriade and Llinàs 1988; Cooper et al. 1991). The modulatory systems release substances that dramatically alter the properties of forebrain networks, and these effects must be considered when trying to understand virtually any function and dysfunction of cerebral cortex. Eclectic approaches are helping to sort out the particular role of each system in specific adaptive aspects of behavior. For example, it is very likely that each monoaminergic and cholinergic system has a unique and different function in the control of various processes that are classically called "arousal" and "attention" (Robbins and Everitt 1995). The mechanisms of modulatory control are exceedingly complex, and each transmitter may act simultaneously at many different subcellular sites. Attempts to synthesize the available data on the roles of neurotransmitters in the control of behavioral state tend to emphasize their modulation of postsynaptic excitability (Steriade and McCarley 1990; McCormick and Bal 1997). However, the same transmitters clearly have potent and specific actions on critical presynaptic terminals of the cortex (Gil et al. 1997a), and presumably of the thalamus as well. A full understanding of modulators and their control of behavioral state must incorporate both sides of the synapse.

ACKNOWLEDGMENTS

Our research was generously supported by the National Institutes of Health, a Fogarty International Research Collaboration Award, the Israel Science Foundation, and the Helen Hay Whitney Foundation.

REFERENCES

Abbott, L. F., Varela, J. A., Sen, K., and Nelson, S. B. (1997). Synaptic depression and cortical gain control. *Science* 275: 220–224.

Agmon, A., and Connors, B. W. (1991). Thalamocortical responses of mouse somatosensory (barrel) cortex in vitro. *Neuroscience* 41: 365–380.

Agmon, A., and Connors, B. W. (1992). Correlation between intrinsic firing patterns and thalamocortical responses of mouse barrel cortex neurons. *J. Neurosci.* 12: 319–330.

Ahissar, E., Haidarliu, S., and Zacksenhouse, M. (1997). Decoding temporally encoded sensory input by cortical oscillations and thalamic phase comparators *Proc. Natl. Acad. Sci. USA* 94: 11633–11638.

Amitai, Y., and Connors, B. W. (1995). Intrinsic physiology and morphology of single neurons in neocortex. In: *Cerebral Cortex*, Vol. 11, E. G. Jones, I. Diamond (eds.), pp 229–331. New York: Plenum.

Aston-Jones, G., Bloom, F. E. (1981). Activity of norepinephrine-containing locus-coeruleus neurons in behaving rats anticipates fluctuations in the sleep-waking cycle. *J. Neurosci.* 1: 876–886.

Bennett, M. K., and Scheller, R. H. (1994). Molecular correlates of synaptic vesicle docking and fusion. *Curr. Opin. Neurobiol.* 4: 324–329.

Bourassa, J., Pinault, D., and Deschenes, M. (1995). Corticothalamic projections from the cortical barrel field to the somatosensory thalamus in rats: a single-fibre study using biocytin as an anterograde tracer. *Eur. J. Neurosci.* 7: 19–30.

Buzsaki, G. (1991). The thalamic clock: emergent network properties. *Neuroscience* 41: 351–364.

Capogna, M., Gahwiler, B. H., and Thompson, S. M. (1995). Presynaptic enhancement of inhibitory synaptic transmission by protein kinases, A and C in the rat hippocampus in vitro. *J. Neurosci.* 15: 1249–1260

Castro-Alamancos, M. A., and Connors, B. W. (1996a). Short-term synaptic enhancement predicts long-term potentiation in neocortex. *Proc. Natl. Acad. Sci. USA* 93: 1335–1339.

Castro-Alamancos, M. A., and Connors, B. W. (1996b). Spatiotemporal properties of short-term plasticity in sensorimotor thalamocortical pathways of the rat. *J. Neurosci.* 16: 2767–2779.

Castro-Alamancos, M. A., and Connors, B. W. (1996c). Behavioral state dynamically modulates short-term plasticity of a thalamocortical pathway. *Science* 272: 274–277.

Castro-Alamancos, M. A., and Connors, B. W. (1996d). Cellular mechanisms of the augmenting response: short-term plasticity in a thalamocortical pathway. *J. Neurosci.* 16: 7742–7756.

Castro-Alamancos, M. A., and Connors, B. W. (1996e). Noradrenergic and cholinergic modulation of augmenting responses in thalamocortical pathways. *Soc. Neurosci. Abstr.* 22: 18.

Castro-Alamancos, M. A., and Connors, B. W. (1997a). Distinct forms of synaptic plasticity in pathways of hippocampus and neocortex. *Proc. Natl. Acad. Sci. USA* 94: 4161–4166.

Castro-Alamancos, M. A., and Connors, B. W. (1997b). Thalamocortical synapses. *Prog. Neurobiol.* 51: 581–606.

Castro-Alamancos, M. A., Donoghue, J. P., and Connors, B. W. (1995). Different forms of synaptic plasticity in somatosensory and motor areas of the neocortex. *J. Neurosci.* 15: 5324–5333.

Castro-Alamancos, M. A., Landisman, C. E., and Connors, B. W. (1997). Mechanisms of facilitation at corticothalamic synapses in the ventrobasal thalamus. *Soc. Neurosci. Abstr.* 23: 574.

Chagnac-Amitai, Y., Luhmann, H., and Prince, D. A. (1990). Burst generating and regular spiking layer 5 pyramidal neurons of rat neocortex have different morphological features. *J. Comp. Neurol.* 296: 598–613.

Chen, C., and Regehr, W. G. (1997). The mechanism of cAMP-mediated enhancement at a cerebellar synapse. *J. Neurosci.* 17: 8687–8694.

Colbert, C. M., and Levy, W. B. (1992). Electrophysiological and pharmacological characterization of perforant path synapses in CA1: mediation by glutamate receptors. *J. Neurophysiol.* 68: 1–8.

Connors, B. W., and Amitai, Y. (1995). Functions of local circuits in neocortex: synchrony and laminae. In *The Cortical Neuron*, I Mody, MJ Gutnick, eds., pp. 123–141. New York, Cambridge University Press.

Connors, B. W., and Amitai, Y. (1997). Making waves in the neocortex. *Neuron* 18: 1–20.

Connors, B. W., and Gutnick, M. J. (1990). Intrinsic firing patterns of diverse neocortical neurons. *Trends Neurosci.* 13: 99–104.

Connors, B. W., Malenka, R. C., and Silva, R. L. (1988). Two inhibitory postsynaptic potentials, and $GABA_A$ and $GABA_B$ receptor-mediated responses in neocortex of rat and cat. *J. Physiol. (Lond.)* 406: 443–468.

Cooper, J. R., Bloom, F. E., and Roth, R. H. (1991). *The Biochemical Basis of Neuropharmacology.* New York, Oxford University Press.

Davis, G. W., and Murphey, R. K. (1994). Long-term regulation of short-term transmitter release properties: retrograde signalling and synaptic development. *Trends Neurosci.* 17: 9–13.

Debanne, D., Guérineau, N., Gähwiler, B. H., and Thompson, S. M. (1996). Paired-pulse facilitation and depression at unitary synapses in rat hippocampus: quantal fluctuation affects subsequent release. *J. Physiol. (Lond.)* 491: 163–176.

Dempsey, E. W., and Morison, R. S. (1943). The electrical activity of a thalamocortical relay system. *Am. J. Physiol.* 138: 283–296.

Donoghue, J. P., Kerman, K. L., and Ebner, F. F. (1979). Evidence for two organizational plans in the somatic sensory motor cortex of the rat. *J. Comp. Neurol.* 183: 647–663.

Eckenstein, F. P., and Baughman, R. W. (1987). The anatomical organization of the cholinergic system in the cerebral cortex. In *Cerebral Cortex*, Vol. 6, Peters, A. and Jones, E. G. eds., pp. 129–160. New York, Plenum Press.

Fee, M. S., Mitra, P. P., and Kleinfeld, D. (1997). Central versus peripheral determinants of patterned spike activity in rat vibrissa cortex during whisking. *J. Neurophysiol.* 78: 1144–1149.

Ferro-Novick, S., and Jahn, R. (1994). Vesicle fusion from yeast to man. *Nature* 370: 191–193.

Ferster, D., and Lindstrom, S. (1985). Augmenting responses evoked in area 17 of the cat by intracortical axon collaterals of cortico-geniculate cells. *J. Physiol. (Lond.)* 367: 217–232.

Gil, Z., and Amitai, Y. (1996a). Adult thalamocortical transmission involves both NMDA and nonNMDA receptors. *J. Neurophysiol.* 76: 2547–2553.

Gil, Z., and Amitai, Y. (1996b). Properties of convergent thalamocortical and intracortical synaptic potentials in single neurons of neocortex. *J. Neurosci.* 16: 6567–6578.

Gil, Z., and Connors, B. W., and Amitai, Y. (1997a). Differential regulation of neocortical synapses by activity and neuromodulators. *Neuron* 19: 679–686.

Gil, Z., and Connors, B. W., and Amitai, Y. (in press). Efficacy of thalamocortical and intracortical synaptic connections: quanta, innervation, and reliability. *Neuron*.

Gray, R., Rajan, A. S., Radcliffe, K. A., Yakehiro, M., and Dani, J. A. (1996). Hippocampal synaptic transmission enhanced by low concentrations of nicotine. *Nature* 383: 713–716.

Hasselmo, M. E. (1995). Neuromodulation and cortical function: modelling the physiological basis of behavior. *Behav. Brain Res.* 67: 1–27.

Hasselmo, M. E., and Bower, J. M. (1992). Cholinergic suppression specific to intrinsic not afferent fiber synapses in rat piriform (olfactory). cortex. *J. Neurophysiol.* 67: 1222–1229.

Herkenham, M. (1986). New perspectives on the organization and evolution of nonspecific thalamocortical projections. In: *Cerebral Cortex*, Vol. 5. E. G. Jones and A. Peters, eds., pp. 403–446. New York, Plenum.

Kahle, J. S., and Cotman, C. W. (1989). Carbachol depresses synaptic responses in the medial but not the lateral perforant path. *Brain Res.* 482: 159–163.

Kamiya, H., and Zucker, R. S. (1994). Residual Ca^{2+} and short-term synaptic plasticity *Nature* 371: 603–606.

Kao, C. Q., and Coulter, D. A. (1997). Physiology and pharmacology of corticothalamic stimulation-evoked responses in rat somatosensory thalamic neurons in vitro. *J. Neurophysiol.* 77: 2661–2676.

Katz, B. (1962). The Croonian Lecture. The transmission of impulses from nerve to muscle, and the subcellular unit of synaptic action. *Proc. R. Soc. Lond. B. Biol. Sci.* 155: 455–477.

Katz, P. S., and Frost, W. N. (1996). Intrinsic neuromodulation: altering neuronal circuits from within. *Trends Neurosci.* 19: 54–61.

Kirkwood, A., Dudek, S. M., Gold, J. T., Aizenman, C. D., and Bear, M. F. (1993). Common forms of synaptic plasticity in hippocampus and neocortex in vitro. *Science* 260: 1518–1521.

Landisman, C. E., Castro-Alamancos, M. A., and Connors, B. W. (1997). Properties of the corticothalamic pathways to the posterior nucleus of the thalamus. *Soc. Neurosci. Abstr.* 23: 574.

LeVay, S., and Gilbert, C. D. (1976). Laminar patterns of geniculocortical projection in the cat. *Brain Res.* 113: 1–19.

Magleby, K. L. (1987). Short-term changes in synaptic efficacy. In: *Synaptic Function*, G. M. Edelman, V. E. Gall, and K. M. Cowan, eds., pp. 21–56. New York. John Wiley & Sons.

Malenka, R. C. (1995). Synaptic plasticity in the neocortex and hippocampus: a comparison. In *The Cortical Neuron*, MJ Gutnick and I Mody, eds., pp. 98–110. New York, Cambridge University Press.

Malenka, R. C., and Nicoll, R. A. (1993). NMDA-receptor–dependent synaptic plasticity: multiple forms and mechanisms. *Trends Neurosci.* 16: 521–527.

Manzoni, O. J., Manabe, T., and Nicoll, R. A. (1994). Release of adenosine by activation of NMDA receptors in the hippocampus. *Science* 265: 2098–2101.

Marder, E. (1996). Neural modulation: following your own rhythm. *Curr. Biol.* 6: 119–121.

Markram, H., and Tsodyks, M. (1996). Redistribution of synaptic efficacy between neocortical pyramidal neurons. *Nature* 382: 807–810.

McCormick, D. A. (1992). Neurotransmitter actions in the thalamus and cerebral cortex and their role in neuromodulation of thalamocortical activity. *Prog. Neurobiol.* 39: 337–388.

McCormick, D. A., and Bal, T. (1997). Sleep and arousal: thalamocortical mechanisms. *Annu. Rev. Neurosci.* 20: 185–215.

McGehee, D. S., and Role, L. W. (1996). Presynaptic ionotropic receptors. *Curr. Opin. Neurobiol.* 6: 342–349.

McGehee, D. S., Heath, M. J., Gelber, S., Devay, P., and Role, L. W. (1995). Nicotinic enhancement of fast excitatory synaptic transmission. *Science* 269: 1692.

Morin, D., and Steriade, S. (1981). Development from primary to augmenting responses in the somatosensory system. *Brain Res.* 205: 49–66.

Morison, R. S., and Dempsey, E. W. (1943). Mechanism of thalamocortical augmentation and repetition. *Am. J. Physiol.* 138: 297–308.

Mountcastle, V. B., Talbot, W. H., Sakata, H., and Hyvarinen, J. (1969). Cortical neuronal mechanisms in flutter-vibration studied in unanesthetized monkeys. Neuronal periodicity and frequency discrimination. *J. Neurophysiol.* 32: 452–484.

Mountcastle, V. B., Steinmetz, M. A., and Romo, R. (1990). Cortical neuronal periodicities and frequency discrimination in the sense of flutter. *Cold. Spring. Harb. Symp. Quant. Biol.* 55: 861–872.

Murthy, V. N., Sejnowski, T. J., and Stevens, C. F. (1997). Heterogeneous release properties of visualized individual hippocampal synapses. *Neuron* 18: 599–612.

Nicolelis, M. A., Baccala, L. A., Lin, R. C., and Chapin, J. K. (1995). Sensorimotor encoding by synchronous neural ensemble activity at multiple levels of the somatosensory system. *Science* 268: 1353–1358.

Nicoll, A., and Blakemore, C. (1993). Single-fibre EPSPs in layer 5 of rat visual cortex in vitro. *Neuroreport* 4: 167–170.

Oliet, S. H., Malenka. R. C., and Nicoll, R. A. (1996). Bidirectional control of quantal size by synaptic activity in the hippocampus. *Science* 271: 1294–1297.

Pierce, J. P., and Lewin, G. R. (1994). An ultrastructural size principle. *Neuroscience* 58: 441–446.

Perkel, D. H., and Bullock, T. H. (1968). Neural coding. *Neurosci. Res. Prog. Bull.* 6: 221–348.

Regehr, W. G., Delaney, K. R., and Tank, D. W. (1994). The role of presynaptic calcium in short-term enhancement at the hippocampal mossy fiber synapse. *J. Neurosci.* 14: 523–537.

Recanzone, G. H., Merzenich, M. M., Schreiner, C. E. (1992). Changes in the distributed temporal response properties of SI cortical neurons reflect improvements in performance on a temporally based tactile discrimination task. *J. Neurophysiol.* 67: 1071–1091.

Rieke, F., Warland, D., de Ruyter van Steveninck, R., and Bialek, W. (1997). *Spikes: Exploring the Neural Code.* Cambridge, MA, MIT Press.

Robbins, T. W., and Everitt, B. J. (1995). Arousal systems and attention. In *The Cognitive Neurosciences*, M. S. Gazzaniga, ed., pp. 703–719. Cambridge, MA, MIT Press.

Rye, D. B., Wainer, B. H., Mesulam, M. M., Mufson, M. F., and Saper, C. P. (1984). Cortical projections arising from the basal forebrain: a study of cholinergic and noncholinergic components employing combined retrograde tracing and immunohistochemical localization of choline acetyltransferase. *Neuroscience* 13: 627–643.

Schikorski, T., and Stevens, C. F. (1997). Quantitative ultrastructural analysis of hippocampal excitatory synapses. *J. Neurosci.* 17: 5858–5867.

Semba, K., and Komisaruk, B. R. (1984). Neural substrates of two different rhythmical vibrissal movements in the rat. *Neuroscience* 12: 761–774.

Sherman, S. M., and Guillery, R. W. (1996). Functional organization of thalamocortical relays. *J. Neurophysiol.* 76: 1367–1395.

Sherman, S. M., and Koch, C. (1986). The control of retinogeniculate transmission in the mammalian lateral geniculate nucleus. *Exp. Brain Res.* 63: 1–20.

Silva, L. R., Amitai, Y., and Connors, B. W. (1991). Intrinsic oscillations of neocortex generated by layer 5 pyramidal neurons. *Science* 251: 432–435.

Simons, D. J. (1978). Response properties of vibrissa units in rat SI somatosensory neocortex. *J. Neurophysiol.* 41: 798–820.

Simons, D. J., and Carvell, G. E. (1989). Thalamocortical response transformation in the rat vibrissa/barrel system. *J. Neurophysiol.* 61: 311–330.

Steriade, M. (1997). Synchronized activities of coupled oscillators in the cerebral cortex and thalamus at different levels of vigilance. *Cereb. Cortex* 7: 583–604.

Steriade, M., and Llinàs, R. R. (1988). The functional states of the thalamus and the associated neuronal interplay. *Physiol. Rev.* 68: 649–742.

Steriade, M., and McCarley, R. W. (1990). *Brainstem Control of Wakefulness and Sleep.* New York, Plenum Press.

Steriade, M., and Timofeev, I. (1997). Short-term plasticity during intrathalamic augmenting responses in decorticated cats. *J. Neurosci.* 17: 3778–3795.

Stevens, C. F., and Wang, Y. (1995). Facilitation and depression at single central synapses. *Neuron* 14: 795–802.

Stratford, K. J., Tarczy-Hornoch, K., Martin, K. A. C., Bannister, N. J., and Jack, J. J. B. (1996). Excitatory synaptic inputs to spiny stellate cells in cat visual cortex. *Nature* 382: 258–261.

Swadlow, H. A. (1995). Influence of VPM afferents on putative inhibitory interneurons in S1 of the awake rabbit: evidence from cross-correlation, microstimulation and latencies of peripheral sensory stimulation. *J. Neurophysiol.* 73: 1584–1599.

Tang, A. C., Hasselmo, M. E. (1994). Selective suppression of intrinsic but not afferent fiber synaptic transmission by baclofen in the piriform (olfactory). cortex. *Brain Res.* 659: 75–81.

Thomson, A. M., and Deuchars, J. (1994). Temporal and spatial properties of local circuits in neocortex. *Trends Neurosci.* 17: 119–126.

Thomson, A. M., and Deuchars, J. (1997). Synaptic interactions in neocortical local circuits: dual intracellular recordings in vitro. *Cereb. Cortex* 7: 510–522.

Tsodyks, M. V., and Markram, H. (1997). The neural code between neocortical pyramidal neurons depends on neurotransmitter release probability. *Proc. Natl. Acad. Sci. USA* 94: 719–723.

Varela, J. A., Sen, K., Gibson, J., Fost, J., Abbott, L. F., and Nelson S. B. (1997). A quantitative description of short-term plasticity at excitatory synapses in layer 2/3 of rat primary visual cortex. *J. Neurosci.* 17: 7926–7940.

White, E. L., and Keller, A. (1989). *Cortical Circuits: Synaptic Organization of the Cerebral Cortex—Structure, Function and Theory.* Boston, Birkhäuser.

Wu, L. G., and Saggau, P. (1997). Presynaptic inhibition of elicited neurotransmitter release. *Trends Neurosci.* 20: 204–212.

Yamamoto, T., Kishimoto, Y., Yoshikawa, H., and Oka, H. (1990). Cortical laminar distribution of rat thalamic ventrolateral fibers demonstrated by the PHA-L anterograde labeling method. *Neurosci. Res.* 9: 148–154.

Zucker, R. S. (1989). Short term synaptic plasticity. *Annu. Rev. Neurosci.* 12: 13–31.

9 Dynamic Representation of Odors by Oscillating Neural Assemblies

Gilles Laurent, Katrina MacLeod, Mark Stopfer, and Michael Wehr

A major goal of modern neuroscience is to understand the various facets of neural coding by brain circuits. Since the pioneering work of Adrian, it has become unambiguously clear that neuronal firing rates usually represent certain attributes of a stimulus. Other results, including Adrian's own (Adrian 1942, 1950), however, indicated that neuronal responses to static sensory stimuli are often temporally structured, suggesting that the time structure of spike trains might also play a role in information coding. Early work in the mammalian olfactory bulb (OB), for example, showed prominent (30 to 80 Hz) oscillations in the electroencephalogram (EEG), riding on slower (5 to 10 Hz) waveforms coupled to sniffing (Adrian 1942; Freeman 1975, 1978, 1992; Gray and Skinner 1988). More recent work in cat and primate visual cortex indicates that pairs of neurons often synchornize and oscillate under very specific stimulation conditions (Eckhorn et al. 1988; Gray and Singer 1989; Singer and Gray 1995; Engel et al. 1991; Jagadeesh et al. 1992). Similarly, work in primate striate cortex suggests that stimulus evoked neuronal responses contain complex temporal features that can be described with a small number of principal parameters (Optican and Richmond 1987; McClurkin et al. 1991a,b; Gawne et al. 1996; Geisler et al. 1991; Heller et al. 1995). In primate frontal cortex, Abeles and co-workers described exquisitely precise sequences of neural activation distributed over several neurons (Abeles 1991; Abeles and Goldstein 1977; Abeles and Gerstein 1988). In some cases, the occurrence of these statistically improbable events is well correlated with the monkey's behavioral task (Vaadia et al. 1995). In auditory cortex, it was recently shown that the degree of pairwise correlation between neurons is sometimes steadily increased during presentation of a pure tone, even though the firing rate of those neurons is no different from that outside of the stimulation period (deCharms and Merzenich 1996). Although neurons, especially in mammalian cortex, appear to be "noisy" because their responses to a constant stimulus are "variable," recent in vitro physiological results show that the mechanisms underlying spike generation can be very precise (Mainen and Sejnowski 1995), providing parts of a potential mechanistic substrate for high-resolution temporal codes (Victor and Purpura 1996).

If information about a stimulus is indeed contained in temporal features of neural activity, is it useful to the animal? In other words, can it be decoded by downstream circuits, and can it be shown that the animal or its brain "cared" about these features? These questions need to be answered before we can convincingly argue that temporal codes are relevant to perception. We have recently developed and studied a preparation in which olfactory stimuli appear to be represented by ensembles of neurons that display both stimulus-evoked oscillatory synchronization and slower, but precise and stimulus-specific, temporal response patterns (Laurent and Davidowitz 1994; Laurent et al. 1996; Wehr and Laurent 1996; Laurent 1996b). We have identified one essential synaptic mechanism responsible for the synchronization of the principal neurons during odor response (MacLeod and Laurent 1996) and can use this knowledge to disrupt specifically and in vivo the temporal features of these neurons' responses while recording from downstream circuits or testing the animal's perceptual state. Using a combination of in vivo electrophysiology and behavioral experiments, we are attempting to determine whether neural synchronization and temporal features of neural activity do indeed play a significant role in olfactory perception.

OLFACTORY MAPS

In 1991, Linda Buck and Richard Axel cloned, from rats, the first putative odorant receptor (OR) genes, thus opening the way to a remarkably detailed description of the projection patterns between nasal epithelium and olfactory bulb (Buck and Axel 1991; Axel 1995; Vassar et al. 1993, 1994; Sullivan et al. 1995; Ressler et al. 1993,1994; Mombaerts et al. 1996; Buck 1996). ORs belong to a large superfamily of G protein–coupled receptors and contain seven hydrophobic domains likely to act as transmembrane *Caenorhabditis elegans* (Sengupta et al. 1996). Insect OR genes remain, to this day, frustratingly elusive. The molecular characterization of these genes has not yet been accompanied by a definitive functional proof that they indeed encode ORs. In situ hybridization and transgenic mouse technology, however, have allowed a detailed description of OR expression patterns and projections to the OB. These studies established the following features. Individual OR neurons (ORNs) appear to express at most a handful of ORs (possibly a single one). ORNs expressing the same OR can be found randomly distributed over large *zones* or horizontal stripes of the nasal epithelium. These zonal expression patterns are bilaterally symmetrical, and virtually identical across conspecifics. ORNs that express ORs of the same subfamily are situated in the same nasal expression zone (Ressler et al. 1993, 1994).

All ORNs that express the same OR gene converge to the same one (or at most two) glomerulus (-i) in the ipsilateral OB (Ressler et al. 1994; Vassar et al. 1994; Mombaert et al. 1996). Because we do not yet know the functional tuning of any of the ORs, the functional *logic* of these projections still remains unknown. It is possible, for example, that the OR projection maps represent "odotopic" or epitope maps (Mori and Shepherd 1994; Mori 1987; Mori and Yoshihara 1995; Hildebrand 1995), that is, maps of the structural features of the odorants. In this respect, recent physiological work by Yokoi et al. (1995), indicating that certain mitral cells in the rabbit OB show a preferred "tuning" to aliphatic alcohols of a certain carbon chain length and lateral inhibition for lengths shorter and longer than the preferred one, suggests that neighboring glomeruli might even represent closely related structural features of odorant molecules. The patterns of projection from epithelium to bulb are bilaterally symmetrical and nearly identical across conspecifics.

These striking results have led some investigators to propose that these OR projection maps represent a "code" for odors (Lewin 1994; Buck 1996; Shepherd 1994). Although possible in principle, we remain skeptical that maps are necessarily an intrinsic part of codes in the nervous system (Laurent 1997). It is indeed difficult to prove that the decoding of neural signals by downstream neurons makes explicit use of the spatial arrangement of their inputs (as a ribosome does when it linearly decodes a strand of messenger RNA, for example). As more information about the odor "tuning" of the ORs becomes available, it will be fascinating to correlate the tuning of receptors to that of their postsynaptic neurons in the bulb, and to understand, at least, the logic of these OR maps.

OLFACTORY PROCESSING

The basic problem that is solved by the olfactory system is to detect (generally) volatile chemicals over a very wide dynamic range (often with thresholds of less than 1 fM), to form "unique" representations of complex, combinatorial multimolecular "objects" (odors), to store these representations, and to allow recognition upon presentation of "noisy" stimuli (pattern completion). In essence, deciphering olfactory codes would amount to understanding one of the most remarkable pattern recognition devices. Our investigations focus on the neural representation of odors in the first and second relay neuropils of the olfactory pathway. Considerable work on the cellular and systems aspects of these circuits in both vertebrates and invertebrates has established the following facts. Odor representation is distributed among many neurons. Imaging experiments in the OB of lower vertebrates, for example, indicate that large numbers of glomeruli are activated by most odors, and that the foci of activation depend little on odor concentration (Kauer 1974; Cinelli and Kauer 1992; Cinelli et al. 1995; Thommesen 1978; Satou 1992; see also Joerges et al. 1997 for honeybees, and Friedrich and Korsching 1997 for zebra fish). The activation patterns in the OB are the same whether the odor is puffed over the entire nasal epithelium or over restricted zones of it (Cinelli et al. 1995). The "tuning" of mitral cells of the generalist olfactory system is generally broad, hard to define in molecular terms, although recent results suggest the existence of a form of molecular tuning to C chain length, at least for aliphatic alcohols (Yokoi et al. 1995; Mori 1987). Mitral cells often display complex multiphasic temporal response patterns (Meredith 1981, 1986, 1992; Meredith and Moulton 1978; Kauer 1974, 1991; Kauer and Moulton 1974; Chaput and Holley 1980) that may depend on odor concentration. Similar findings have been made with insect pheromone-sensitive neurons (Christensen and Hildebrand 1987, Christensen et al. 1989, 1993, 1995; Burrows et al. 1982). Odor presentation often leads to oscillatory field potential responses. This has now been established in the OB of vertebrates (Adrian 1942; Freeman 1992; Gray 1994; Gray and Skinner 1988), in the procerebral lobe of the terrestrial mollusc *Limax maximus* (Gelperin and Tank 1990; Delaney et al. 1994; Kleinfeld et al. 1994), and in the antennal lobe (AL) of locusts (Laurent and Davidowitz 1994).

Among these features, one of the most intriguing is the almost universal finding of stimulus-induced oscillatory synchronization (Gray 1994). Such a phenomenon, also observed in the visual (Eckhorn et al. 1988, Singer and Gray 1995) and sensorimotor (Murthy and Fetz 1992) system of mammals, was first proposed by Milner (1974) to be a means to "bind" the neural elements of cell assemblies (as defined theoretically by Hebb in the 1940s). Further theoretical work by von der Malsburg and Schneider (1986) suggested that oscillations might offer a substrate for figure-ground segmentation in the visual system, whereby neurons encoding figure and ground could be segregated by their respective phase relative to a common oscillatory "clock." Though much experimental work followed this idea (Eckhorn et al. 1988, Singer and Gray 1995), little direct support for this hypothesis has been published thus far. Gelperin's work with *Limax* procerebral lobe (Gelperin and Tank 1990; Delaney et al. 1994; Kleinfeld et al. 1994) shows that odors cause a collapse of a phase gradient that is observed at rest over the width of the procerebral lobe, possibly related to an odor-evoked change in the attentive state of the animal. A precise role for oscillatory synchronization of neural assemblies (if any), however, remains to be firmly established.

Structure of the Insect Olfactory System and Relations to the Vertebrate System

Though fascinating in its own right, work with arthropod and molluscan olfactory systems is made all the more relevant to mammalian (including human) neuroscience by the striking similarity between the vertebrate and invertebrate olfactory systems. Indeed, both architectural design and neuronal physiology appear similar in most respects, leading Hildebrand and Shepherd (1997) to state that "it seems that a common set of neural mechanisms have evolved across phyla for detecting and discriminating among olfactory stimuli." Among these similarities are the following: (1) absorption and transport of odorants by lymph or mucus (nose or antenna), and the common presence of olfactory binding proteins, whose effect is to enhance ORN response; (2) transduction via activation of G protein–coupled second messenger pathways: cyclic adenosine monophosphate (cAMP) in vertebrates, inosital 1,4,5-triphosphate (InsP$_3$) and diacylglycerol (DAG) in insects, and possibly (though not convincingly proved yet) both in certain vertebrate and invertebrate species; (3) generalist and specialist odorant pathways: moths, for example, possess a macroglomerular complex in their AL that receives exclusive input from pheromone-tuned ORNs on the antenna (Kanzaki et al. 1989; Almaas et al. 1991; Christensen et al. 1993; Hansson et al. 1991; Homberg et al. 1988; Lee and Strausfeld 1990); similarly, pheromonal olfactory signals in vertebrates project from a vomeronasal organ to a specialized "accessory" OB; (4) convergence of ORNs to a first relay formed of a glomerular neuropil: OB in vertebrates; AL in insects (Masson and Mustaparta 1990) and crustaceans (Mellon et al. 1992); (5) local dendrodendritic circuits between inhibitory local interneurons (granule and periglomerular cells in vertebrates; local neurons, or LNs, in insects) and projection neurons (mitral and tufted cells in vertebrates; projection neurons, or PNs, in insects) (Jahr and Nicoll 1982; Christensen et al. 1993; MacLeod and Laurent 1996; Ache et al. 1993); (6) odor-evoked field potential oscillations in OB and AL (see below); (7) divergent projection patterns from OB and AL to second relay, associated with olfactory memory functions: piriform cortex in vertebrates, mushroom body in insects (Haberly and Bower 1989; Davis 1993; Hammer and Menzel 1995; Homberg et al. 1988); (8) odor-evoked temporal response patterns in principal cells of the OB and AL (Meredith 1992; Kauer 1974; Laurent and Davidowitz 1994).

It thus seems that most of the integrative principles gathered from any of these systems have an analog in most of (if not all) the others. For example, our recent demonstration of the role of LN-mediated inhibition in generating oscillatory synchronization of PNs in the insect AL (MacLeod and Laurent 1996) directly supports mechanistic models (as yet not directly confirmed experimentally) of circuit dynamics in the mammalian OB (Freeman 1992; Rall et al. 1966; Gray 1994). We believe, therefore, that despite mechanistic differences (such as, e.g., the precise nature of the neurotransmitter systems used), the integrative principles derived from work with insects will prove to be directly applicable to an understanding of vertebrate olfaction.

SPATIOTEMPORAL ODOR RESPONSES OF LOCUST ANTENNAL LOBE NEURONS

Spatial Features

When an airborne odor is puffed onto one antenna of a locust, a subgroup of PNs and LNs in its ipsilateral AL are activated (figures 9.1, and 9.2A). The size of the PN subgroup is estimated to be about 10% to 15% of the total complement (i.e., around 80 to 100 of 830 PNs) and appears not to depend greatly on whether the odor is mono- or multimolecular (Laurent and Davidowitz 1994). Individual PNs can respond to, and hence participate in

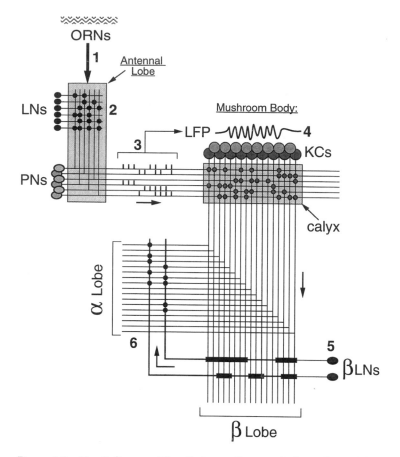

Figure 9.1 Circuit diagram of the olfactory pathway in the locust brain. Odors are transduced by arrays of olfactory receptor neurons (ORNs) in the antenna (1). ORNs activate ensembles of local and projection neurons (LNs and PNs) in the antennal lobe. LNs inhibit PNs (2) via a fast picrotoxin-sensitive GABAergic synapse. This inhibitory synapse is (at least in part) responsible for the oscillatory synchronization of the PNs that respond to an odor. PNs responding to a given odor usually display specific and reliable slow temporal activity patterns (3) superimposed on these oscillatory responses. These patterns are neuron- and odor-specific. The coactivation of PNs during an odor response causes synchronized and rhythmic EPSPs in Kenyon cells (KCs), the intrinsic neurons of the mushroom body. These synchronized EPSPs (caused by direct connections between PN axon collaterals and KC spiny dendrites in the calyx) can be detected extracellularly as an odor-evoked 20-Hz oscillatory local field potential (LFP) in the calyx (4). Arrays of KCs are so activated and send synchronized action potentials down their axons. These axons bifurcate into the so-called α and β lobes. In the β lobe, KC axons contact extrinsic neurons (β lobe neurons (5), which send axonal terminals to the α lobe (6). It is not known whether a reciprocal arrangement of projections exist between α and β lobes. β and α Lobe neurons can thus be used as a "readout" of this olfactory coding circuit.

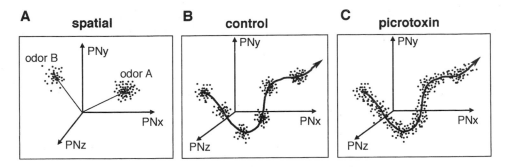

Figure 9.2 Possible odor-encoding schemes. Each axis represents activity along three of the n dimensions used for encoding, where n can be thought of as the number of independent projection neurons (PNs) in one antennal lobe. Each diagram is therefore an idealized projection of the n-dimensional odor representation onto a three-dimensional D (or three-PN) space. (A) The representation is static, and each odor is represented by a cloud of points in a region of PN space. The clouds of points represents (intertrial) noise in the representation of each odor. (B) The representation of each odor is dynamic and is updated at regular time intervals—in our case, at each cycle of the population oscillation. An odor is thus represented by a (discretized) trajectory in this space (see Wehr and Laurent 1996; Laurent et al. 1996; Laurent 1997). (C) In the presence of the GABA receptor antagonist picrotoxin (PCT), the PNs desynchronize (leading to the disappearance of the 20-Hz local field potential oscillations) but retain their slow and odor-specific response patterns (see MacLeod and Laurent 1996; Stopfer et al. 1997). The representation thus remains dynamic, but is not precisely updated by neurons whose spikes occur at regular 50-ms intervals. Under these conditions, fine odor discrimination is impaired (Stopfer et al. 1997).

representing, different odors, even if these odors do not share molecular compounds. These "spatial" representations are thus overlapping and combinatorial (Laurent 1996ab). If the AL were a noise-free system, if PNs could be described simply as responding or not responding to an odor, and if downstream decoding networks could differentiate two PN ensembles that differed only by one PN, the number of possible combinations (and therefore odor representations) would be astronomical: 830!/730! * 100!, that is, around $17 * 10 \wedge 130$. The three conditions listed above, however, are unlikely to apply to brain circuits.

Temporal Features

Odor responses of locust AL PNs contain the following overlapping temporal features.

Oscillations The responses of PNs to odors contain 20- to 30-Hz membrane potential oscillations composed of fast alternating excitatory (EPSPs) and inhibitory postsynaptic potentials (IPSPs) (Laurent and Davidowitz 1994). The spikes produced by a PN are thus often periodic (see below). The IPSPs are caused by γ-aminobutyric acid (GABA)–mediated inputs (Christensen et al. 1993; Leitch and Laurent 1996) from connected LNs which oscillate at the same frequency, with a 90-degree phase lead over the PNs (MacLeod and Laurent 1996). Blocking the GABAergic synapse between LNs and PNs with picrotoxin (PCT) selectively desynchronizes all AL neurons. Individual PNs receive inputs from many LNs, for hyperpolarizing a LN during an odor response does not significantly alter the oscillatory response of a postsynaptic PN (Laurent and Davidowitz 1994; MacLeod and Laurent 1996).

Synchronization   The PNs that respond to the same odor fire in synchrony. Their synchronized spikes provide periodic input to the postsynaptic mushroom body Kenyon cells, producing 20- to 30-Hz local field potential (LFP) oscillations in the mushroom body calyx. Every odor, but not air alone, evokes such bursts of LFP oscillations, whose frequency is independent of the odor. These oscillations can also be seen as subthreshold 20- to 30-Hz oscillations of membrane potential in the Kenyon cells (Laurent and Naraghi 1994; Laurent and Davidowitz 1994).

Phase   The phase of PN spikes relative to the LFP oscillations (or to other responding PNs) varies around a constant mean which is stimulus-independent. Spike phase, therefore, contains no information about odor identity (Laurent and Davidowitz 1994; Laurent 1996b; Wehr and Laurent 1996).

Phase-Locking   Not all the successive spikes produced by a PN in response to an odor phase-lock to the LFP. The ones that do, however, occur in relatively precise temporal windows during the odor response. The length and timing of these windows differ across neurons for an odor, and across odors for one neuron. Consequently, any two neurons that respond to the same odor may produce phase-locked spikes during a few cycles only of the ensemble response, or even never fire synchronized spikes together (Laurent et al. 1996).

Slow Temporal Patterns   Superimposed on these fast odor-evoked oscillatory responses are slow temporal patterns. Indeed, individual PNs usually respond to an odor with a specific spike profile, composed of several successive periods of activity and silence. Different PNs respond differently to the same odor, and individual PNs respond differently to different odors (Laurent et al. 1996).

Precision   The ordering of PN spikes in these oscillatory temporal patterns is very precise. Indeed, the response of a PN to two odors, A and B, may differ only by the rank order of these spikes; they can, for example, occur with nonzero probabilities in cycles 1, 2, and 3 of the LFP oscillation for odor A and in cycles 2, 3, and 4 for odor B. This indicates that a rate code that considers spike number alone misses information contained in the timing of the spikes within the oscillatory response (Wehr and Laurent 1996).

Inter-PN Coupling The firing probability of a PN during a given cycle of its response is coupled to its firing probability in a different cycle of the same trial. Similarly, the firing probability of a PN during a given cycle is linked to the firing probability of other PNs recorded simultaneously in this or a different cycle of the same trial (Wehr and Laurent 1996). In other words, the firing behaviors of different PNs are not independent during an odor response, and the encoding of odors must therefore be studied in the context of a complex circuit dynamics in which PNs probably influence each other.

A SPATIOTEMPORAL CODING HYPOTHESIS

A simple mean rate decoding scheme which assigns significance only to mean firing rates and discards spike timing yields a fraction only of the information about odor identity that is contained in the spike trains (Wehr and Laurent 1996). In other words, we demonstrated that odor-specific information is contained in precise spatial and temporal aspects of PN firing. We therefore propose that space and time (i.e., which neurons and when they are activated) are essential dimensions of the code for odors. The spatial aspects are contained in the identities of the activated PNs (10% to 15% of the total number of available PNs for most odors). The temporal aspects involve two interlocked phenomena: (1) the transient and periodic synchronization of active PNs and (2) the "evolution" of the odor-coding assemblies along an odor-specific "trajectory" during an odor response (figure 9.2B). In this hypothesis, the oscillation can be seen as a "clock" at whose rate the spatial representation is updated during a single odor response (Laurent et al. 1996; Wehr and Laurent 1996; Laurent 1996b). What is now needed is evidence that both spatial and temporal aspects of the representation are indeed used by the brain for odor learning, recognition, or discrimination.

While the idea that sensory stimuli can be represented combinatorially by distributed ensembles of coarsely tuned neurons is not new (see, e.g., Georgopoulos 1995 and Salinas and Abbott 1994 for representation of hand movement in primate motor cortex, or Wilson and McNaughton 1993 for representation of behavioral space in rat hippocampus), the hypothesis that spike timing or oscillations might play a role in stimulus encoding has received rather little hard experimental support (Bialek et al. 1991; Heller et al. 1995; Abeles 1981; Abbott et al. 1996; O'Keefe and Recce 1993; Gray 1994). We think, therefore, that a convincing demonstration (or falsification) of this proposed scheme will require, among other things, that the temporal features of the stimulus representation be manipulated, and that the effects of specific manipulations be tested on downstream circuits and behavior.

MECHANISTIC FEATURES AND THEIR PRACTICAL CONSEQUENCES

The synchronization and phase-locking of AL PNs during odor responses can be blocked selectively by local injection of the GABA receptor chloride channel blocker PCT into the AL (MacLeod and Laurent 1996). This manipulation blocks the fast IPSPs caused by LNs onto PNs but not the slow and odor-specific temporal patterns seen in PNs during odor responses, even when these appear to be caused by long-lasting synaptic inhibition (MacLeod and Laurent 1996). This suggests that the slow temporal patterns are shaped by mechanisms that are independent of the activation of this GABA receptor type. Other mechanisms include other types of GABA receptors (note that $GABA_B$ receptors are not known in insects and that phaclophen, a $GABA_B$ receptor antagonist, had no effect on the temporal patterns; MacLeod and Laurent, in preparation); other neurotransmitters, such as histamine (McClintock and Ache 1989), though cimetidine and pirylamine had effects only at very high concentrations; ionic pumps (though long-lasting hyperpolarizations do not always follow spike bursts; Laurent et al. 1996); nitric oxide (Gelperin 1994; Müller and Buchner 1993); temporal patterning of the antennal afferent input; and finally, complex dynamical behavior of the highly interconnected AL circuits.

Our finding that fast local inhibition is essential to produce oscillatory synchronization of AL networks agrees with recent in vitro results showing that inhibitory feedback shapes oscillatory synchronization in mammalian hippocampus (Traub et al. 1996ab, Whittington et al. 1995, Wang and Buzsaki 1996), thalamus (Bal and McCormick 1996; van Vreeswijk et al. 1995), and cerebral cortex (Lytton and Sejnowski 1991; Connors and Amitai 1997). Our results in locusts, however, were obtained in vivo and in non-anesthetized animals, and showed that the response tuning of PNs was not altered by PCT-mediated desynchronization. It is to our knowledge the only preparation thus far in which oscillations in a specific circuit can be abolished in vivo, conditions essential to testing the role of neural synchronization for stimulus learning and discrimination.

Behavioral Role of Oscillatory Synchronization for Odor Discrimination

To test the possible importance of oscillatory synchronization (and thus of the temporal codes they appear to carry) for odor discrimination, we used honeybees (Stopfer et al. 1997), which can be trained to extend their mouthparts (proboscis) in response to specific odors after a few associative forward pairings of these odors with a sucrose reward (proboscis extension, or PE, conditioning) (Kuwabara 1957; Bitterman et al. 1983; Menzel 1990; Smith and Menzel 1989; Hammer and Menzel 1995).

A first set of experiments was designed to establish whether odor presentation to the antenna of a bee produces the same neural phenomena in its ALs and mushroom bodies as those observed in locusts. These experiments indeed demonstrated that many of the phenomena described above for locusts also apply to bees. Namely, odors evoke synchronized (30 Hz) oscillations of AL neurons and phase-locked oscillations of field potential in the ipsilateral mushroom body calyx; these synchronized oscillations are blocked by PCT application, whereas the slow temporal response patterns of PNs are not altered by PCT (Stopfer et al. 1997). PCT can therefore be used in the honeybee as a selective agent to abolish oscillatory synchronization of PNs during odor conditioning (figure 9.2C).

In a second set of experiments, performed in collaboration with Drs. Brian Smith and Seetha Bhagavan (Ohio State University, Columbus), we tested the importance of oscillatory synchronization for odor learning and discrimination, using PCT injection into, or selective application onto, the ALs. We used a PE conditioning assay to test whether picrotoxin could disrupt olfactory discrimination (Bitterman et al. 1983; Smith and Menzel 1989). When forager honeybees experience forward pairing of an odor (conditioned stimulus, or CS) with sucrose reinforcement, their PE response to that specific odor increases dramatically for forty-eight hours or more. This increase is selectively due to associative learning mechanisms (Menzel 1990). In addition, the conditioned response generalizes to some extent to odors that are structurally similar to the conditioned odorant (Smith and Menzel 1989). For example, once conditioned to an aliphatic alcohol (e.g., 1–hexanol), bees show a somewhat heightened response to other, structurally similar alcohols (e.g., 1–octanol). This generalization response is never as strong as the response to the CS itself, but it is higher than the generalization response to structurally dissimilar odorants (e.g., terpenes). We reasoned that if oscillatory synchronization plays a role in odor learning or discrimination, PCT application to the AL should diminish the ability of bees to discriminate odors and therefore should increase odor generalization.

Animals were divided into two groups, a control (saline-treated) group and a test (PCT-treated) group, and the drugs were applied blind (Stopfer et al. 1997). We used a recovery interval of ten minutes between drug treatment and conditioning. Both PCT- and saline-treated groups learned the CS-sucrose pairing equally well, showing a maximal response by conditioning trial 5. Sixty minutes after conditioning, the two groups were given extinction trials with the CS, a similar odor (S), and a dissimilar odor (D). The number of animals in each group that responded with a PE to CS, S, or D was measured. Saline-treated animals responded significantly more often to the CS than they did to S, indicating discrimination of the two related odors. PCT-treated animals, by contrast, failed to discriminate the CS from S. Like the saline-treated controls, however, PCT-treated bees could discriminate the dissimilar odor, geraniol, from the two aliphatic alcohols (CS and S). We concluded that PCT had no significant nonspecific effects on learning, but rather that PCT affected certain odor discrimination tasks specifically (Stopfer et al. 1997).

CONCLUSIONS

These results suggest that neural synchronization plays a role in fine sensory discrimination tasks, that is, ones that require the separation of stimuli whose (spatial) neural representations probably overlap greatly (see results of imaging experiments in honeybee ALs by Joerges et al. 1997, for example). Synchronization, and hence the associated temporal features of the codes for odors, however, appears unimportant for the discrimination of dissimilar stimuli (i.e., ones less likely to have spatially overlapping neural representations). Because the effect of PCT was limited to the conditioning period, and because discrimination of dissimilar odors was always possible sixty minutes after conditioning, it is concluded that PCT-induced desynchronization did not impair odor learning per se. Rather, PCT (and thus desynchronization) appeared to impair the separation of the neural representations of two related odor stimuli, of which one was stored in memory in a form that lacked its natural oscillating temporal features. Synchronization of PN assemblies may therefore be important in helping to reduce the overlap between the neural representations of related stimuli, possibly by using the temporal aspects of their representations (Laurent et al. 1996; Wehr and Laurent 1996) as separable features. These behavioral results provide direct support for the hypothesis presented above, proposing that spike timing and synchronization are important parameters for odor sensation or perception. How these features are read out, however, remains unknown.

It is thus now important to further document the nature of these temporal representations and to determine the mechanisms which underlie their putative decoding by downstream networks. This will require the identification of neuronal populations in or downstream of the mushroom bodies, and the description of their sensitivity to the temporal structure of their inputs from the ALs. The realization that temporal features of spike trains might play a significant role in information coding in the brain is becoming more widespread than it once was. This insect preparation (and, hopefully, soon, others) will allow direct experimental tests of the causal relationship that may exist between dynamical codes and perception. If stimulus representations in the brain rely on spatiotemporal codes, it is likely that the mechanisms for pattern learning and recognition should be adapted to such dynamic encoding and decoding tasks too. Finding what these mechanisms are may not be so utopian (see chapter 10) and should be fascinating.

ACKNOWLEDGMENTS

This work has been supported by grants from the National Science Foundation and the Sloan Center for Theoretical Neuroscience, California Institute of Technology to G. L. Many thanks also to our friends Brian H Smith and Seetha Bhagavan for their crucial collaboration on the honeybee experiments.

REFERENCES

Abbott, L. F., Rolls, E. T., Tovee, M. J. (1996). Representational capacity of face coding in monkeys. *Cereb. Cortex* 6: 498–505.

Abeles, M. (1991). *Corticonics. Neural Circuits of the Cerebral Cortex*. Cambridge, UK: Cambridge University Press.

Abeles, M., and Gerstein, G. (1988). Detecting spatiotemporal firing patterns among simultaneously recorded single neurons. *J. Neurophysiol.* 60: 909–924.

Abeles, M., and Goldstein, M. H. (1977). Multispike train analysis. *Proc. IEEE* 65: 762–773.

Ache, B. W., Hatt, H., Breer, H., Boekhoff, I., and Zufall, F. (1993). Biochemical and physiological evidence for dual transduction pathways in lobster olfactory receptor neurons. *Chem. Senses* 18: 523.

Adrian, E. D. (1942). Olfactory reactions in the brain of the hedgehog. *J. Physiol. (Lond.)* 100: 459–473.

Adrian, E. D. (1950). The electrical activity of the mammalian olfactory bulb. *Electroencephalogr. Clin. Neurophysiol.* 2: 377–388.

Almaas, T. J., Christensen, T. A., and Mustaparta, H. (1991). Encoding of different features of an olfactory stimulus by the sex pheromone receptors in *Heliothis zea*. *J. Comp. Physiol. [A]* 169: 249–258.

Axel, R. (1995). The molecular logic of smell. *Sci. Am.* 1273: 154–159.

Bal, T., and McCormick, D. A. (1996). What stops synchronized thalamocortical oscillations? *Neuron* 17: 297–308.

Bhagavan, S., and Smith, B. H. (1997). Olfactory conditioning in the honey bee, *Apis mellifera*: effects of odor intensity. *Physiol. Behav.* 61: 107–117.

Bialek, W., Rieke, F., de Ruyter van Steveninck, R. R., Warland, D. (1991). Reading a neural code. *Science* 252: 1854–1857.

Bitterman, M. E., Menzel, R., Fietz, A., Schäfer, S. J. (1983). Clameal conditioning of proboseir extension in honeybees (Apis mellifera). *Comp. Psychol.* 97: 107–119.

Buck, L. (1996). Information coding in the vertebrate olfactory system *Annu. Rev. Neurosci.* 19: 517–544.

Buck, L., and Axel, R. (1991). A novel multigene family may encode odorant receptors: a molecular basis for odorant recognition. *Cell* 65: 175–187.

Burrows, M., Boeckh, J., and Esslen, J. (1982). Physiology and morphology properties of interneurons in the deutocerebrum of male cockroaches which respond to female pheromone. *J. Comp. Physiol. [A]* 145: 447–457.

Chaput, M., and Holley, A. (1980). Single unit responses of olfactory bulb neurons to odor presentation in awake rabbits. *J. Physiol. Paris* 76: 551–558.

Christensen, T. A., and Hildebrand, J. G. (1987). Male-specific, sex pheromone–selective projection neurons in the antennal lobes of the moth *Manduca sexta*. *J. Comp. Physiol. [A]* 160: 553–569.

Christensen, T. A., Hildebrand, J. G., Tumlinson, J. H., and Doolittle, R. E. (1989). Sex pheromone blend of *Manduca sexta*: responses of central olfactory interneurons to antennal stimulation in male moths. *Arch. Insect Biochem. Physiol.* 10: 281–291.

Christensen, T. A., Waldrop, B. R., Harrow, I. D., Hildebrand, J. G. (1993). Local interneurons and information processing in the olfactory glomeruli of the moth *Manduca sexta*. *J. Comp. Physiol. [A]* 173: 385–399.

Christensen, T. A., Harrow, I. D., Cuzzocrea, C., Randolph, P. W., and Hildebrand, J. G. (1995). Distinct projections of two populations of olfactory receptor axons in the antennal lobe of the sphinx moth *Manduca sexta*. *Chem. Senses* 20: 313–323.

Cinelli, A. R., and Kauer, J. S. (1992). Voltage-sensitive dyes and functional activity in the olfactory pathway. *Annu. Rev. Neurosci.* 15: 321–351.

Cinelli, A. R., Hamilton, K. A., and Kauer, J. S. (1995). Salamander olfactory bulb neuronal activity observed by video-rate voltage-sensitive dye imaging. 3—Spatial and temporal properties of responses evoked by odorant stimulation. *J. Neurophysiol.* 73: 2053–2071.

Connors, B. W., and Amitai, Y. (1997). Making waves in the neocortex *Neuron* 18: 347–349.

Davis, R. L. (1993). Mushroom bodies and *Drosophila* learning. *Neuron* 11: 1–14.

deCharms, R. C., and Merzenich, M. M. (1996). Primary cortical representation of sounds by the coordination of action potential timing. *Nature* 381: 610–613.

Delaney, K. R., Gelperin, A., Fee M. S., Flores, J. A., Gervais, R., Tank, D. W., and Kleinfeld, D. (1994). Waves and stimulus modulated dynamics in an oscillating olfactory network. *Proc. Natl. Acad. Sci. USA* 91: 669–674.

Dulac, C., and Axel, R. (1995). A novel family of genes encoding putative pheromone receptors in mammals. *Cell* 83: 195–206.

Eckhorn, R., Bauer, W., Jordan, W., Brosch, M., Kruse, W., Munk, M., Reitboeck, H. J. (1988). Coherent oscillations: a mechanism of feature linking in the visual cortex? *Biol. Cybern.* 60: 121–130.

Engel, A. K., König, P., Kreiter A. K., Singer, W. (1991). Interhemispheric synchronization of oscillatory neuronal responses in cat visual cortex. *Science* 252: 1177–1179.

Freeman, W. J. (1975). *Mass Action in the Nervous System.* New York, Academic Press.

Freeman, W. J. (1978). Spatial properties of an EEG event in the olfactory bulb and cortex. *Electroencephalogr. Clin. Neurophysiol.* 44: 586–605.

Freeman, W. J. (1992). Nonlinear dynamics in olfactory infromation processing. In *Olfaction, a Model System for Computational Neuroscience,* J. L. Davis and H. Eichenbaum, eds., pp. 225–249. Cambridge, MA., MIT Press.

Friedrich, R. W., and Korsching, S. I. (1997). Combinatorial and chemotopic odorant coding in the zebrafish olfactory bulb visualized by optical imaging. *Neuron* 18: 737–752.

Gawne, T. J., Kjaer, T. W., Hertz, J. A., and Richmond, B. A. (1996). Adjacent visual cortical complex cells share about 20% of their stimulus-related information. *Cereb. Cortex* 6: 482–489.

Geisler, W. S., Albrecht, D. G., Salvi, R. J., and Saunders, S. S. (1991). Discrimination performance of single neurons: rate and temporal-pattern information. *J. Neurophysiol.* 66: 334–362.

Gelperin,, A. (1994). Nitric oxide mediates network oscillations of olfactory interneurons in a terrestrial mollusc. *Nature* 369: 61–63.

Gelperin, A., and Tank, D. W. (1990). Odor-modulated collective network oscillations of olfactory interneurons in a terrestrial mollusc. *Nature* 345: 437–440.

Georgopoulos, A. P. (1995). Current issues in directional motor control. *Trends Neurosci.* 18: 506–510.

Gray, C. M. (1994). Synchronous oscillations in neuronal systems: mechanisms and functions. *J. Comput. Neurosci.* 1: 11–38.

Gray, C. M., and Singer, W. (1989). Stimulus-specific neuronal oscillations in orientation columns of cat visual cortex. *Proc. Natl. Acad. Sci. USA* 86: 1698–1702.

Gray, C. M., and Skinner, J. E. (1988). Centrifugal regulation of neuronal activity in the olfactory bulb of the waking rabbit as revealed by reversible cryogenic blockade. *Exp. Brain Res.* 69: 378–386.

Haberly, L. B., and Bower, J. M. (1989). Olfactory cortex: model circuit for study of associative memory. *Trends Neurosci.* 12: 258–264.

Hammer, M., and Menzel, R. (1995). Learning and memory in the honey-bee. *J. Neurosci.* 15: 1617–1630.

Hansson, B. S., Christensen, T. A., and Hildebrand, J. G. (1991). Functionally distinct subdivisions of the macroglomerular complex in the antennal lobe of the male sphinx moth *Manduca sexta. J. Comp. Neurol.* 312: 264–278.

Heller, J., Hertz, J. A., Kjaer, T. W., Richmond, B. J. (1995). Information flow and temporal coding in primate pattern vision. *J. Comput. Neurosci.* 2: 175–193.

Hildebrand, J. G. (1995). Analysis of chemical signals by nervous systems. *Proc. Natl. Acad. Sci. USA* 92: 67–74.

Hildebrand, J. G., and Shepherd, G. M. (1997). Mechanisms of olfactory discrimination: converging evidence for common principles across phyla. *Annu. Rev. Neurosci.* 20: 595–631.

Homberg, U., Montague, R., and Hildebrand, J. G. (1988). Anatomy of antenno-cerebral pathways in the brain of the sphinx moth *Manduca sexta. Cell Tissue Res.* 254: 255–281.

Jagadeesh, B., Gray, C. M., and Ferster, D. (1992). Visually evoked oscillations of membrane potential in cells of cat visual cortex. *Science* 257: 552–554.

Jahr, C. E., and Nicoll, R. A. (1982). An intracellular analysis of dendrodendritic inhibition in the turtle in vitro olfactory bulb. *J. Physiol. (Lond.)* 326: 213–234.

Joerges, J., Kuttner, A., Galizia, C. G., and Menzel, R. (1997). Representation of odors and odor mixtures visualized in the honeybee brain. *Nature* 387: 285–288.

Kanzaki, R., Arbas, E. A., Strausfeld, N. J., and Hildebrand, J. G. (1989). Physiology and morphology of projection neurons in the antennal lobe of the male moth *Manduca sexta. J. Comp. Physiol. [A]* 165: 427–453.

Kauer, J. S. (1974). Response patterns of amphibian olfactory bulb neurones to odor stimulation. *J. Physiol (Lond.)* 243: 695–715.

Kauer, J. S. (1991). Contributions of topography and parallel processing to odor coding in the vertebrate olfactory pathway. *Trends Neurosci.* 14: 79–85.

Kauer, J. S., and Moulton, D. G. (1974). Responses of olfactory bulb neurones to odour stimulation of small nasal areas in the salamander. *J. Physiol. (Lond.)* 243: 717–737.

Kleinfeld, D., Delaney, K. R., Fee, M. S., Flores, J. A., Tank, D. W., and Gelperin, A. (1994). Dynamics of propagating waves in the olfactory network of a terrestrial mollusc: an electrical and optical study. *J. Neurophysiol.* 72: 1402–1419.

Kuwabara, M. (1957). Bildung des bedingten Reflexes von Pavlovs Typus bei der Honigbiene, *Apis mellifica. J. Fac. Sci. Hokkaido Univ. (Ser. 6 Zool.)* 13: 458–464.

Laurent, G. (1996a). Odor images and tunes. *Neuron* 16: 473–476.

Laurent, G. (1996b). Dynamical representation of odors by oscillating and evolving neural assemblies. *Trends Neurosci.* 19: 489–496.

Laurent, G. (1997). Olfactory processing: maps, time and codes. *Curr. Opin. Neurol.* 7: 547–553.

Laurent, G., and Davidowitz, H. (1994). Encoding of olfactory information with oscillating neural assemblies. *Science* 265: 1872–1875.

Laurent, G., and Naraghi, M. (1994). Odorant-induced oscillations in the mushroom bodies of the locust. *J. Neurosci.* 14: 2993–3004.

Laurent, G., Wehr, M., and Davidowitz, H. (1996). Temporal representation of odors in an olfactory network. *J. Neurosci.* 16: 3837–3847.

Lee, J. K., and Strausfeld, N. J. (1990). Structure, distribution and number of surface sensilla and their receptor cells on the olfactory appendage of the male moth *Manduca sexta. J. Neurocytol.* 19: 519–538.

Leitch, B., and Laurent, G. (1996). GABAergic synapses in the antennal lobe and mushroom body of the locust olfactory system. *J. Comp. Neurol.* 372: 487–514.

Lewin, B. (1994). On neuronal specificity and the molecular basis of perception *Cell* 79: 935–943.

Lytton, W. W., and Sejnowski, T. J. (1991). Simulations of cortical pyramidal neurons synchronized by inhibitory interneurons. *J. Neurophysiol.* 66: 1059–1079.

McClintock, T. S., and Ache, B. W. (1989). Histamine directly gates a chloride channel in lobster olfactory receptor neurons *Proc. Natl. Acad. Sci. USA* 86: 8137–8141.

MacLeod, K., and Laurent, G. (1996). Distinct mechanisms for synchronization and temporal patterning of odor-encoding neural assemblies. *Science* 274: 976–979.

Mainen, Z., and Sejnowski, T. J. (1995). Reliability of spike timing in neocortical neurons. *Science* 268: 1502–1506.

Masson, C., and Mustaparta, H. (1990). Chemical information processing in the olfactory system of insects. *Physiol. Rev.* 70: 199–245.

McClurkin, J. W., Gawne, T. J., Optican, L. M., and Richmond, B. J. (1991a). Lateral geniculate neurons in behaving primates. II. Encoding information in the temporal shape of the response. *J. Neurophysiol.* 66: 794–808.

McClurkin, J. W., Gawne, T. J., Richmond, B. J., Optican, L. M., and Robinson, D. L. (1991b). Lateral geniculate neurons in behaving primates. I. Responses to two-dimensional stimuli. *J. Neurophysiol.* 66: 777–793.

Mellon, D., Alones, V., and Lawrence, M. D. (1992). Anatomy and fine structure of neurons in the deutocerebral projection pathway of the crayfish olfactory system. *J. Comp. Neurol.* 321: 93–111.

Menzel, R. (1990). In *Neurobiology of Comparative Cognition*, R. P. Kesner and D. S. Olton, eds., pp. 237–292. Hillsdale, NJ, Erlbaum.

Meredith, M. (1981). The analysis of response similarity in single neurons of the goldfish olfactory bulb using amino acids as odor stimuli. *Chem. Senses* 6: 277–293.

Meredith, M. (1986). Patterned response to odor in mammalian olfactory bulb: the influence of intensity. *J. Neurophysiol.* 56: 572–597.

Meredith, M. (1992). Neural circuit computation: complex patterns in the olfactory bulb. *Brain Res. Bull.* 29: 111–117.

Meredith, M., and Moulton, D. G. (1978). Patterned response to odor in single neurons of goldfish olfactory bulb: influence of odor quality and other stimulus parameters. *J. Gen. Physiol.* 71: 615–643.

Milner, P. (1974). A model for visual shape recognition. *Psychol. Rev.* 81: 521–535.

Mombaert, P., Wang, F., Dulac, C., Chao, S. K., Nemes, A., Mendelshon, M., Edmondson, J., and Axel, R. (1996). Visualizing an olfactory sensory map. *Cell* 87: 675–686.

Mori, K. (1987). Membrane and synaptic properties of identified neurons in the olfactory bulb. *Prog. Neurobiol.* 29: 275–320.

Mori, K., and Shepherd, G. M. (1994). Emerging principles of molecular signal processing by mitral/tufted cells in the olfactory bulb. *Semin. Cell Biol.* 5: 65–74.

Mori, K., and Yoshihara, Y. (1995). Molecular recognition and olfactory processing in the mammalian olfactory system. *Prog. Neurobiol.* 45: 585–619.

Müller, U., and Buchner, E. (1993). Histochemical localization of NADPH-diaphorase in the adult *Drosophila* brain: is nitric oxide a neuronal messenger also in insects? *Naturwissenschaft* 80: 524–526.

Murthy, V. N., and Fetz, E. E. (1992). Coherent 25–35 Hz oscillations in the sensorimotor cortex of the awake behaving monkey. *Proc. Natl. Acad. Sci. USA* 89: 5670–5674.

O'Keefe, J., and Recce, M. (1993). Phase relationship between hippocampal place units and the EEG theta-rhythm. *Hippocampus* 3: 317–330.

Optican, L. M., and Richmond, B. J. (1987). Temporal encoding of two-dimensional patterns by single units in primate inferior temporal cortex. III. Information theoretic analysis. *J. Neurophysiol.* 57: 162–178.

Rall, W., Shepherd, G. M., Reese, T. S., and Grightman, M. W. (1966). Dendro-dendritic synaptic pathway for inhibition in the olfactory bulb. *Exp. Neurol.* 14: 44–56.

Ressler, K. J., Sullivan. S. L., and Buck, L. B. (1993). A zonal organization of odorant receptor gene expression in the olfactory epithelium. *Cell* 73: 597–609.

Ressler, K. J., Sullivan. S. L., and Buck, L. B. (1994). Information coding in the olfactory system: evidence for a stereotyped and highly organized epitope map in the olfactory bulb. *Cell* 79: 1245–1255.

Salinas, E., and Abbott, L. F. (1994). Vector reconstruction from firing rates. *J. Comput. Neurosci.* 1: 89–107.

Satou, M. (1992). Synaptic organization, local neuronal circuitry, and functional segregation of the teleost olfactory bulb. *Prog. Neurobiol.* 34: 115–142.

Shepherd, G. M. (1994). Discrimination of molecular signals by the olfactory receptor neuron. *Neuron* 13: 771–790.

Sengupta, P., Chou, J. H., and Bargman, C. J. (1996). *odr-10* encodes a seven transmembrane domain olfactory receptor required for responses to the odorant diacetyl. *Cell* 84: 899–909.

Singer, W., and Gray, C. M. (1995). Visual feature integration and the temporal correlation hypothesis. *Annu. Rev. Neurosci.* 18: 555–586.

Smith, B. H., and Menzel, R. (1989). An analysis of variability in the Ceding motor program of the honey bee: the role of learning in releasing a model action pattern. *Ethology* 82: 68–81.

Stopfer, M., Bhagavan, S., Smith, B. H., and Laurent, G. (1997). Impaired odor discrimination on desynchronization of odor encoding neural assemblies. *Nature* 390: 70–74.

Sullivan. S. L., Bohm, S., Ressler, K. K., Horowitz, L. F., and Buck, L. B. (1995). Target-independent pattern specification in the olfactory epithelium. *Neuron* 15: 779–789.

Thommesen, G. (1978). The spatial distribution of odor-induced potentials in the olfactory bulb of char and trout (Salmonidae). *Acta Physiol. Scand.* 102: 414–426.

Traub, R. D., Whittington, M. A., Colling, S. B., Buzsaki, G., and Jefferys, J. G. R. (1996a). Analysis of gamma rhythms in the rat hippocampus in vitro and in vivo. *J. Physiol. (Lond.)* 493: 471–484.

Traub, R. D., Whittington, M. A., Stanford, I. M., and Jefferys, J. G. R. (1996b). A mechanism for generation of long-range synchronous fast oscillations in the cortex. *Nature* 383: 621–624.

Vaadia, E., Haalman, I., Abeles, M., Bergman, H., Prut, Y., Slovin, H., and Aertsen, A. (1995). Dynamics of neuronal interactions in monkey cortex in relation to behavioral events. *Nature* 373: 515–518.

van Vreeswijk, C., Abbott, L. F., and Ermentrout, G. B. (1995). When inhibition, not excitation synchronizes neural firing. *J. Comput. Neurosci.* 1: 313–322.

Vassar, R., Ngai, J., and Axel, R. (1993). Spatial segregation of odorant receptor expression in the mammalian olfactory epithelium. *Cell* 74: 309–318.

Vassar, R., Chou, S. K., Sitcheran, R., Nuñez, J. M., Vosshall, L. B., and Axel, R. (1994). Topographic organization of sensory projections to the olfactory bulb. *Cell* 79: 981–991.

Victor, J. D., and Purpura, K. P. (1996). Nature and precision of temporal coding in visual cortex: a metric-space analysis. *J. Neurophysiol.* 76: 1310–1326.

Von der Malsburg, C., and Schneider, W. (1986). A neural cocktail-party processor. *Biol. Cybern.* 54: 29–40.

Wang, X-J., and Buzsaki, G. (1996). Gamma oscillation by synaptic inhibition in a hippocampal interneuronal network model. *J. Neurosci.* 16: 6402–6413.

Wehr, M., and Laurent, G. (1996). Odour encoding by temporal sequences of firing in oscillating neural assemblies. *Nature* 384: 162–166.

Whittington, M. A., Traub, R. D., and Jeffreys, J. G. R. (1995). Synchronized oscillations in interneuron networks driven by metabotropic glutamate receptor activation. *Nature* 373: 612–615.

Wilson, M. A., and McNaughton, B. L. (1993). Dynamics of the hippocampal ensemble code for space. *Science* 261: 1055–1058.

Yokoi, M., Mori, K., and Nakanishi, S. (1995). Refinement of odor molecule tuning by dendrodendritic synaptic inhibition in the olfactory bulb. *Proc. Natl. Acad. Sci. USA* 92: 3371–3375.

10 Frequency-Dependent Synaptic Transmission in the Neocortex

Henry Markram, Misha Tsodyks, Yun Wang, and Ascher Uziel

Frequency-dependent synaptic transmission is a prominent property of synapses in the peripheral and central nervous systems of a large variety of animals (Feng 1941; Liley and North 1953; del Castillo and Katz 1954; Parnas and Atwood 1966; Pinsker et al. 1970; Takeuchi 1958; Zucker 1989; Laurent and Sivaramakrishnan 1992; Davis and Murphey 1993; Katz et al. 1993; Thomson and Deuchars 1994). This property suggests that synapses do not simply act as transmission devices, but as computational elements capable of transmitting a limited subset of information contained within the presynaptic action potential train. Frequency-dependent synaptic transmission has been considered extensively in simple organisms (see also Hutter 1952; Liley 1956; Hubbard 1963; Thies 1965; Betz 1970; Magleby and Zengel 1976, 1982; Magleby 1979) and in particular has been central to an extensive characterization of the cellular basis of learning and memory and simple behavior in *Aplysia* (Pinsker et al. 1970; Byrne 1978; Carew et al. 1981; Gingrich and Byrne 1985; Buonomano et al. 1990; Ciaccia et al. 1992). Despite all these studies, except in a very few cases (Grossberg 1969; Liaw and Berger 1996; Markram and Tsodyks 1996), frequency-dependent synaptic transmission has essentially been ignored in virtually every concept developed for information processing, learning, and memory in the mammalian brain, and frequency-dependent synaptic transmission is mostly overlooked when interpreting phenomena observed in in vitro and in vivo experiments. This oversight may have a tremendous cost, since frequency dependence of transmission could allow the construction of a vast repertoire of transmission codes as a function of the activation states of neurons and hence could be fundamental to information processing in the nervous system, as well as learning and memory processes. This chapter describes an attempted revival of the study of frequency dependence with a new direction and a new approach. The aim is to determine the function of frequency dependence in the nervous system, not only to study its properties and dissect its mechanics. This approach has recently guided experiments and yielded data that pose a serious challenge to current views of information transmission by synapses, synaptic plasticity, and information processing in neuronal networks.

In this chapter we begin by considering the new experimental techniques that have made a systematic study of frequency-dependent synaptic transmission possible. We then move to consider previous approaches to studying frequency-dependent synaptic transmission and the approach we chose to adopt. A method used to quantify frequency dependence which recently revealed interesting properties of frequency-dependent synapses is then provided. The next section derives what are referred to as "synaptic transfer functions" of frequency-dependent synapses and illustrates the relationship between transfer functions and various synaptic parameters and how these synaptic parameters dictate the transmission capability of synapses. Next we examine synaptic plasticity in the context of frequency-dependent transmission and show that there are four basic classes of synaptic plasticity in which transmission of specific ranges of presynaptic action potential (AP) frequencies can be regulated. This section also proposes that synaptic modifications are governed according to a supraalgorithm termed the "synaptic plasticity code." The final section deals with the latest and less accessible issue of how to incorporate frequency-dependent synaptic transmission into concepts of information processing within networks of neurons as a step toward understanding the function of frequency dependence in vivo.

WHOLE-CELL RECORDING FROM SYNAPTICALLY COUPLED NEURONS

Synaptically coupled recordings in cortical slices (figure 10.1) have revealed a mosaic of frequency-dependent properties displayed at connections between specific classes of neurons (Thomson et al. 1989, 1993a,b, 1995, 1996; Thomson and Deuchars 1994; Deuchars and Thomson 1995, 1996; Thomson 1997; Thomson and West 1993; Stratford et al. 1996). This finding points out that generalizing results obtained in one synaptic pathway is not justified. A more thorough approach is required whereby synaptic connections between any two classes of neurons are considered potentially unique. Recordings between coupled neurons offer the best approach to establishing not only particular synaptic properties but also the comparative anatomy of cortical microcircuits (Somogyi et al. 1983; Buhl et al. 1997; Deuchars et al. 1994; Thomson and Deuchars 1994; Markram et al. 1997a). In order to study plasticity of frequency-dependent synapses it is also necessary to be able to isolate a defined synaptic pathway systematically. This approach is enabled by the recent application of video-enhanced infrared differential interference contrast (IR-DIC) microscopy in brain slices to visually preselect neurons for recordings (figure 10.1; Stuart et al. 1993; Markram et al. 1997a).

The advantages of this approach are that a predefined synaptic pathway can be studied systematically, that whole-cell recordings can be obtained from both pre- and postsynaptic neurons enabling precise control over the AP activity patterns in the coupled neurons, and that the detailed microanatomy and putative number and location of synaptic contacts can be determined.

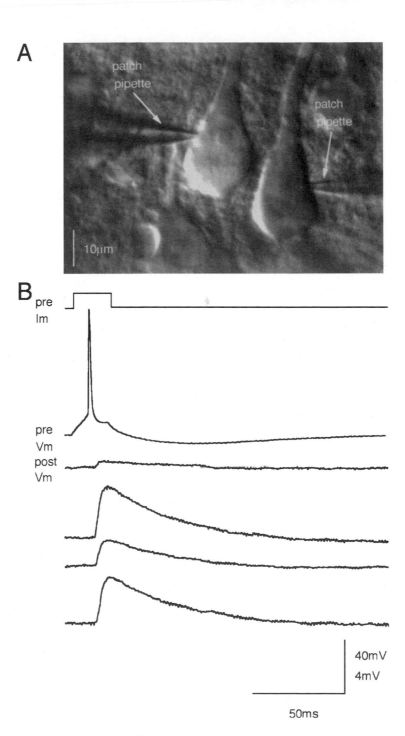

Figure 10.1 Infrared differential interference contrast photomicrograph of a pair of thick-tufted layer 5 pyramidal neurons from which whole-cell patch-clamp recordings were obtained. An action potential evoked in one neuron resulted in excitatory synaptic responses in the other.

The disadvantages of this approach are that recordings are restricted to neurons within about 120 μm of the surface of the slice, that in most cases experiments are restricted to juvenile animals since the surface neurons do not survive as well in adult slices (perhaps due to sectioning of their more extensive axonal and dendritic arbors), and that washout of essential constituents required for synaptic modifications restricts the duration and number of different control protocols that can be tested in the same pair.

Some of the disadvantages may be overcome. For example, synaptically coupled recordings have been obtained in adult rats (A. Gupta and H. Markram, in preparation) and in kittens up to 19 weeks of age (K. Stratford, personal communication). Nystatin-, amphotericin-, or gramicidin- perforated patch recordings of synaptically coupled neurons can be performed to eliminate the problems with washout, but in many cases the associated difficulties (slow perforation, decaying quality of perforation, spontaneous break-in), combined with the difficulties of obtaining synaptically coupled recordings, render this approach useful only for a select set of control experiments.

Optimizing sectioning of slices is an essential step to studying transmission in a defined synaptic pathway. The extensive body of information covering the morphological features of neurons, as well as the known afferent pathways, can be used initially to choose the optimal angle for sectioning of the slices. The subsequent steps are as follows:

1. ***Establishing criteria for identifying neurons of interest.*** In some cases identifying neurons of interest may be easy using IR-DIC microscopy alone (e.g., identifying the thick-tufted neurons in layer 5), but in some cases this is not trivial (e.g., distinguishing pyramidal neurons from bipolar or even from basket cells in the upper layers) and in other cases this may be impossible (e.g., distinguishing different subtypes of interneurons). Biocytin-loading and postexperiment analysis of the morphology can help to obtain a selection criterion that yields more reliable recording of a specific type of neuron, but other techniques, such as genetic engineering of cell-specific expression of green fluorescent protein, will be required to maximize preselection.

2. ***Visual preselection of potential synaptically coupled pairs using IR-DIC microscopy.*** IR-DIC images can also be used to select the best slices for paired recordings. The best slice is the one in which the plane of sectioning is optimal for maximal axonal arborization near the target neuron. The most important criterion is to ensure that the main axon is not cut for 100 to 200 μm depending on how many collaterals emerge from the main axon. Typically, close-neighbor neurons (e.g., pyramidal neurons) are contacted from collaterals branching within 100 to 200 μm of the soma.

3. ***Reconstructing neurons loaded with biocytin.*** An essential step in establishing the preparation for recording a specific synaptic connection is to perform a detailed morphological analysis of biocytin-loaded neurons and identify the locations of putative contact sites. This allows estimation of the extent to which the axonal and dendritic arbors are optimal to enable maxi-

mal probability of synaptic coupling and maximal synaptic innervation per connection.

APPROACHES TO STUDYING FREQUENCY-DEPENDENT SYNAPSES

Frequency-dependent synaptic transmission has been studied using several different approaches. A biophysical approach has been used to examine the detailed properties of frequency dependence with the aim of establishing the various processes governing frequency dependence (Liley and North 1953; del Castillo and Katz 1954; Liley 1956; Thies 1965; Betz 1970; Pinsker et al. 1970; Magleby 1973, 1979; Magleby and Zengel 1976, 1982; Zucker 1989). This approach involves a wide spectrum of stimulation protocols to observe and extract the various components of facilitation, their different time constants and amplitudes. The advantage of this approach is that fine detail concerning the properties of frequency dependence can be established. The disadvantage is that numerous different protocols are required to extract this information which is not always possible since changes in synaptic properties could be triggered by the stimulation protocols themselves. A second approach is to construct a model of frequency dependence. This model can be based on biophysical properties (Krausz and Friesen 1977; Magleby 1987; Magleby and Zengel 1982; Gingrich and Byrne 1985; Ciaccia et al. 1992; Destexhe et al. 1994; Liaw and Berger 1996; Bertram et al. 1996) or can be phenomenological (Markram et al. 1998b; Tsodyks and Markram 1997). The advantage of this approach is that the main properties of frequency-dependent transmission can be determined using only one or a very few stimulation protocols. The disadvantage of this approach is that it is not always feasible to capture all the fine detail of the frequency dependence.

A third approach has been to apply nonlinear systems analysis where Wiener kernels are used to characterize the transmission (Krausz and Friesen 1977; Abbott et al. 1997). The advantage of this approach is that it can predict or reproduce data from a particular connection even more accurately than models can, since it captures more of the nonlinearities (see Krausz and Friesen 1977). The disadvantage of this approach is that it is not straightforward to relate the success of the model to specific synaptic properties. A fourth approach has been to examine the changes in the statistics of transmission, particularly changes in the coefficient of variation (CV) during high-frequency stimulation in the framework of the quantal model (del Castillo and Katz 1954; Takeuchi 1958; Thies 1965; Betz 1970; Byrne 1978; Korn et al. 1984, 1986). The advantage of this approach is that it can potentially be used to establish the role of the probability of release (Pr) in frequency dependence. The disadvantage of this approach is that it is not always trivial to determine the source of changes in CV (Faber and Korn 1991) since it rests on several assumptions and is subject to several inaccuracies because single-sweep responses must be analyzed reliably (see Faber and Korn 1991; Redman 1990).

A PHENOMENOLOGICAL MODEL OF FREQUENCY-DEPENDENT SYNAPTIC TRANSMISSION

The Tsodyks-Markram (TM) Model

The phenomenological model constructed by Tsodyks and Markram (Tsodyks and Markram 1997; Markram et al. 1998a) represents an integration of previous experiments on synaptic depression, showing that depression is analogous to a refractory period of neurotransmitter release, and on experimental and theoretical analyses of synaptic depression and facilitation. The model can be described as follows:

1. The synapse has an absolute synaptic efficacy (A), defined as the maximum response produced at the recording site (usually the soma) if all active sites released transmitter simultaneously (i.e., when Pr is 1 at all release sites).

2. The presynaptic AP utilizes some fraction of the A, defined as the utilization of synaptic efficacy parameter (U).

3. U changes for each AP. The running value of U is referred to as u.

4. Each AP causes a pulsed transient increase in U by an amplitude of ($U(1 - u)$).

5. u decays with a time constant of τ_{facil}.

6. The response is equivalent to the effective synaptic efficacy (E), which inactivates virtually instantly (τ_{inac}).

7. The inactive synaptic efficacy (I) recovers with a time constant of τ_{rec} to add to the pool of recovered synaptic efficacy (R).

The kinetic equations for the three states of the model that simulate depression are:

$$\frac{dR}{dt} = \frac{1}{\tau_{rec}} - U \cdot R \cdot \delta(t - t_{AP}), \tag{1}$$

$$\frac{dE}{dt} = -\frac{A}{\tau_{inac}} + U \cdot R \cdot \partial(t - t_{AP}), \tag{2}$$

$$I = 1 - R - E. \tag{3}$$

Facilitation is included as

$$u_{n+1} = u_n \exp\left(\frac{-\Delta t}{\tau_{facil}}\right) + U\left(1 - u_n \exp\left(\frac{-\Delta t}{\tau_{facil}}\right)\right). \tag{4}$$

The four sets of parameters, A, U, τ_{rec} and τ_{facil} therefore can describe the most salient features of both facilitating and depressing synapses. Under certain circumstances, more specific experiments and modifications to the model may be required to capture finer details of frequency dependence. For example, the model employs only single time constants for facilitation and depression. Facilitation can be characterized by at least four time constants (Magleby and Zengel 1982; Zucker 1989; Bertram et al. 1996) and depression between neocortical pyramidal neurons by at least two time constants (Thomson and West 1993; H. Markram, unpublished data). These time constants may have to be incorporated when examining discharge responses in which they contribute significantly and in cases where modifications may regulate specific subcomponents of the depression or facilitation selectively. The model also assigns the amplitude of facilitation the same value as U, but this implicitly assumes that the degree of facilitation is determined by the same mechanism as that which determines the initial Pr at low frequencies. This equivalence is, however, not necessary and amplitude can be made a specifc parameter. It is also possible that the various subcomponents of facilitation and depression have different amplitudes. The basic TM model is therefore a first-line approach given the available data. The mathematical complexity and hence the difficulty of fitting single-axon experimental results increases markedly as multiple time constants with different amplitudes are considered.

Stimulation Protocols to Derive Model Parameters for Frequency-Dependent Synapses

A major advantage of the phenomenological approach is that the average response to a high-frequency train is normally sufficient to derive the model parameters that would then reproduce synaptic responses for any AP train. The value of this advantage depends on how well the average response represents the true mean. The number of sweeps required to obtain an average that would be within 5% of the true mean is; $(\sigma/0.05 \cdot \mu)^2$ where σ is the standard deviation and μ is the true mean. For single-axon data it is not always possible to obtain sufficient sweeps for a near-true-mean response. This error can be offset by examining more excitatory postsynaptic potentials (EPSPs) within the train or several different frequencies, since a best fit is made through all available amplitudes. The model could even be applied to the average amplitudes measured from single-sweep responses to Poisson trains of presynaptic APs at different frequencies. The amplitudes of EPSPs during high-frequency trains are measured by subtracting an exponentially decaying trace to correct for the decaying voltage of the preceding EPSP. This is a small correction for depressing synapses, but can be large for facilitating synapses.

The model is then applied to iteratively determine the optimal parameters that would simulate the successive EPSP amplitudes for the AP train used as a test stimulus. For display purposes only, voltage responses are simulated in a "point neuron," with an arbitrary input resistance and an experimentally determined membrane time constant. The fitting routine is programmed to iterate until a minimum error (E) is reached. E for each EPSP in the train is given by $\mathrm{EPSP}_{\mathrm{experiment}} - \mathrm{EPSP}_{\mathrm{predicted}}$ and total $E = \sqrt{E_1^2 + E_2^2 + \cdots E_n^2}$, where E_1 to E_n represents the error contribution of each EPSP in the train. The iteration then yields the value of the model parameters A, U, τ_{rec} and τ_{facil}.

Relationship Between Parameters of the TM Model and Those of the Quantal Model

Few models are likely to capture such pertinent descriptors of synaptic transmission as those of the quantal model of transmission (see Redman 1990; Stevens 1993). It is therefore important to establish the relationship between the phenomenological parameters and those of the quantal model.

The Parameter A The parameter A is equivalent to the quantal size (q) multiplied by the number of release sites (n) and an electrotonic attenuation factor (X). Current-clamp recording from the soma yields A at the recording site. For somatic recordings this reflects the potential of the synaptic input to directly influence AP discharging. Voltage-clamp recordings would reveal A at the synapses, which could be used to determine the average q.

The Parameter U U is equivalent to the Pr if frequency dependence is determined only by presynaptic factors, such as vesicle depletion, AP-evoked Ca^{2+} channel inactivation, or AP axonal conduction failure. If postsynaptic receptor desensitization contributes to frequency dependence, then U is equivalent to Pr added to a postsynaptic component. The postsynaptic component is likely to depend on multiple parameters at the synapse that determine the extent to which postsynaptic receptors are saturated (see Jones and Westbrook 1996). U would also reflect the activation of voltage-dependent conductances during high-frequency trains and hence alternate voltage-clamp and current-clamp experiments can be used to isolate such conductances. Most single-axon synaptic responses are, however, small in amplitude and hence the kinetics of frequency dependence are hardly affected (Markram 1997). U is therefore a functional parameter that relates to the specific properties of the frequency dependence expressed by the connection between any two neurons.

The Parameter τ_{rec} The parameter τ_{rec} can be determined either directly from the experimental traces or derived from the model fit of the experimental traces. The biophysical correlate of recovery from depression could be vesicle depletion (Liley and North 1953; Zucker 1989) or recovery from a functional refractory period of release due to, for example, progressive decrease in AP-evoked Ca^{2+} influx (Klein et al. 1980; Zucker 1989), desensitization of the Ca^{2+}-induced release machinery, or recovery from an axonal refractory period.

The Parameter τ_{facil} Most theories of facilitation involve residual Ca^{2+} in the terminal. The specific mechanisms underlying various time constants for facilitation, and the differing amplitudes of these time constants, as well as their apparent independence, are less clear (see Magleby and Zengel 1982). According to data from the neuromuscular junction, τ_{facil} could represent an average over the first two faster time constants of facilitation and part of augmentation (Magleby and Zengel 1982).

Advantages of the TM Model

There are several advantages to adopting a phenomenological model to study frequency dependence. (1) The difficulty of recording and measuring single synaptic responses is overcome since only the average response is required for analysis. (2) The phenomenological approach allows analysis of frequency dependence without debatable assumptions of the release process which is required in the statistical analyses of single synaptic responses (see Faber and Korn 1991; Redman 1990). A separation from the precise biophysical mechanisms of release is therefore possible. This is important since a full characterization of the biophysics of neurotransmitter release is likely to evolve at the rate of molecular characterization of the building blocks of the presynaptic terminal. (3) A full characterization of the phenomena is able to point to the most likely biophysical mechanisms that underlie the change. (4) The formulation can be used to explore the properties of transmission mathematically to reveal properties of synapses that are relevant to how they transfer information contained in presynaptic AP trains. This may allow the construction of elementary building blocks to bridge the gap between synaptic transmission and information processing and between synaptic plasticity and learning and memory.

QUANTIFYING FREQUENCY-DEPENDENT PROPERTIES

The major problem with frequency-dependent synaptic transmission is that it seems too complex to deal with. It is therefore important to establish a means of analyzing frequency dependence in a quantitative manner. The simplest way to do this is to examine the relationship between the amplitudes of EPSPs, or inhibitory postsynaptic potentials (IPSPs), that reach a steady-state (termed $EPSP_{St}$) for different frequencies of stimulation. This frequency-response relationship has yielded novel properties of both depressing and facilitating synapses (Tsodyks and Markram 1997; Markram et al. 1998a).

The Limiting Frequency (λ)

When depressing synapses are driven at progressively higher frequencies, then $EPSP_{St}$ decrease progressively. However, at a specific frequency, termed the limiting frequency (λ), an intriguing phenomenon emerges—$EPSP_{St}$ begin to decrease inversely proportional to the frequency (r) (Tsodyks and Markram 1997; Markram et al. 1998a) (figure 10.2).

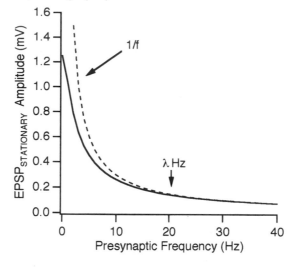

A Depressing Synapses

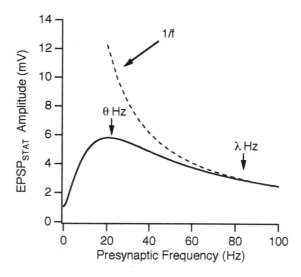

B Facilitating Synapses

Figure 10.2 Frequency dependence of facilitating and depressing synaptic connections. Represented are the curves that were used to fit experimental data (not shown). (A) The frequency-$EPSP_{St}$ relationship for depressing synaptic connections. The dashed lines show the 1/f curve and the frequency of convergence is termed the limiting frequency, λ. B, The Frequency-$EPSP_{St}$ relationship for facilitating synaptic connections. The dotted lines show the 1/f curve and the frequency at the peak is termed the peak frequency, θ.

$$EPSP_{st} \approx \frac{A}{r \cdot \tau_{rec}}. \tag{5}$$

This 1/f rule of synaptic depression has been indirectly referred to by assuming that the product of the frequency and of the amplitudes of $EPSP_{St}$ saturates (Grossberg 1969). The limiting frequency is a characteristic frequency of synapses since it reflects a specific relationship between neurotransmitter release and recovery from depression and, if present, facilitation. For depressing synapses,

$$\lambda \approx \frac{1}{U \cdot \tau_{rec}}. \tag{6}$$

Facilitating synapses also obey the 1/f rule, but at much higher frequencies. The formulation to determine λ for facilitating synapses is more complex (see Tsodyks et al. 1998). Typical values of l are 5 to 30 Hz for depressing synapses and 70 to 130 Hz for facilitating synapses.

The Peak Frequency (θ)

When facilitating synapses are stimulated at progressively higher frequencies, $EPSP_{St}$ first increase and then decrease. The resulting frequency-response relationship is described by a bell-shaped curve (figure 10.3). This behavior is absent from depressing synapses because it is generated by the simultaneous facilitation of u and growing depression (decrease in R) at higher values of u. Independent changes in facilitation and depression have also been reported for neuromuscular junction synapses (Magleby and Zengel 1976). The peak of the bell-shaped curve is a characteristic feature of a given facilitating synapse and is defined as the *peak frequency* (Markram et al. 1998a). θ can be derived from the model equations by finding the frequency where the product of u and R are at a maximum. The relationship between θ and the model parameters can be approximated for any facilitating synapse;

$$\theta \approx \frac{1}{\sqrt{U \cdot \tau_{rec} \cdot \tau_{facil}}}. \tag{7}$$

Typical values of θ range from 3 to 30 Hz for connections from neocortical pyramidal neurons to interneurons in layers 2 to 3, 4, and 5 (Markram et al. 1998a).

By incorporating additional time constants and different amplitudes for the various components of depression and facilitation, further characteristic features of the frequency-response relationship of synapses can be determined. These characteristic parameters of frequency-dependent synapses can also be used to quantify the impact of synaptic modifications in terms of changes in λ or θ. Changes in λ or θ in turn allow quantification of the impact of synaptic modifications on the information transmission capacity of synapses.

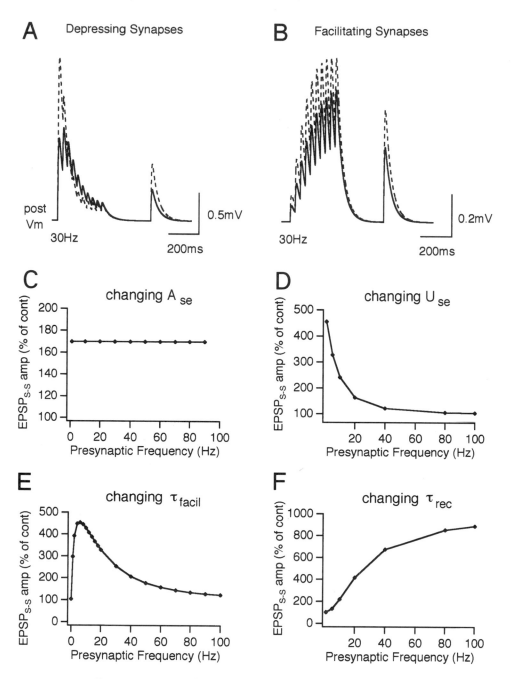

Figure 10.3 Four classes of synaptic plasticity at single facilitating-type synapses. A and B show differences in synaptic responses to trains of action potentials before and after U is increased. Plotted are the differences in the steady-state EPSPs for different frequencies of presynaptic action potentials following a change in one of the synaptic parameters. (C) A was increased from 1.0 to 1.7 mV. A was 1 and U was 0.4. (D) U was increased from 0.03 to 0.05. A_{se} was 1, τ_{rec} was 150 ms, and τ_{rec} was 600 ms. (E) τ_{facil} was decreased from 600 to 200 ms. A was 2, U was 0.03 and τ_{rec} was 150 ms. (F) τ_{rec} was decreased from 150 ms to 75 ms. U was 0.03, τ_{rec} and τ_{facil} was 600 ms.

TRANSFER FUNCTIONS OF FREQUENCY-DEPENDENT SYNAPSES

The phenomenological model can be used to derive mathematical descriptions of the features of the presynaptic APs transmitted to postsynaptic neurons; defined as synaptic transfer functions. These transfer functions provide a means of quantifying the information transmission capacity of synapses. Such an approach is essential since the information transmission is complex and history- or state-dependent as opposed to a simple linear transfer of presynaptic discharge rates.

To derive the various forms of a transfer function for a given synaptic connection, the average postsynaptic response at time t after arbitrary changes in presynaptic discharge rates $r(t')$ at times $t' < t$ of a Poisson AP train is computed and the linearity of the response with respect to the increment in discharge rate is assessed. Details of the calculations are presented in Tsodyks et al. 1998. The frequency ranges in which synapses transmit specific features of the presynaptic APs are referred to as signaling regimes.

A Signaling Regime for Derivatives of Presynaptic Discharge Rates

Beyond λ, it is no longer possible to transmit the absolute discharge rates since the product of the frequency and $EPSP_{St}$ saturates. The frequency range near and above λ therefore contains only a sublinear regime of signaling. This signaling regime exists for both depressing and facilitating synapses, but for facilitating synapses the regime is at much higher frequencies due to higher ranges of λ. The main feature that is transmitted in this signaling regime is changes in frequencies [derivatives of discharge rates, $r(t)$]. The form of the transfer function for this frequency range is;

$$r(t) \int_{-\infty}^{t} dt'e - \int_{t'}^{t} r(t'') \, dt'' = 1 + \frac{r'}{r^2} + \frac{3(r')^2}{r^4} + \frac{r''}{r^3} + \cdots. \tag{8}$$

A Signaling Regime for Discharge Rates

The frequency range below λ contains a progressively higher contribution of the absolute discharge rate of the presynaptic neuron until it becomes dominant in the range around θ. This signaling regime is referred to as a linear regime and the form of the transfer function is simply the discharge rate, $r(t)$. This signaling regime also exists for depressing synapses, but their linear regime is in a narrow range of low frequencies (less than 1 Hz).

A Signaling Regime for Integrated AP Activity

A supralinear signaling regime also exists for facilitating synapses in the frequency range between 0 and θ. In this regime the postsynaptic response reflects not only the presynaptic discharge rate but also the total number of

APs. This is an intriguing property since it enables facilitating synapses to "count" the number of APs in a burst. More precisely, the presynaptic rate is amplified by a facilitating factor equivalent to the integral of discharge rates weighted with a decaying kernel of time constant, τ_{facil}. The form of the transfer function for this frequency range is

$$r(t) \int_{-\infty}^{t} r(t')e^{-(t-t')/\tau_{facil}} \, dt' \tag{9}$$

which can be approximated by multiplying the discharge rate by the number of APs emitted during the preceding time window of τ_{facil}.

These analyses demonstrate that the values of q and l determine the *content* of information that can be transmitted between neurons via APs. It follows then that plasticity of frequency dependence, also referred to as "redistribution of synaptic efficacy," serves to alter the content of information transmitted between neurons as opposed to the gain of transmission (Markram and Tsodyks 1996).

HETEROGENEITY IN THE VALUES OF MULTIPLE SYNAPTIC PARAMETERS

A single neuron may contact hundreds or thousands of target neurons. Understanding the heterogeneity in the properties of these connections is not only crucial to understanding how synapses are involved in information processing within neural networks but also what effect modifying specific synaptic properties would have on information processing and hence how synaptic plasticity relates to learning and memory. Differential facilitation and depression of synaptic transmission via the same axon has been reported in several simple organisms (Parnas and Atwood 1966; Laurent and Sivaramakrishnan 1992; Davis and Murphey 1993; Katz et al. 1993; Cooper et al. 1995; Frost and Katz 1996). In the neocortex, dual recordings have also revealed depressing synaptic responses from pyramidal neurons to interneurons and facilitating synaptic responses from pyramidal neurons to interneurons (Thomson et al. 1993a,b; Thomson 1997). Recently, triple and quadruple cell recordings revealed directly that differential synaptic transmission via the same axon is a prominent feature of synaptic transmission in the neocortex (Markram et al. 1998a). The main findings and interpretations are the following:

1. Synaptic connections established via the same axon and in many cases via the same collateral from a pyramidal neuron onto a homogeneous class of pyramidal neurons differ significantly in the number and location of synapses on the dendrites as well as A, U, and as τ_{rec}.

2. Synaptic connections established via the same axon from a pyramidal neuron onto a pyramidal neuron and an interneuron can display depression onto the pyramidal neuron and facilitation onto the interneuron.

3. Synaptic connections onto two interneurons can display differential facilitation and depression.

4. Synaptic responses generated by connections established from three pyramidal neurons of the same morphological class onto a single interneuron all display facilitation of transmission, but the connections differ greatly in their values of A, U, τ_{rec}, and τ_{facil}, as well as their numbers of synaptic contacts. In 65% of cases the synapse from one neuron was established on the same dendritic branch as the synapse formed by the other convergent input connection, indicating that differential synaptic properties can arise even when contacts are formed on the same dendritic branch.

These studies support previous conclusions that the type of pre- and postsynaptic neuron determines the class of frequency dependence of synapses and further suggest that the precise values of the synaptic parameters are determined by the unique interaction between the two neurons in the context of the network. This alludes to an enormous "plastic potential" and strongly supports the notion that synaptic plasticity involves much more than merely changing the gain of synapses. These findings also indicate that the synaptic representations conveyed to each of the potentially thousands of targets neurons are potentially unique—the transfer functions are unique —which suggests that information processing in neural networks is considerably more complex than previously imagined.

PLASTICITY OF FREQUENCY-DEPENDENT SYNAPSES

A Potential for Multiple Mechanisms and Phenomena of Synaptic Plasticity at Single Synapses

At least four different parameters determine the properties of synaptic transmission, each in a unique manner (Markram et al. 1988b). It follows then that there are at least four classes of synaptic modifications. Briefly, the four classes of synaptic plasticity that are produced are (1) a frequency-independent change in synaptic transmission by changing A; (2) a selective regulation of low-frequency synaptic transmission by changing U; (3) a selective regulation of intermediate frequencies by changing τ_{facil}; and (4) a selective regulation of high frequency synaptic transmission by changing τ_{rec}.

A Frequency-Independent Change in Synaptic Transmission by Changing A Modulation of postsynaptic receptor efficacies (McNaughton 1982; Kauer et al. 1988; Bashir et al. 1991) is a straightforward potential mechanism to change the absolute synaptic strength since a uniform, frequency-independent change in all synaptic responses would be observed. This can be quantified as an increase in A and the phenomena could be referred to as, for example, long-term potentiation-a (LTP$_a$) and long-term depression-a (LTD$_a$). It is essential to confirm changes in A by monitoring the change in synaptic responses to an irregular train of afferent stimuli, since it is possible that the change is only uniform for the particular frequency used in the test pulse. Adding more receptors will increase A if sufficient transmitter is released to saturate receptors or if receptor clustering is rearranged (Xie et al. 1997). Postsynaptic receptor desensitization could be important during high-frequency stimulation (Jonas 1993; Jonas et al. 1994; Jonas and Spruston 1994; Jones and Westbrook 1996) and would confound the effects of adding receptors. Both A and U would tend to change if receptors are added under these conditions. Determining whether receptors are saturated and whether there is any postsynaptic component of frequency dependence is therefore necessary in order to understand the effects of changing postsynaptic receptor numbers and distributions.

Adding or modulating postsynaptic N-methyl-D-aspartate (NMDA) receptors could also change A, but if postsynaptic NMDA receptors contribute to the value of U, then U would be voltage dependent and adding these receptors would change U at depolarized potentials.

Opening new active sites within a single terminal or a newly matured synapse would change A, but it seems unlikely that this would be accompanied by an exact jump to the mean of the kinetic parameters of the other synapses or release sites of the connection, and therefore will probably also be accompanied by changes in U, τ_{rec}, and τ_{facil}. Synaptic responses at all frequencies will therefore be altered, but not necessarily uniformly.

A Selective Regulation of Low-Frequency Synaptic Transmission by Changing U Changing Pr is readily distinguished from virtually all other types of synaptic changes since changing Pr is actually a mechanism to selectively regulate low-frequency synaptic transmission, which can be quantified as a change in U and termed, for example, LTP$_u$ or LTD$_u$. This is because at high frequencies, Pr either decreases to converge at low values regardless of the initial Pr (presynaptic mechanism of depression) (Thies 1965; Betz 1970) or Pr becomes irrelevant since recovery from synaptic depression becomes the rate-limiting step (postsynaptic mechanism of depression).

A Selective Regulation of Intermediate-Frequency Synaptic Transmission by Changing τ_{facil} A change in τ_{facil} results in LTP$_f$ or LTD$_f$. The phenomenon is unique and is expressed as a change in transmission over only an intermediate range of frequencies, unlike those caused by changing U (low frequencies) or τ_{rec} (high frequencies). It is also possible that both the amplitudes and time constants of multiple components of facilitation could be modulated (see Magleby and Zengel 1976) producing LTP$_{f[n(m)]}$ where n would indicate which component of facilitation is affected $(1, 2 \ldots n)$, and m would indicate whether either the amplitude (a) or time constant, (t) changed. The biophysical targets are not clear, but could include changing the buffer capacity of the terminal for Ca^{2+}, as well as direct modulation of the affinities for Ca^{2+} binding to the release machinery.

A Selective Regulation of High-Frequency Synaptic Transmission by Changing τ_{rec}   Changing τ_{rec} is a powerful potential mechanism for regulating high-frequency synaptic transmission (termed, e.g., LTP_d and LTD_d). The biophysical mechanisms responsible for determining τ_{rec} could include, for example, modulating the rate of vesicle recycling, the rate of AP-evoked Ca^{2+} channel inactivation, blockade of axon conduction failure, or reduction in the desensitization rate of Ca^{2+} induced release.

Experimental Evidence for Distinct Types of Synapses

The effect of changing synaptic properties largely depends on whether the synapse is a depressing type or a facilitating type. Are these distinctions justified? Whether facilitation or depression is expressed is usually considered to depend only on Pr. While Pr can certainly determine whether facilitation or depression is displayed, some evidence indicates that there may also be distinct depressing-type and facilitating-type synapses. (1) Depression is observed at all synaptic connections between layer 5 pyramidal neurons regardless of U (range, 0.1 to 0.95 Markram and Tsodyks 1996; Tsodyks and Markram 1997; see also Markram et al. 1997a for Pr ranges). (2) Lowering external $[Ca^{2+}]:[Mg^{2+}]$ to produce up to 90% failures from about 5% unmasks a small amount of facilitation in some connections (two of four tested), but cannot convert synaptic responses into those that remotely resemble those produced by the connection from pyramidal neurons to interneurons (H. Markram, unpublished). (3) Incorporating facilitation into the model does not improve the fit to experimental traces even when U is very low.

Experimental Evidence for Redistribution of Synaptic Efficacy

Heterogeneity of the values of the various synaptic parameters is not the only evidence for plasticity of frequency dependence. (1) Hebbian pairing of pre- and postsynaptic neurons results in a selective increase in low-frequency synaptic transmission (Markram and Tsodyks 1996) due to a change in U (Tsodyks and Markram 1997). (2) Presynaptic regulation of Pr, which is typically considered as a mechanism to block or enhance transmission between neurons, actually changes U. (3) Changes in paired-pulse ratios in LTP experiments inadvertently demonstrates redistribution of synaptic efficacy (Christie and Abraham 1994; Jung and Larson 1994; Schulz et al. 1995; Choi and Lovinger 1997; Schulz 1997; Torii et al. 1997). (4) Recent experiments suggest that the initial stage of LTD_a, of facilitating synapses from pyramidal neurons to interneurons, is preceded by a selective loss of facilitation (LTD_f) (A. Gupta and H. Markram, in preparation). (5) Selective changes in both the amplitudes and time constants of subcomponents of facilitation that could correspond to LTP_{f3a}, LTD_{f3t}, and LTP_{f4t} have been observed at the neuromuscular junction (Magleby and Zengel 1976).

A "Synaptic Plasticity Code"

Analysis of the phenomenological model reveals that an intricate and complex relationship exists between the various parameters to determine how each parameter would influence transmission under different conditions. For example, when τ_{facil} is changed, then the change has a maximum effect over an intermediate range of frequencies. The amplitude of this effect on transmission, and the precise frequency range of over which the effect is exerted, would depend on the values of U and τ_{rec}. Similarly, the smaller U is for facilitating synapses, the less important τ_{rec} is, or the larger τ_{facil} is, the more important τ_{rec} becomes since depression is more readily engaged. It seems unlikely therefore that the mechanisms which regulate one synaptic parameter would operate independently of the existing value and changes in the other parameters. This alludes to an apparent need for a "synaptic plasticity code" to coordinate modifications of specific parameters since modulating any one parameter depends on the value of the others.

There is also some experimental evidence that could already point to a "synaptic plasticity code." The conditions driving U, but not those driving (Markram et al. 1997a; Senn et al. 1997) A, τ_{facil}, and τ_{rec}, are known for the synaptic connections between neocortical pyramidal neurons. One prediction is that the same conditions that cause LTP_u would also trigger LTP_a if a metabotropic receptor were simultaneously activated. Some evidence pointing in this direction is provided by a study where AP activity only in the presence of neurotrophins results in structural changes (McAllister et al. 1995) and a recent report indicated that two different forms of LTD can be produced with the same stimulation protocol depending on whether a metabotropic receptor is activated or not (Kemp and Bashir 1997).

How Many Algorithms for Synaptic Plasticity Are There?

It is usually assumed that algorithms are universal for all synaptic connections (for review, see Fregnac and Shulz 1994). Given the complexity of pre- and postsynaptic interactions and the large potential types of synapses, the only reasonable assumption is that there are as many algorithms as there are classes of pre- and postsynaptic neurons—that is, potential classes of synapses. At least the two broad classes of depressing and facilitating synapses exist and recent evidence suggests that the rules for synaptic modifications are different for these two connections. For example, repetitive stimulation with brief high-frequency bursts (typically used as test pulses) induces LTD_a in facilitating synapses (in preparation), which is not observed at depressing synapses between pyramidal neurons.

Markram et al.

NETWORK COMPUTATION WITH FREQUENCY-DEPENDENT SYNAPSES

The Mystery of Recurrent Network Architecture

The recurrent architecture of neural networks, inferred by Hebb from the work of the early anatomists, is perhaps the most mysterious of all neuronal designs. It captured Hebb's imagination and he proposed that this could enable reverberations of activity which could "hold" representations for a short period of time (short-term memory) until changes in the strength of synaptic coupling could change to deposit the memory trace for long-term retrieval (long-term memory) (Hebb 1949; see also Amit 1996). What Hebb did not consider, however, was how these reverberations could survive when neurons are connected by frequency-dependent synapses since this essentially allows the functional architecture of synaptic coupling strength to change markedly on the time scale of milliseconds. Initial simulations indicate that only very special (if at all) conditions would support reverberations. Recurrence in networks with frequency-dependent connections will also not simply act to amplify internal activity for a longer period of time than it takes the synapses to depress (Douglas et al. 1995).

The mystery of recurrence is therefore not solved. The network of layer 5 pyramidal neurons is massively recurrent with first-, second-, and higher-order reciprocal feedback, suggesting that the "echo" of a single neuron's activity can return to the neuron after integration at several different layers (Markram 1997). What message is returning to these neurons and why? The computational function in quantitative terms of such parallel multilayered feedback is not known (see Hebb 1949; Amit 1989; Sutton and Barto 1990; Hertz et al. 1991; Churchland and Sejnowski 1992; Fregnac and Shulz 1994; Gluck and Myers 1997). Recordings from three and four neurons in layers 2 and 3 also revealed highly complex connections between neurons. A local neocortical microcircuit that would make up a neocortical column is therefore a massively recurrent circuit. This does not only apply to excitatory connections; inhibitory neurons are also enveloped within the meshwork of recurrent connections and can even be reciprocal onto the neuron that provides excitation. In other words, at the microcircuit level, hierarchical flow of processed information will be rapidly diluted and each neuron may exist potentially at many levels of integration depending on the topography of the stimulus as well as the history of activity.

The Concept of "Per Action Portential Synaptic Efficiency"

The activation of a subset of neurons within a network initially results in a feedforward response and then other neurons in the network are excited via the recurrent connections. It would seem possible that a fraction of the synaptic responses generated by the recurrent connection will be "wasted" in that they will not contribute to discharging postsynaptic neurons since these target neurons could either be in a refractory period of activity or too far from threshold to discharge. On the other hand, it is possible that as the recurrent connections facilitate reintegration of information, that the activity of the neurons in the network become orchestrated. The extreme of such an orchestration is where each AP from each neuron discharges at the precise moment so that its synaptic output at all its synapses is optimally effective. This would represent an incredible computational feat in which each neuron's activity becomes optimally orchestrated with every other neuron in the network and would therefore be an extremely ordered and efficient state of the network. It is proposed that the "per action potential synaptic efficiency" (PAP_{se}) increases following a stimulus (A. Uziel, H. Markram, and M. Tsodyks, in preparation) and that PAP_{se} could be a measure of the efficiency by which a neural network performs a specific computation. Various algorithms for quantifying PAP_{se} can be formulated and are not considered further here.

Iterations Between Synaptic Transfer Functions and Action Potential Activity Patterns as a Mechanism of Orchestrating Neuronal Network Activity

At the onset of a stimulus, the neurons in a network are driven by the feed-forward input from a distant area—that is, the network has not computed anything using the recurrent connections (see also Grossberg 1980). As time passes, the network is able to compute, involving more and more integration via its recurrent connections. What are the consequences of repeatedly feeding the APs emitted by the circuit back into the circuit? The mathematical analysis of frequency-dependent synapses reveals that AP activity patterns would alter the forms of synaptic transfer functions of each synapse in a unique manner. In recurrent networks, the changed forms of synaptic transfer functions would influence subsequent AP activity patterns in the network and iterations of AP activity patterns and synaptic transfer functions therefore seems inevitable. Differential signaling via the same axon within recurrent networks may therefore allow transfer functions of each synapse to fine-tune the network AP response through repetitive iterations and hence cause an increase in PAP_{se} following a stimulus.

The Effect of Plasticity of Frequency Dependence on Neural Network Dynamics

Plasticity of frequency-dependent synapses is a complex issue where it seems likely that multiple mechanisms, phenomena, and algorithms for plasticity exist even at single synapses. Synaptic modifications can be seen as a change in at least one or more of the four parameters, A, U, τ_{rec}, and τ_{facil}. This effect can be translated into changes in the higher-level functional parameters, λ and θ, which in turn provides a means of assessing the change in the various forms of the synaptic transfer functions of the synapses. When considering the several thousand synapses formed by each axon, then synaptic plasticity could serve to regulate the precise forms of the transfer functions for each synapse. This could change the sequence in which the iterations are performed or change the step size of iterations (in preparation; Markram 1997) and hence optimize the speed of network processing using recurrent interconnections to allow more "in-depth" integration of the stimulus. In other words, synaptic modifications could enable progressively more of the information embedded within the interconnections to be incorporated into the network response within the time allowed before the next stimulus imposes its feedforward information.

REFERENCES

Abbott, L. F., Varela, J. A., Sen, K., and Nelson, S. B. (1997). Synaptic depression and cortical gain control. *Science* 275: 220–224.

Abeles, M. (1991). *Corticonics.* New York, Cambridge University Press.

Amit, D. J. (1989). *Modeling Brain Function.* New York, Cambridge University Press.

Amit, D. J. (1996). The Hebbian paradigm reintegrated: local reverberations as internal representations. *Behav. Brain Res.* 18.

Bashir, Z. I., Alford, S., Davies, S. N., Randall, A. D., and Collingridge, G. L. (1991). Long-term potentiation of NMDA receptor–mediated synaptic transmission in the hippocampus. *Nature* 349: 156–158.

Bertram, R., Sherman, A., and Stanley, E. F. (1996). Single-domain/bound calcium hypothesis of transmitter release and facilitation. *J. Neurophysiol.* 75: 1919–1931.

Betz, W. J. (1970). Depression of transmitter release at the neuromuscular junction of the frog. *J. Physiol. (Lond.)* 206(3): 629–644.

Buhl, E. H., Tamas, G., Szilagyi, T., Stricker, C., and Paulsen, O. S., P. (1997). Effect, number and location of synapses made by single pyramidal cells onto aspiny interneurones of cat visual cortex. *J. Physiol. (Lond.)* 500: 689–713.

Buonomano, D. V., Baxter, D. A., and Byrne, J. H. (1990). Small networks of empirically derived adaptive elements simulate some high-order features of classical conditioning. *Neural Networks* 3: 507–523.

Byrne, J. (1978). Analysis of the synaptic depression contribution to habituation of gill-withdrawal reflex in *Aplysia californica. J. Neurophysiol.* 48: 431–438.

Carew, T. J., Walters, E. T., and Kandel, E. R. (1981). Classical conditioning in a simple withdrawal reflex in *Aplysia californica. J. Neurosci.* 1: 1426–1437.

Choi, S., and Lovinger, D. M. (1997). Decreased probability of neurotransmitter release underlies striatal long-term depression and postnatal development of corticostriatal synapses. *Proc. Natl. Acad. Sci. USA* 94: 2665–26670.

Christie, B. R., and Abraham, W. C. (1994). Differential regulation of paired-pulse plasticity following LTP in the dentate gyrus. *Neuroreport* 5: 385–388.

Churchland, P. S., and Sejnowski, T. J. (1992). *The Computational Brain.* Cambridge, MA, MIT Press.

Ciaccia, P., Maio, D., and Vacca, G. P. (1992). An analytical short- and long-term memory model of presynaptic plasticity. *Biol. Cybern.* 67: 335–345.

Cooper, R. L., Marin, L., and Atwood, H. L. (1995). Synaptic differentiation of a single motor neuron: conjoint definition of transmitter release, presynaptic calcium signals, and ultrastructure. *J. Neurosci.* 15: 4209–4222.

Davis, G. W., and Murphey, R. K. (1993). A role for postsynaptic neurons in determining presynaptic release properties in the cricket CNS: evidence for retrograde control of facilitation. *J. Neurosci.* 13: 3827–3838.

del Castillo, J., and Katz, B. (1954). Statistical factors involved in the neuromuscular facilitation and depression. *J. Physiol.* 124: 574–585.

Desmond, J. E., and Moore, J. W. (1988). Adaptive timing in neural networks: the conditioned response. *Biol. Cybern.* 58: 405–415.

Destexhe, A., Mainen, Z. F., and Sejnowski, T. J. (1994). Synthesis of models for excitable membranes, synaptic transmission and neuromodulation using a common kinetic formalism. *J. Comput. Neurosci.* 1(3): 195–230.

Deuchars, J., and Thomson, A. M. (1995). Single axon fast inhibitory postsynaptic potentials elicited by a sparsely spiny interneuron in rat neocortex. *Neuroscience* 65: 935–942.

Deuchars, J., and Thomson, A. M. (1996). CA1 pyramid-pyramid connections in rat hippocampus in vitro: dual intracellular recordings with biocytin filling. *Neuroscience* 74: 1009–1108.

Deuchars, J., West, D. C., and Thomson, A. M. (1994). Relationships between morphology and physiology of pyramid-pyramid single axon connections in rat neocortex in vitro. *J. Physiol. (Lond.)* 3: 423–435.

Douglas, R. J., Koch, C., Mahowald, M., Martin, K. A., and Suarez, H. H. (1995). Recurrent excitation in neocortical circuits. *Science* 269: 981–985.

Faber, D. S., and Korn, H. (1991). Applicability of the coefficient of variation method for analyzing synaptic plasticity. *Biophys. J.* 60: 1288–1294.

Feng, T. P. (1941). Studies on the neuromuscular junction. XXVI. The changes of the end-plate potential during and after prolonged stimulation. *Chin. J. Physiol.* 16: 341–372.

Fregnac, Y., and Shulz, D. (1994). Models of synaptic plasticity and cellular analogs of learning in developing and adult visual cortex. In *Advances in Neuronal and Behavioral Development*, Vol. 4, V. A. Casagrande and P. G. Shinkman, eds., pp. 149–235. NU Ablex. New Jersey.

Frost, W. N., and Katz, P. S. (1996). Single neuron control over a complex motor program. *Proc. Natl. Acad. Sci. USA* 93: 422–426.

Gingrich, K. J., and Byrne, J. (1985). Simulation of synaptic depression, posttetanic potentiation, and presynaptic facilitation of synaptic potentials from sensory neurons mediating gill-withdrawal reflex in Aplysia. *J. Neurophysiol.* 53: 652–669.

Gluck, M. A., and Myers, C. E. (1997). Psychobiological models of hippocampal function in learning and memory. *Annu. Rev. Psychol.* 48: 481–514.

Grossberg, S. (1969). On the production and release of chemical transmitters and related topics in cellular control. *J. Theorl. Biol.* 22: 325–364.

Grossberg, S. (1980). How does a brain build a cognitive code? *Physiol. Rev.* 87: 1–51.

Hebb, D. O. (1949). *The Organization of Behavior*. New York, John Wiley & Sons.

Hertz, J., Krogh, A., and Palmer, R. G. (1991). *Introduction to the Theory of Neural Computation* New York, Adison-Wesley.

Hubbard, J. I. (1963). Repetitive stimulation at the neuromuscular junction, and the mobilization of transmitter. *J. Physiol.* 169: 641–662.

Hutter, O. F. (1952). Post-tetanic restoration of neuromuscular transmission blocked by *d*-tubocurarine. *J. Physiol.* 118: 216–227.

Jonas, P. (1993). Glutamate receptors in the central nervous system. *Ann. N Y Acad. Sci.* 707: 126–135.

Jonas, P., and Spruston, N. (1994). Mechanisms shaping glutamate-mediated excitatory post-synaptic currents in the CNS. *Curr. Opin. Neurobiol.* 4: 366–372.

Jonas, P., Racca, C., Sakmann, B., Seeburg, P. H., and Monyer, H. (1994). Differences in Ca^{2+} permeability of AMPA-type glutamate receptor channels in neocortical neurons caused by differential GluR-B subunit expression. *Neuron* 12: 1281–1289.

Jones, M. V., and Westbrook, G. L. (1996). The impact of receptor desensitization on fast synaptic transmission. *Trends Neurosci.* 19: 96–101.

Jung, M. W., and Larson, J. (1994). Further characteristics of long-term potentiation in piriform cortex. *Synapse* 18: 298–306.

Katz, P. S., Kirk, M. D., and Govind, C. K. (1993). Facilitation and depression at different branches of the same motor axon: evidence for presynaptic differences in release. *J. Neurosci.* 13: 3075–3089.

Kauer, J. A., Malenka, R. C., and Nicoll, R. A. (1988). A persistent postsynaptic modification mediates long-term potentiation in the hippocampus. *Neuron* 1: 911–917.

Kemp, N., and Bashir, Z. I., (1977). Long-term depression of synaptic transmission in the CA1 region of the adult rat hippocampus in vitro. *J. Physiol. (Lond.)* 504P: P212–P212.

Klein, M., Shapiro, E., and Kandel, E. R. (1980). Synaptic plasticity and the modulation of the Ca^{2+} current. *J. Exp. Biol.* 89: 117–157.

Korn, H., Faber, D. S., Burnod, Y., and Triller, A. (1984). Regulation of efficacy at central synapses. *J. Neurosci.* 4: 125–130.

Korn, H., Faber, D. S., and Triller, A. (1986). Probabilistic determination of synaptic strength. *J. Neurophysiol.* 55: 402–421.

Krausz, H. I., and Friesen, O. (1977). The analysis of nonlinear synaptic transmission. *J. Gen. Physiol.* 70: 244–265.

Laurent, G., and Sivaramakrishnan, A. (1992). Single local interneurons in the locust make central synapses with different properties of transmitter release on distinct postsynaptic neurons. *J. Neurosci.* 12: 2370–2380.

Liaw, J. S., and Berger, T. W. (1996). Dynamic synapse: a new concept of neural representation and computation. *Hippocampus* 6: 591–600.

Liley, A. W. (1956). The quantal components of the mammalian end-plate potential. *J. Physiol. (Lond.)* 133: 571–587.

Liley, A. W., and North, K. A. K. (1953). An electrical investigation of the effects of repetitive stimulation on mammalian neuromuscular junction. *J. Neurophysiol.* 16: 509–527.

Magleby, K. L. (1973). The effect of repetitive stimulation on transmitter release at the frog neuromuscular junction. *J. Physiol. (Lond.)* 234: 327–352.

Magleby, K. L. (1979). Facilitation, augmentation, and potentiation of transmitter release. *Prog. Brain Res.* 49: 175–182.

Magleby, K. L. (1987). Short-term changes in synaptic efficacy. In *Synaptic Function*, G. M. Edelman, W. E. Gall, and Cowman, eds., pp. 21–56. New York, John Wiley & Sons.

Magleby, K. L., and Zengel, J. E. (1976). Long term changes in augmentation, potentiation, and depression of transmitter release as a function of repeated synaptic activity at the frog neuromuscular junction. *J. Physiol. (Lond.)* 257: 471–494.

Magleby, K. L., and Zengel, J. E. (1982). A quantitative description of stimulation-induced changes in transmitter release at the frog neuromuscular junction. *J. Gen. Physiol.* 80: 613–638.

Markram, H. (1997). A network of tufted layer 5 pyramidal neurons. *Cereb. Cortex* 7: 523–533.

Markram, H., and Tsodyks, M. (1996). Redistribution of synaptic efficacy between neocortical pyramidal neurons [see comments]. *Nature* 382: 807–180.

Markram, H., Lübke, J., Frotscher, M., Roth, A., and Sakmann, B. (1997a). Physiology and anatomy of synaptically coupled connections between thick tufted pyramidal neurons in the developing rat neocortex. *J. Physiol. (Lond.)* 500: 4009–4440.

Markram, H., Lubke, J., Frotscher, M., and Sakmann, B. (1997b). Regulation of synaptic efficacy by coincidence of postsynaptic APs and EPSPs. *Science* 275: 213–215.

Markram, H., Wang, Y., and Tsodyks, M. (1998a). Differential synaptic signaling via the same axon of neocortical pyramidal neurons. *Proc. Natl. Acad. Sci. USA* 95: 5323–5328.

Markram, H., Gupta, A., Wang, Y., Uziel, A., and Tsodyks, M. (1998b). Information processing in neural networks with frequency-dependent synapses. *Neurobiol. Learn. Mem.* 70: 101–112.

Markram, H., Tsodyks, H., and Pikus, D. (1998c). Potential for multiple mechanisms, phenomena and algorithms for synaptic plasticity at single synapses. *J. Neuropharmacol.* 37: 489–500.

McAllister, A. K., Lo, D. C., and Katz, L. C. (1995). Neurotrophins regulate dendritic growth in developing visual cortex. *Neuron* 15: 791–803.

McNaughton, B. L. (1982). Long-term synaptic enhancement and short-term potentiation in rat fascia dentata act through different mechanisms. *J. Physiol. (Lond.)* 324: 249–262.

Parnas, I., and Atwood, H. L. (1966). Phasic and tonic neuromuscular systems in the abdominal extensor muscles of the crayfish and rock lobster. *Comp. Biochem. Physiol* 18: 701–723.

Pinsker, H., Kandel, E. R., Castellucci, V., and Kupfermann, I. (1970). An analysis of habituation and dishabituation in *Aplysia*. *Adv. Biochem. Psychopharmacol.* 2: 351–373.

Redman, S. (1990). Quantal analysis of synaptic potentials in neurons of the central nervous system. *Physiol. Rev.* 70: 165–198.

Schulz, P. E. (1997). Long-term potentiation involves increases in the probability of neurotransmitter release. *Proc. Natl. Acad. Sci. USA* 94: 5888–5893.

Schulz, P. E., Cook, E. P., and Johnston, D. (1995). Using paired-pulse facilitation to probe the mechanisms for long-term potentiation (LTP). *J. Physiol. Paris* 89: 3–9.

Senn, W., Tsodyks, M., and Markram, H. (1997). An algorithm for synaptic plasticity based on exact timing of pre- and post-synaptic action potentials. *Lect. Notes Comput. Sci.* 1327: 121–126.

Somogyi, P., Kisvarday, Z. F., Martin, K. A., and Whitteridge, D. (1983). Synaptic connections of morphologically identified and physiologically characterized large basket cells in the striate cortex of cat. *Neuroscience* 10: 261–294.

Stevens, C. F. (1993). Quantal release of neurotransmitter and long-term potentiation. *Neuron* 10: 55–63.

Stevens, C. F., and Wang, Y. (1995). Facilitation and depression at single central synapses. *Neuron* 14: 795–802.

Stratford, K. J., Tarczy Hornoch, K., Martin, K. A., Bannister, N. J., and Jack, J. J. (1996). Excitatory synaptic inputs to spiny stellate cells in cat visual cortex. *Nature* 382: 258–261.

Stuart, G. J., Dodt, H.-U., and Sakmann, B. (1993). Patch-clamp recordings from the soma and dendrites of neurons in brain slices. *Pflugers Arch.* 490: 511–518.

Sutton, R. S., and Barto, A. G. (1990). Toward a modern theory of adaptive networks: expectation and prediction. *Psychol. Rev.* 88: 135–170.

Takeuchi, A. (1958). The long lasting depression in neuromuscular transmission of frog. *Jpn. J. Physiol.* 8: 102–113.

Thies, R. E. (1965). Neuromuscular depression and the apparent depletion of transmitter in mammalian muscle. *J. Neurophysiol.* 212: 431–446.

Thomson, A. M. (1997). Activity-dependent properties of synaptic transmission at two classes of connections made by rat neocortical pyramidal axons in vitro. *J. Physiol. (Lond.)* 502: 131–147.

Thomson, A. M., and Deuchars, J. (1994). Temporal and spatial properties of local circuits in neocortex. *Trends Neurosci.* 17: 119–126.

Thomson, A. M., and West, D. C. (1993). Fluctuations in pyramid-pyramid excitatory postsynaptic potentials modified by presynaptic firing pattern and postsynaptic membrane potential using paired intracellular recordings in rat neocortex. *Neuroscience* 54: 329–436.

Thomson, A. M., Girdlestone, D., and West, D. C. (1989). A local circuit neocortical synapse that operates via both NMDA and non-NMDA receptors. *Br. J. Pharmacol.* 96: 406–408.

Thomson, A. M., Deuchars, J., and West, D. C. (1993a). Large, deep layer pyramid-pyramid single axon EPSPs in slices of rat motor cortex display paired pulse and frequency-dependent depression, mediated presynaptically and self-facilitation, mediated postsynaptically. *J. Neurophysiol.* 70: 2354–2369.

Thomson, A. M., Deuchars, J., and West, D. C. (1993b). Single axon excitatory postsynaptic potentials in neocortical interneurons exhibit pronounced paired pulse facilitation. *Neuroscience* 54: 347–360.

Thomson, A. M., West, D. C., and Deuchars, J. (1995). Properties of single axon excitatory postsynaptic potentials elicited in spiny interneurons by action potentials in pyramidal neurons in slices of rat neocortex. *Neuroscience* 69: 727–738.

Thomson, A. M., West, D. C., Hahn, J., and Deuchars, J. (1996). Single axon IPSPs elicited in pyramidal cells by three classes of interneurones in slices of rat neocortex. *J. Physiol. (Lond.)* 496: 81–102.

Torii, N., Tsumoto, T., Uno, L., Astrelin, A. V., and Voronin, L. L. (1997). Quantal analysis suggests presynaptic involvement in expression of neocortical short- and long-term depression. *Neuroscience* 79: 317–321.

Tsodyks, M., and Markram, H. (1997). The neural code between neocortical pyramidal neurons depends on neurotransmitter release probability. *Proc. Natl. Acad. Sci. USA* 94: 719–723.

Tsodyks, M., Pawelzik, K., and Markram, H. (1998). Neural networks with dynamic synapses. *Neural Comput.* 10: 821–835.

Xie, X., Liaw, J. S., Baudry, M., and Berger, T. W. (1997). Novel expression mechanism for synaptic potentiation: alignment of presynaptic release site and postsynaptic receptor. *Proc. Natl. Acad. Sci. USA* 94: 6983–6988.

Zalutsky, R. A., and Nicoll, R. A. (1990). Comparison of two forms of long-term potentiation in single hippocampal neurons. *Science* 248: 1619–1624.

Zucker, R. S. (1989). Short-term synaptic plasticity. *Annu. Rev. Neurosci.* 12: 13–31.

11 Neurobiological Substrates of Associative Memory: A Limbic-Cortical Dialogue

François S. Roman, Franck A. Chaillan, Bruno Truchet, and Bernard Soumireu-Mourat

Modifications of synaptic efficacy in distributed neural networks in the brain could be the result of learning and memory processes. From neuropsychological observations in humans, it was possible to distinguish different subtypes of long-term memories (for a review, see Squire and Zola 1996). While implicit memory is spared in monkeys and humans with hippocampal lesions (Squire 1986; Squire and Zola-Morgan 1988), explicit memory is deeply impaired, although memory from the past is spared.

From these data, it appears that the hippocampus is mainly involved in the training, acquisition, and consolidation processes, while cortical areas are required to store long-term memories. In order to study the nature and properties of synaptic modifications following learning and memory in limbic and cortical structures, rats were trained in an olfactory associative task which has several interesting behavioral, anatomical, and electrophysiological features. Briefly, rats can perform an olfactory task as well as primates trained with visual cues (Slotnick and Katz 1974; Slotnick 1994). Furthermore, the dichotomy of memory features discussed above can be observed with this task (Roman et al. 1993b; Chaillan et al. 1997).

The anatomy of the olfactory system is relatively simple. There is only one synapse between the olfactory bulb (OB) and the piriform cortex (Pir Cx) and between the OB and the entorhinal cortex (Ent Cx) (Witter et al. 1991). Both cortices are connected (monosynaptically and polysynaptically) to the hippocampus, a structure which is well-known to be involved in learning and memory since the original neuropsychological observations of Scoville and Milner (1957). In addition, olfactory information reaches the dendate gyrus (DG) specifically via the lateral perforant path (Witter et al. 1991). Moreover, the Pir Cx is much simpler than the neocortex, and the projections from the OB generate a dense but restricted terminal field in a cell-sparse dendritic layer (Valverde 1965), a situation that allows extracellular recording of monosynaptic responses. Thus, electrical stimulation of the lateral olfactory tract (LOT) evokes monosynaptic and polysynaptic field potentials in the Pir Cx and DG, respectively (Haberly and Price 1977; Wilson and Steward 1978), while stimulation of the lateral perforant path, originating from the lateral Ent Cx, evokes monosynaptic field potentials in the DG.

The combined electrophysiological and behavioral experiments presented in this chapter were designed to study what types of synaptic plasticity could be observed in cortical and limbic structures following learning and memory processes. The time courses of these synaptic modifications were analyzed in order to discriminate the chronological events which allow associative memories to be stored in the brain.

EXPERIMENTAL STRATEGY AND METHODS

The three experiments presented in this chapter were performed to test the modulation of synaptic plasticity in one cortical area, the Pir Cx, and in one limbic structure, the dentate gyrus in its rostral portion, resulting from physiologically meaningful olfactory cues in an olfactory association task.

In experiment 1, one group of animals (n = 7) without surgery was trained to discriminate two natural odors, one arbitrarily designated as positive and the other as negative. The discrimination training was an associative Go–No Go learning task. Rats had to approach the odor and water ports detected by a photoelectric circuit only when the positive odor was presented for ten seconds. Responses to the odor designated as positive were rewarded with 0.1 mL of water. Responses to the designated negative (i.e., unrewarded) odor resulted in a ten-second presentation of a nonaversive light. Individual trials were presented in a quasi-random fashion and both odors were presented at most for ten seconds. A new trial was started only when the subject left the corner and, in any case, not earlier than fifteen seconds after the termination of either water or light delivery. A daily session consisted of sixty trials with an intertrial interval of fifteen seconds. Animals were tested every day for five days between 0800 and 1400. Correct responses were Go for the positive odor and No Go for the negative. Incorrect responses were Go for the negative odor and No Go for the positive odor.

The others groups were implanted with two bipolar stainless steel stimulating electrodes located in the LOT. One electrode was used to apply a patterned stimulation consisting of 36-ms bursts of four pulses (at 100 seconds^{-1}) delivered with an interburst interval of 160 ms which elicited a robust sniffing reaction. These rats (n = 7) were trained to discriminate between the patterned electrical stimulation (so-called olfactomimetic stimulations, or OMS) and a natural odor. A monopolar platinum recording electrode was implanted in the ipsilateral layer I of the Pir Cx to record the monosynaptic field potential elicited by LOT stimulation. The training paradigm with the implanted rats was the same as above except that the positive odor was replaced by the patterned electrical stimulation distributed through one stimulating electrode referred to as the active electrode (AE), the other one being used as a control electrode (CE).

One group of naive animals with implants in LOT and Pir Cx (n = 6) was given the same amount of experience (five sessions) with the patterned electrical stimulation of the LOT, natural odor, water, and light rewards with no association.

In experiment 2, rats were implanted in the LOT and DG according to Wilson and Steward (1978), and two groups of animals were trained, one using the conditioned paradigm (n = 10) and the other, the pseudoconditioned paradigm (n = 6). This experiment was set to evaluate the potential involvement of the dorsal hippocampus in our discrimination olfactory training.

In experiment 3, the following implantations were used to determine synaptic efficacy of the monosynaptic input to the DG from the lateral Ent Cx: one stimulating electrode, used to apply the patterned electrical stimulation, was implanted into the LOT, while the other was implanted into the lateral perforant path to elicit monosynaptic evoked potentials by single pulses in DG. Two groups of six implanted rats were trained either with the conditioned or the pseudoconditioned procedure.

RESULTS

Experiment 1

The nonimplanted control group increased their percentage of correct responses across the five learning sessions, reaching a correct response level of more than 80% on session 5 (figure 11.1A). From the chance level in

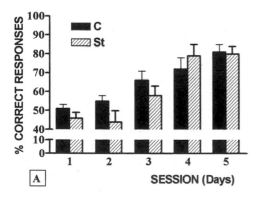 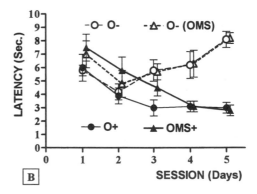

Figure 11.1 Mean performance ($\pm$SE) obtained across five sixty-trial sessions, by two different groups of control and stimulated rats. (A) Mean percentage of correct responses. The animals of the control group (C) were trained to discriminate between two natural odors. The conditioned group (St) had to discriminate between patterned electrical stimulation as a positive cue and a natural odor as a negative cue. (B) Mean latency. The control animals had to respond to the natural positive cue (O+) associated with a water reward and not respond to the natural negative cue (O−) associated with a nonaversive light. For the conditioned group, the patterned electrical stimulations or olfactomimetic stimulation (OMS) was associated with a water reward as a positive cue. The negative cue (O−) was a natural odor.

Neurobiological Substrates of Associative Memory

session 1 (approximatively 50%), a significant improvement in performance was observed in session 3 and in sessions 4 and 5, a substantial increase in percent correct indicating that correct responses for both odors were consistently produced.

The latency analyses indicated that the discrimination started from the third session when the rats learned to withhold a prepotent response during the delivery of negative odor (figure 11.1B).

The responses of the conditioned group submitted to discrimination between patterned stimulation as a positive cue vs. natural odor as a negative cue indicated that rats were able to learn this problem.

A slight improvement in percent correct was observed in session 3. Then in sessions 4 and 5, a statistically significant correct response level of 80% was obtained. Thus a statistically significant difference between the latencies obtained with the OMS vs. the negative natural odor was obtained only from the fourth session (analysis of variance, or ANOVA—$F(1, 12) = 152.4$; $P < .001$).

The comparison of behavioral performance between these two groups of rats did not reveal a significant difference in percentage of correct responses across sessions (multivariate ANOVA, or MANOVA—$F(4, 48) = 1.56$; ns) or in a particular session (ANOVA—$F(1, 12) \leq 3272$; ns).

There was no significant difference between pooled latencies throughout the learning sessions (MANOVA—$F(4, 104) = 1, 41$; ns). However, as can be observed in figure 11.1B, the stimulated group started to respond to artificial or natural odor at a higher level and a statistically significant difference was obtained during this session (ANOVA—$F(1, 26) = 18.43$; $P < .001$). Then, for the following sessions, no significant difference between the two groups was observed and from session 4 all the rats responded similarly to the natural or artificial cues.

The changes in field potentials when the patterned electrical stimulation was used instead of the positive odor are reported in figure 11.2A. Although a substantial increase in the percentage of change in slope was observed before the start of the third training session, a statistically significant change in field potential slope evoked by the AE was present prior to the fourth session ($P < .05$; compare the responses collected prior to the fourth session with the baseline collected prior to the first session; Mann-Whitney U-test, two-tailed). During the following session, twenty-four hours later, synaptic efficacy increased prior to the session (session 5) and remained elevated until the end of the training session. An example of this modification is shown in figure 11.2C. A highly significant correlation was found between the change in the slope of responses evoked by AE stimulation as well as in response latency differences across sessions (n = 91; $r = .59$; $P < .001$). The slope of the responses evoked by stimulation of the CE, through which only single pulses were delivered before and after every session, did not change significantly across the five sessions. The results obtained with naive pseudoconditioned rats are reported on figure 11.2B. A more pronounced reversal

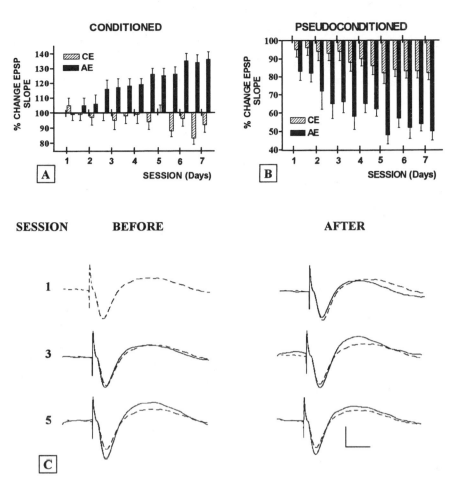

Figure 11.2 Changes in monosynaptic field potentials evoked by lateral olfactory tract stimulation and recorded in the piriform cortex before and after each learning session. Each bar represents the mean value of the slope of twenty evoked responses. (A) Mean percentage of change of field potential slope for the conditioned animals trained to discriminate between electrical patterned stimulation and a natural odor. The slope of the field potentials evoked by the active electrode (AE), used to apply the patterned electrical stimulation, developed a progressive long-term potentiation across the seven learning sessions. The slope of the field potentials evoked by the control electrode (CE) exhibited a slight but significant long-term depression (LTD) during the last sessions. (B) Mean percentage of change of field potential slope for the pseudoconditioned animals. Water, nonaversive light, natural odor, and patterned electrical stimulation were presented without any association. Both field potentials evoked by the active (AE) and control (CE) electrodes developed a rapid LTD; meanwhile the AE evoked potentials exhibited a greater depression. (C) Examples of averaged field potentials recorded before (1, dashed baseline) and after (solid line) sessions 1, 3, and 5. Calibration bars: 1 mV, 10 ms.

Neurobiological Substrates of Associative Memory

phenomenon was observed with the AE and a statistically significant depression was present from the start of the third session ($P < .01$; Mann-Whitney U-test, two-tailed). A similar phenomenon was recorded with the CE but the difference was only statistically significant at the end of the fifth session ($P < .05$).

Experiment 2

In experiment 2, the same parameters were used for the training, and polysynaptic potentials were recorded in DG following LOT stimulation as described by Wilson and Steward (1978); however, whereas they observed responses with a 20-ms latency following high intensities of stimulation (in the millivolt range), we observed small responses with a 40-ms latency following low-intensity stimulation (less than 50 μV). This polysynaptic field potential evoked in the DG increased tremendously earlier during the second session when the rats started to make associations without significant discrimination between the two cues ($P < .01$; Mann-Whitney U-test, two-tailed) (figure 11.3A). This increase was still present and significant twenty-four hours later ($P < .05$). The peak amplitude latency of these polysynaptic potentials was around 60 ms. An example of the change observed for this polysynaptic field potential recorded in DG across the five training sessions is shown in figure 11.3C. No significant changes in polysynaptic field potential recorded by the CE were observed except at the end of the first and at the beginning of the fifth session ($P < .05$).

The analyses of the polysynaptic field potential recorded with the pseudo-conditioned group did not reveal any change across the five sessions for either the AE or the CE (figure 11.3B).

Experiment 3

As in the other two experiments, conditioned rats exhibited similar behavioral performance, starting to make significant discriminations from the fourth session. A statistically significant modification of the slope of the monosynaptic field potential recorded in the DG following single-pulse stimulation of the lateral perforant path was observed earlier than for the Pir Cx and was even more pronounced than that of the polysynaptic field potential recorded in DG. Indeed a statistically significant increase of the synaptic efficacy appeared at the end of the first training session ($P < .002$) and represented a 30% increase in slope. However, and in contrast to the long-term potentiation (LTP) observed in the two previous experiments, this increase was not maintained twenty-four hours later (figure 11.4A). Rather, an opposite phenomenon, that is, a substantial depression of the monosynaptic field potential, appeared from the beginning of the second session ($P < .002$). This depression remained until the end of the session, and the slope of the field potential decreased session after session to reach approxi-

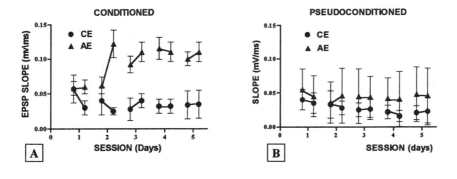

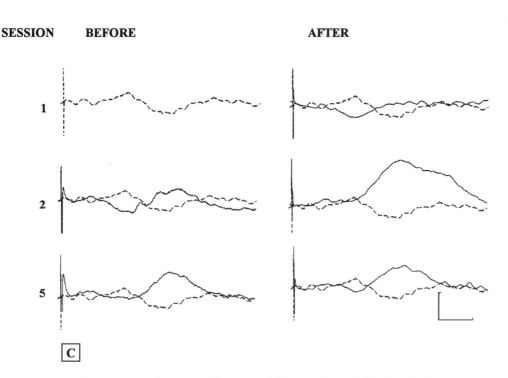

Figure 11.3 Changes in polysynaptic field potentials evoked by lateral olfactory tract stimulation and recorded in the dentate gyrus before and after each learning session. Each point represents the mean value of the slope of twenty evoked responses. (A) Mean slope of the field potentials evoked by the active (AE) and control (CE) electrodes of the conditioned rats. The AE field potentials developed a significant potentiation immediately after learning session 2. No significant changes appeared for the field potentials evoked by the CE. (B) Mean slope of the field potentials evoked by the AE and CE electrodes of the pseudoconditioned rats. Neither significant potentiation nor depression of the field potentials evoked by AE or Ce was observed. (C) Example of averaged polysynaptic field potentials recorded before (1, dashed baseline) and after (solid line) sessions 1, 2, and 5. Calibration bars: 0.2 mV, 40 ms.

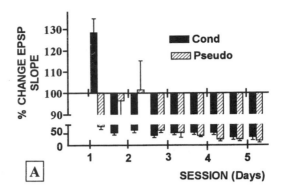

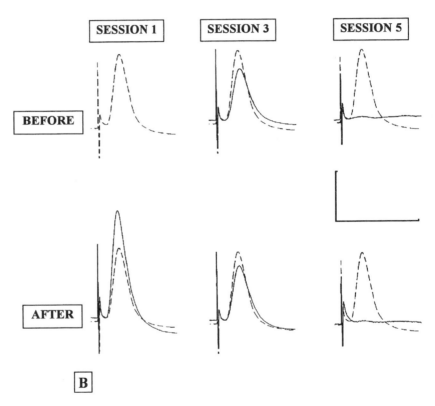

Figure 11.4 Changes in monosynaptic field potentials evoked by lateral perforant path stimulation and recorded in the dentate gyrus before and after each learning session. Each bar represents the mean value of the slope of twenty evoked responses. (A) Mean percentage changes in the slope of field potentials for the active electrode of the conditioned (Cond) and pseudoconditioned (Pseudo) animals. (B) The field potentials of the conditioned animals exhibited long-term potentiation only after learning session 1. The next day, before session 2, the field potentials expressed a long-term depression which was maintained during the following sessions. The depression expressed by the field potentials of the pseudoconditioned was significant only before session 3. This depression was increased during the following sessions. Calibration bars: 1 mV, 20 ms.

matively 30% of the baseline value at the end of the five training sessions ($P < .002$). An example of the potentiation followed by a significant long-term depression (LTD) is shown in figure 11.4C.

In pseudoconditioned rats, a nonstatistically significant decrease was observed at the end of the first session (figure 11.4B). In session 2, prior to and after the training session, the values were similar to the baseline value, while a statistically significant depression started prior to the third session ($P < .05$). This depression was amplified at the end of the session and during the following sessions. At the end of the fifth training session, the slope of monosynaptic field potential represented only about 20% of baseline values ($P < .002$).

In experiment 1, as for the discrimination with two natural odors, stimulated animals were able to discriminate between the positive electrical patterned stimulation and the negative natural odor, and only a slight difference in the time course of learning was seen between these two groups. During exploratory sniffing, rats inhale at a frequency of 4 to 7 Hz and these inhalations become synchronized with hippocampal electroencephalographic (EEG) theta rythms and presumably with activity in other olfactory structures (Macrides et al. 1982; Eeckman and Freeman 1990). It is not surprising that no statistically significant difference was observed between the behavioral performance of both groups of rats. Previous results showed that when rats were trained on a series of two natural odors, an immediate and extremely stable LTP was induced as soon as one of the natural odors was replaced by the electrical patterned stimulations (Roman et al. 1987). The results obtained in experiment 1 showed a gradual increase in synaptic efficacy (i.e., LTP) in Pir Cx while rats were learning the meaning of the electrical stimulations without previous learning. In pseudoconditioned rats submitted to these patterned stimulations, the opposite of the increase in synaptic efficacy (i.e., a homosynaptic LTD) was observed. In addition, a somewhat identical phenomenom of depression, but heterosynaptic in this case, was recorded with the CEs in both experiments. All of these experiments suggest that both LTP and LTD phenomena participate in the formation of associative memories in Pir Cx.

In experiment 2, the time course of the increase in polysynaptic field potentials recorded in DG was quite different. Whereas conditioned rats started to make consistant (session 3), then significant (session 4) cue-reward associations in late sessions, the maximal increase in synaptic efficacy appeared during the second training session. No electrophysiological change for the AEs and CEs was recorded in the DG of the pseudoconditioned animals, suggesting that the polysynaptic potentiation was specifically linked to the learning context. The onset latency of this field potential excluded identification of precisely which synapses are modified in this limbic structure or elsewhere in the brain. Nevertheless, these early modifications in synaptic efficacy in this limbic circuit suggest that thay play an important role in learning processes. These data are to be related to the observations of De

Curtis et al. (1991) who identify a reverberant activation of the entorhinal (cortex)-hippocampal-entorhinal (cortex) circuit following a single electrical stimulation of the LOT in vitro.

In experiment 3, the monosynaptic potential recorded in DG by stimulation of the lateral perforant path prior to and after each training session exhibited a substantial increase in synaptic efficacy only following the first training session. This potentiation observed just after the session did not remain twenty-four hours later and, conversely, an LTD developed session after session. In pseudoconditioned animals this short-term potentiation was not seen and the LTD phenomenon started to appear forty-eight hours later (i.e., during session 3).

Taking all the data together, we propose as a working hypothesis the existence of a sequential dialogue between the limbic (and particularly the hippocampus) and cortical structures involving at least the Pir Cx and Ent Cx.

Olfactory information originating from the olfactory bulb travels through the Pir Cx, then the lateral Ent Cx before reaching the hippocampus in the DG. In the early stages, a short-term potentiation observed in DG in conditioned rats (experiment 3) represents the first event related with the first cue-reward associations. Without long-term synaptic modifications, this early activation in DG could allow a sustained reverberant activation of the entorhinal (cortex)-hippocampal-entorhinal (cortex) circuit and long-term modifications of synaptic efficacy in this neural network. At later stages, this could allow the gradual storage of significant olfactory information in a defined set of potentiated cortical synapses, as seen with the gradually developing LTP recorded in the Pir Cx. The temporary but necessary potentiation of monosynaptic field potential in DG followed by a polysynaptic LTP, which decreased when associations were significantly performed, while a long-term increase in synaptic efficacy appeared in Pir Cx, represent synaptic modifications in good agreement with neuropsychological observations in humans. Indeed, as reported since the first observation in H.M. by Scoville and Milner (1957), then reviewed more recently by Squire and Zola (1996), amnesic patients in whom the limbic structures and specifically the hippocampus are affected cannot make new memories of the explicit type while memories from the past are preserved. In our experiment, it appears that the limbic circuit was imperatively involved only during the phases of learning and acquisition processes allowing the formation of long-term memory in a specific cortical territory (i.e., olfactory cortex). As the patterned stimulation by itself (Racine et al. 1983; Roman et al. 1987) or in pseudoconditioned rats (Roman et al. 1993a, Chaillan et al. 1996) did not produce the synaptic efficacy increase supporting long-term memory storage, it is suspected that the limbic circuits related to the olfactory system play an important role in reducing a tonic inhibition of target cells in the Pir Cx (Hasselmo and Bower 1991; Barkai and Hasselmo 1994). In addition, previous work in which the horizontal diagonal band of Broca, which is reciprocally connected with the Pir

Cx and hippocampus, or the hippocampus proper was partially damaged, revealed drastic impairments in learning and memory processes in this olfactory associative task (Roman et al. 1993b; Chaillan et al. 1997).

In conclusion, the dialogue between the limbic and cortical structures, via parallel neural networks, is sequential with a reverberant activation of the connected circuitries. The consecutive resulting synaptic modifications appeared chronologically segregated in time and space in these territories, and to generate a persistent trace only in a specific cortical neural network located for the olfactory system, at least in Pir Cx.

REFERENCES

Barkai, E., and Hasselmo, M. E. (1994). Modulation of input/output function of rat piriform cortex pyramidal cells. *J. Neurophysiol.* 72: 644–658.

Chaillan, F. A., Devigne, C., Diabira, D., Khrestchatisky, M., Roman, F. S., Ben-Ari, Y., and Soumireu-Mourat, B. (1997). Neonatal γ-ray irradiation impairs learning and memory of an olfactory associative task in adult rats. *Eur. J. Neurosci.*, 9: 884–894.

Chaillan, F. A., Roman, F. S., and Soumireu-Mourat, B. (1996). Modulation of synaptic plasticity in the hippocampus and piriform cortex by physiologically meaningful olfactory cues in an olfactory association task. *J. Physiol. Paris* 90: 343–347.

De Curtis, M., Pare, D., and Llinas, R. R. (1991). The elctrophysiology of the olfactory-hippocampal circuit in the isolated and perfused adult mammalian brain in vitro. *Hippocampus* 1: 341–354.

Eeckman, F. H., and Freeman, W. J. (1990). Correlation between unit firing and EEG in the rat olfactory system. *Brain Res.* 528: 238–244.

Haberly, L. B., and Price, J. L. (1977). The axonal projection patterns of the mitral and tufted cells of the olfactory bulb in the rat. *Brain Res.* 129: 152–157.

Hasselmo, M. E., and Bower, J. M. (1991). Selective suppression of afferent but not intrinsic fiber synaptic transmission by 2–amino-4–phosphonobutyric acid (AP4) in piriform cortex. *Brain Res.* 548: 248–255.

Macrides, F., Eichenbaum, H., and Forbes, W. (1982). Temporal relationship between sniffing and the limbic theta rhythm during odor discrimination reversal learning. *J. Neurosci.* 2: 1705–1717.

Racine, R. J., Milgram, N. M., and Hafner, S. (1983). Long-term potentiation phenomena in the rat limbic forebrain. *Brain Res.* 260: 217–231.

Roman, F. S., Staubli, U., and Lynch, G. (1987). Evidence for synaptic potentiation in a cortical network during learning. *Brain Res.* 418: 221–226.

Roman, F. S., Chaillan, F. A., and Soumireu-Mourat, B. (1993a). Long-term potentiation in rat piriform cortex following discrimination learning. *Brain Res.* 601: 265–272.

Roman, F. S., Simonetto, I., and Soumireu-Mourat, B. (1993b). Learning and memory of odor-reward association: selective impairment following horizontal diagonal band lesions. *Behav. Neurosci.* 107: 72–81.

Scoville, W. B., and Milner, B. (1957). Loss of recent memory after bilateral hippocampal lesions. *J. Neurol. Neurosurg. Psychiatry* 20: 11–21.

Slotnick, B. M. (1994). The enigma of olfactory learning revisited. *Neuroscience* 58: 1–12.

Neurobiological Substrates of Associative Memory

Slotnick, B. M., and Katz, H. M. (1974). Olfactory learning set formation in rats. *Science* 185: 796–798.

Squire, L. R. (1986). Mechanisms of memory. *Science* 232: 1612–1619.

Squire, L. R., and Zola, S. M. (1996). Structure and function of declarative and nondeclarative memory systems. *Proc. Natl. Acad. Sci. USA* 93: 13515–13522.

Squire, L. R., and Zola-Morgan, S. (1988). Memory: brain systems and behavior. *Trends Neurosci.* 11: 170–175.

Valverde, F. (1965). Studies on the piriform lobe. Cambridge, Massachusetts, Harvard University Press, 1–129.

Wilson, R. C., and Steward, O. (1978). Polysynaptic activation of the dentate gyrus of the hippocampal formation: an olfactory input via the entorhinal cortex. *Exp. Brain Res.* 33: 523–534.

Witter, M. P., Groenewegen, H. J., Lopes Da Silva, F. H., and Lohman, A. H. M. (1991). Functional organization of the extrinsic and intrinsic circuitry of the parahippocampal region. *Prog. Neurobiol.* 33: 161–253.

12 The Purkinje Local Circuit as an Example of a Functional Unit in the Nervous System

Gilbert A. Chauvet and Pierre Chauvet

It has long been known that the cerebellum responds differently according to the region activated (Holmes 1917; Chambers and Sprague 1951, 1955; Allen and Tsukahara 1974). Clinical observations have shown that specific cerebellar areas are involved in various motor abnormalities. Classically, the findings are described in terms of structure and function, that is, given structures of the cerebellum correspond to specific functions. Obviously, this terminology covers a broad spectrum of physiological functions and the numerous couplings existing between them make it difficult to give a rigorous description of any specific set of functions. This has led to the several ambiguous hypotheses and statements found in the literature. For example, Bloedel (1994) attempts to investigate the problem of how the cerebellum operates on the basis of the idea that functional heterogeneity is related to structural homogeneity. In this chapter we address this important question. The functions, which correspond to actions varying with time, are described by dynamical systems. These functions are generated by mechanisms operating between physical structures. From a formalized point of view, though it is convenient to distinguish between functions in terms of observed phenomena, for example, eye movement, posture coordination, and so forth, all the motor functions are more or less coupled and must be described as a whole. At first sight, the complexity of this approach might appear discouraging. However, a specific formalism (Chauvet 1993b, 1996) may be used to simplify the complicated organization of the functions.

The above problem may be stated in mathematical terms as follows. The physiological function is represented by a mathematical function denoted by ψ depending on time and space. For example, the "posture equilibrium" function is represented by the mathematical function $\psi(r, t)$, that is, neuronal activity at point r and at time t in physical space. In order to describe the "eye movement" function simultaneously, a convenient method consists in addressing the "posture equilibrium" function by subscript 1, and the "eye movement" function by subscript 2. Coupling between these movements means that $\psi_1(r, t)$ and $\psi_2(r, t)$ are two coupled functions, and the global movement may be described by the vector $\underline{\psi}(r, t)$ composed of the two components $\psi_1(r, t)$ and $\psi_2(r, t)$. This is exactly the same as saying that the knowledge of activity $\underline{\psi}(r, t)$ in the domain of definition of variable r, say D_r, is the parceling of a physiological function in different regions of the cerebellum. Within this representation, how can the operation performed by the cerebellum be described? The output $\underline{\psi}(r, t)$ results from inputs onto the domain D_r, and the basic physiological mechanisms in this domain. Briefly, anatomy and physiology are the two basic sciences providing knowledge of the global function performed by the observed structure. The geometrical location of neurons in D_r and their connectivity, together with the physiological mechanisms of each cell type in this domain, are necessary and sufficient to determine the operation of the network in this domain.

From this point of view, functional heterogeneity coupled with structural homogeneity corresponds to a nonuniform activity $\underline{\psi}(r, t)$ over a supposed "uniform" domain D_r. As shown below, it is not actually a uniform domain, but rather a repetitive pattern of neural networks (which we have called "Purkinje units") that gives the cerebellar cortex an important functional property regarding the global output activity. Obviously, nonuniform activity is not really a property of the system. Indeed, were this the case it would be most surprising given the innumerable mechanisms in the cells that generate the output! These specific properties, if they exist, need to be determined. In fact, no specific hypotheses need be made and the properties of the nervous tissue should be derived from the *constraints observed*, that is, the anatomical structures and the local physiological mechanisms. One such property is the coordination of movement determined by the behavior of the global system. How are the outputs $\psi_1(r, t)$ and $\psi_2(r, t)$ coupled? This raises another related issue: *how*, in anatomical and physiological terms, is a set of spatiotemporal patterns actually learned and memorized for the execution of a specific task (Braitenberg et al. 1997)? These issues call for the resolution of three problems: (1) the learning and memorization of a spatiotemporal pattern; (2) the precise definition of a coordinated movement; and (3) the learning and memorization of coordinated spatiotemporal patterns in view of executing a particular task. The nature of these problems is essentially dynamic since we have to consider the spatiotemporal variations of patterns created by neurons possessing the specific properties of connectivity, cellular location, and learning.

We first have to identify the specific biological constraints that exist in all nervous tissues, here called real neural networks: (1) the hierarchical structural organization: from the bottom to the top level, the molecular machinery, the synapses, the dendritic spines, the neurons, and the assemblies of neurons. For example, in the case of the cerebellar cortex, granule cells are associated in networks (called Purkinje units or local Purkinje circuits as described below) and such networks are associated in a supernetwork of Purkinje units; (2) the topological organization, that is, the specific interneuronal connectivity; and (3) the "learning rules," which reflect the properties of individual neurons at the molecular level as, for example, in long-term depression (LTD).

Then we have to decide which kind of property is essential to an explanation of how the cerebellum operates. As mentioned above, such properties of real neural networks should be based on anatomical description and observed physiological mechanisms. One of them is the stability of the function observed, that is, the fact that the physiological function exists (tends toward a limit, remains within a given interval, and so on), which depends on both the local mechanisms and the local circuitry. This raises major difficulties in the modeling of real neural networks. Our approach has two major advantages over classic computational models (Tyrrell and Willshaw 1992), and pattern associators (Albus 1971; Fujita 1982; Marr 1969; Melkonian et al. 1982). On the one hand, it allows integration of anatomical and physiological data, and on the other, it provides a description of function, for example, coordination of movement, in terms of the dynamics of processes based on the geometry of the structure, for example, the cerebellar cortex. Along these lines, Braitenberg et al. (1997) offer an interesting functional interpretation of the role of the cerebellum in movement control in the light of available histologic knowledge. They introduce the tidal wave concept based on the existence of a beam of parallel fibers, which is considered as the computational unit of the cerebellar cortex. However, as we shall see, a sound mathematical model is required for the deduction of the spatiotemporal properties of the cerebellar function.

In this chapter, we argue that the Purkinje unit is the functional unit of the cerebellar cortex. The method proposed may also be used for the determination of other functional units in the central nervous system. The functional unit is first rigorously defined in the framework of the hierarchical representation of nervous tissue. We then deal with the following points:

1. The definition of a Purkinje unit is geometrical (Chauvet 1986) and functional (Chauvet and Chauvet 1993). A set of Purkinje units may correspond to a microzone (Ito 1984).

2. The stability of the function, taking into account the internal dynamics due to the propagation time lags inside the unit and between two units, determines the conditions for the structural definition of the unit (Chauvet and Chauvet 1996).

3. The variational learning rules (VLRs; table 12.1), which apply between units and govern the coordination of movement through excitatory or inhibitory interactions between Purkinje units, are deduced from neuronal learning rules (Chauvet 1995). As part of these learning rules, the hypothesis of synaptic plasticity with respect to granule cells has revealed a rich variety of learning behavior. The same types of learning probably occur during development, as well as in adulthood, through signals transported by the climbing fibers which ensure convergence toward the targets (Chauvet and Chauvet 1995).

Table 12.1 Variational learning rules

At the level of neurons, covariance rule (Chauvet 1986):

$$\frac{dw_{ij}}{dt}(t) = \alpha_{ij} E_j(t - \tau)(S_i(t) - \bar{S}_i(t)) \tag{1}$$

At the level of Purkinje units (Chauvet 1995):

If

$|dH_0| \gg |dG_0|$, $\mathrm{sgn}(dH_0) = cste$,

H_0 bounded   and $\lim\limits_{t \to \infty} dH_0 = 0$

$|dH| \gg |dG|$, $\mathrm{sgn}(dH) = cste$, $\qquad\qquad$ (2)

H bounded   and $\lim\limits_{t \to \infty} dH = 0$

synaptic efficacies vary according to

$dH_0 > 0 \Rightarrow dX < 0$ with

$(U_i = 1 \Rightarrow d\sigma_i > 0$ and $U_i = 0 \Rightarrow d\sigma_i < 0)$

$dH_0 < 0 \Rightarrow dX > 0$ with $\qquad\qquad$ (3)

$(U_i = 1 \Rightarrow d\sigma_i < 0$ and $U_i = 0 \Rightarrow d\sigma_i > 0)$

and

$dH > 0 \Rightarrow dY > 0$ with

$(dX < 0 \Rightarrow d\mu_p > 0$ and $dX > 0 \Rightarrow d\mu_p < 0)$

$dH < 0 \Rightarrow dY < 0$ with $\qquad\qquad$ (4)

$(dX < 0 \Rightarrow d\mu_p < 0$ and $dX > 0 \Rightarrow d\mu_p > 0)$

for a presented pattern $\underline{U}$

---

4. The coupling between units increases the stability of the global system, in keeping with the general theory (Chauvet 1993b).

5. These results, substantiated by analysis of the movements of a robot executing a specific task (Daya and Chauvet 1996), suggest that the cerebellum can be usefully considered a major part of the sensorimotor system (Chauvet and Chauvet 1994).

Finally, we discuss our results in the light of present controversies concerning the working of the cerebellum.

DEFINITION OF A FUNCTIONAL UNIT

The definition of a functional unit in a biological system obviously requires that the biological system be first adequately defined. In the case of nervous tissue, the specific constraints enumerated above, that is, the structural hierarchy (molecules, synapses, network), topology (connectivity), and functional hierarchy (learning rules), must be taken into account for the representation.

Neural networks may be intuitively described in several ways. For example, Wu et al. (1994) and Dickinson (1995) distinguish between dedicated and distributed network models (figure 12.1). However, there is nothing to choose between them except that the structure-function relationship seems

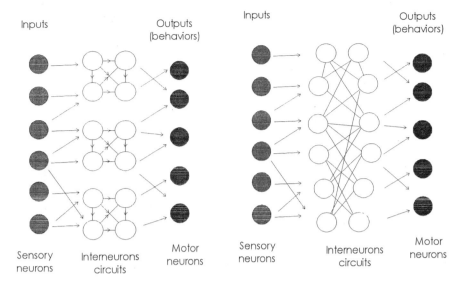

Figure 12.1 Dedicated (left) and distributed (right) networks. (From Wu et al. 1994; and Dickinson 1995.)

to be more intimate in the former than in the latter. Another possibility is the hierarchical network shown in figure 12.2 (Chauvet 1993a), in which a property emerges from one level to appear at a higher level in a new structure. As we shall see, this leads to a rigorous definition of a functional unit. As a preliminary to identifying the essential property, that is, synaptic efficacy, of the new structure (the Purkinje unit), let us recall the basic concepts underlying this representation.

We have proposed a general formalism for representing the functional organization of biological systems (Chauvet 1996). This is based on three main concepts: (1) the *functional interaction* between two structural units, the source (e.g., the emitting neuron) and the sink (e.g., the target neuron); (2) the *space scale* to define the structural hierarchy; and (3) the *time scale* to define the functional hierarchy.

This representation offers at least two major advantages: (1) the possibility of decomposing a biological system into its functions, that is, its mechanisms, with the corresponding structures that generate these functions; and (2) the establishment of couplings between the functions. Indeed, the most difficult problem that arises in the formalization of physiological processes is that of obtaining a "clean" system, that is, a rigorous definition of the system considered as being isolated.

A major complication in formalizing a biological system is the nature, functional or structural, of the level of organization. As shown in figure 12.3, such a definition can be given in the context of the relation between the two kinds of organization, structural and functional, existing in biological systems.

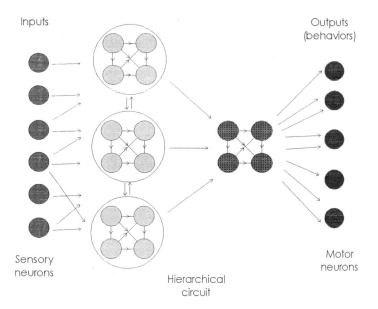

Figure 12.2 A hierarchical network (Chauvet 1993a). Properties emerge from the lower level and appear at the higher level inside a new structure. This new structure is called a functional unit if and only if it has a specific function.

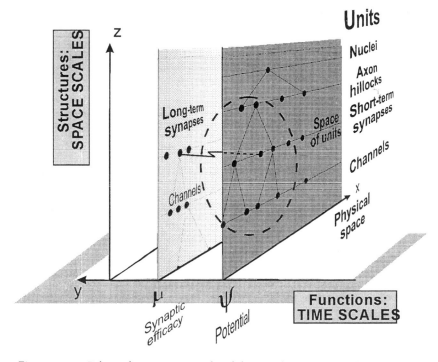

Figure 12.3 Relation between structural and functional organizations: functions defined by their time scales are shown on the y-axis; structures defined by their space scales are shown on the z-axis; at each of these levels, structural units, belonging to a given space scale for a given time scale, are shown on the x-axis. It should be noted that in this formal representation the physical distances in natural space have no meaning. (From Chauvet, 1996)

An operational, that is, mathematical, description of this relation is rather difficult and requires a specific formalism which we have called the "S-propagator formalism" (Chauvet 1996). In fact, it is easy to conceive that structure is related to a space scale, and that the process (i.e., function), which is mathematically described by a dynamical system, is related to time scales. Because these dynamical systems are defined through the corresponding structures, there is a relation between space scales and time scales, that is, between structural organization and functional organization.

The *functional interaction* is introduced between sources and sinks. This concept is general and represents, for example, the action of one neuron on another, as well as, though less obviously, the action of one group of neurons on another group. The *space scale* is associated with the different self-included structures such as synapse, neuron, network, group of networks (which is the Purkinje unit network as shown below); the *time scale* is associated with the duration of the processes that are generated by the structural units (the duration of synaptic efficacies). This less obvious definition leads to activity processes generated by neurons, synaptic efficacy modulation generated by synapses, processes generated by groups of neurons, and so on. An important issue is the identification of the relation between hierarchical structures and hierarchical processes and the possible consequences of this identification on the existence of specific learning rules at the higher levels.

On these bases, we may define the functional unit as a *structural unit having its own function at a higher level of organization*. For example, in figure 12.2, the functional unit (represented as a unique object compared of four round objects on the right) has a new function which emerges, that is, is derived mathematically, from the properties at the lower level. According to the given definitions for the construction of the biological system (figure 12.3), the functional unit has its own time scale.

This is the abstract conceptualization of the problem presented here. We will now take the cerebellar cortex as an example and extend the results to the nervous system in general. The principal result may be expressed as follows: *the determination of the functional unit in the nervous system is derived from the relation between the hierarchical structural and functional organizations, that is, from the knowledge of "what does what."* Thus, we first have to identify the group of neurons, then the function accomplished by this network, and finally the properties that emerge in the set of networks. The expected results are shown in table 12.2. The aim of this chapter is to give a mathematical proof of these results.

THE PURKINJE LOCAL CIRCIUT AS THE BASIC STRUCTURE

An element of the cerebellar cortex is presented in figure 12.4, where the five types of cell are shown with their connections and their approximate numbers (underlined). Given the geometrical structure of the cerebellar cortex,

Table 12.2 Corresponding structures and functions with the expected property at different levels of complexity for the cerebellum

Structure	Function	Property
Purkinje cell	Synaptic modifiability	Hebbian learning rule
Purkinje unit = Purkinje local circuit	Learning and memory of patterns	Variational learning rule
Generalized Purkinje unit = set of Purkinje units	Learning and memory of coordinated patterns	Stability of the function increased by the association of Purkinje units
Purkinje domain = Purkinje network associated with cerebellar deep nucleus neurons	Learning and memory of coordinated patterns	Increased learning capacity
Sensorimotor system	Integration of sensory signals and coordinated patterns	Motor control

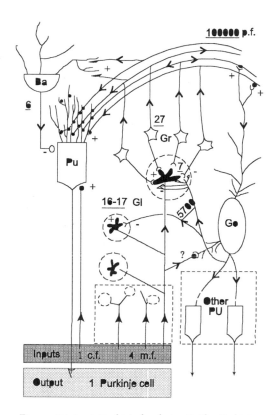

Figure 12.4 A Purkinje local circuit (the Purkinje unit) in the cerebellar cortex. Numbers of type cells are underlined. Ba, basket cell; Gr, granule cell; Gl, glomerulus; Go, Golgi; Pu, Purkinje cell; p.f., parallel fiber; c.f., climbing fiber; m.f., mossy fiber; PU, Purkinje unit. Dashed circles are glomeruli. Inhibitory connections are designated by white circles, and excitatory connections by dark circles. (From Chauvet, 1986)

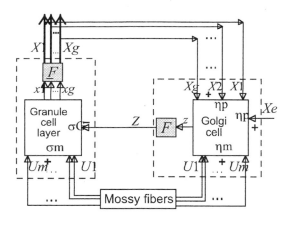

$$X = X(\, U, \, Xe \,)$$

Figure 12.5 The granule cell subsystem is composed of the granule cell layer and the Golgi cell. Inputs come from the mossy fibers and are denoted as U_i. Outputs are denoted as X_i. Output from the Golgi cell is Z. The nonlinear transformation is $\underline{F}$, and before transformation small letters are used (z and x_i). The two other inputs for the Golgi cell are V (climbing fiber) and Xe, the "external context" that comes from other Purkinje units. (From Chauvet et al., 1995)

the Purkinje unit has been defined as follows (Chauvet 1986): a granule cell, denoted gc, belongs to the unit containing the nearest Purkinje cell it contacts. Then gc is considered to belong to a specific unit numbered k if the following conditions apply: gc has synapses with at least one Purkinje cell of the unit k, the distance between gc and the Purkinje cells corresponds to the smallest distance between gc and any Purkinje cell it contacts outside the unit, and gc has synapses with at least one Golgi cell of the unit k. The basket and stellar cells included in unit k are those that are contacted by the granule cells of unit k and connected to the Purkinje cell of unit k. This unit may be separated into two subsystems, that is, the granule cell neural network and the Purkinje cell subsystem (PCS), as shown in figures 12.5 and 12.6.

This geometrical definition is obviously incomplete. Admitting that the function of the cerebellar cortex is learning and retrieving space-time patterns (Chapeau-Blondeau and Chauvet 1991), satisfactory cerebellar operation requires that *the output of the system remain within physiological limits and that the modifiable synaptic efficacies be asymptotically stable to ensure learning ability.*

These necessary conditions for the stability of the observed function involve parameters such as the number of cells, the value of the synaptic efficacy, and so on, all of which contribute to the determination of the Purkinje unit.

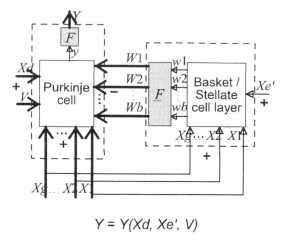

Purkinje cell subsystem

$$Y = Y(Xd, Xe', V)$$

Figure 12.6 The Purkinje cell subsystem is composed of a Purkinje cell and of the basket and stellate cell layer connected with this Purkinje cell. Inputs are the outputs X1 of the granule cell subsystem (on the right). There are three other inputs: Xe' and Xd from the other Purkinje units (the "external context" for the basket cells and the Purkinje cell, respectively), and V carried along the climbing fiber. The output of the system is Y. The nonlinear transformation is F, and before transformation small letters are used (z and xi). (From Chauvet et al., 1995)

The First Level of Structural Organization: The Neuron. Input-Output Relation

The output S of a neuron is considered to be equal to a normalized short-term mean frequency. It is given as a function of its inputs by

$$S(t) = F[s_0 + {}^t \underline{w} \underline{E}(t - \tau)]$$

where the second term of the sum is the scalar product between $\underline{w}$ and $\underline{E}$, where $\underline{w}$ is the vector of n synaptic weights w_i, and $\underline{E}(t - \tau)$ is the vector of n inputs E_i at time $t - \tau$. τ is the assumed processing delay of the neuron and s_0 is a basic activity. We consider for F two kinds of function: a "linear" function, where F is the identity on positive reals and zero on negative reals; a nonlinear but continuous function defined by a sigmoid: $F(s) = (1 + e^{-a(s-b)})^{-1}$ with $a > 0$ and $b > 0$. Then, the output $\underline{S}(t)$ of a layer of neurons that are not interconnected is $\underline{F}[\underline{s_0} + W\underline{E}(t - \tau)]$ where **W** is the matrix of the synaptic weights.

The LTD of synaptic efficacy w_{ij} for the synapse in neuron j that receives the input E_j is assumed to depend on the difference between the signal and its long-term mean value, which itself depends on molecular processes (Chauvet 1988) in the presynaptic terminal. In our model, only the synapses between parallel fibers and Purkinje cells are considered to be modifiable. Then, the input-output relation (Chauvet 1986) is

$$\frac{dw_{ij}}{dt}(t) = \alpha_{ij}E_j(t - \tau)(S_i(t) - \bar{S}_i(t))$$

where α_{ij} is a plasticity coefficient, equal to a negative real, and $\bar{S}_i$ is the long-term mean value which takes into account of a memory effect (Uttley 1979).

The Second Level of Structural Organization: The Purkinje Unit. Input-Output Relation

Activity in the Granule Cell Subsystem   The granule cell subsystem (GCS) includes a layer of g granule cells and a layer of go Golgi cells. These cells are not interconnected in their layer. The subsystem inputs are (see figure 12.5): a pattern $\underline{U}$ of m real elements in [0, 1] that represent information propagated along the m mossy fibers; and the *external context* $\underline{X}_e$ representing activities propagated along the parallel fibers connected with the Golgi cells which do not issue from this unit. The output of the GCS before the transformation by F is the vector $\underline{x}$ and after the transformation is the vector $\underline{X}$ of g activities X_i along the parallel fibers, which are the outputs of the granule layer. Delays of propagation are assumed inside the loop constituted by the granule cell and the Golgi cell.

Activity in the Purkinje Cell Subsystem   The PCS includes a layer of b basket or stellate cells, and a layer of p Purkinje cells which are not interconnected in their layer. It receives as inputs (see figure 12.6) (1) the vector $\underline{X}$ of activities X_i, which is the output of the granule cell subsystem; (2) the external contexts $\underline{X}_{e'}$ and $\underline{X}_d$, which are activities propagated along parallel fibers connected, respectively, with the basket cells and the Purkinje cell, and issuing from other Purkinje units; and (3) the vector of climbing fibers V_i. The output activity along the Purkinje cell axon is the main output of the unit, and is denoted as Y_i. The signal y_i is the output of the Purkinje cell before transformation by F. Delays of propagation are assumed inside the pathways between granule cells, Purkinje cells, and basket cells.

Function of the Purkinje Unit: Condition for Learning and Retrieving
Retrieving occurs in a unit when it is not in learning phase, that is, the Purkinje unit is studied around its steady state. Since the synaptic weights between parallel fibers and the Purkinje cell are constant, the error signal V is null, and the inputs X_e, X_d, and $X_{e'}$ do not depend on time. This state may therefore be called the "resting state" of the unit. Since delays of propagation occur inside the Purkinje unit, certain conditions must be satisfied for pattern retrieval. In other words, given the inputs to the Purkinje unit (*external contexts* defined by H_0 and H, which involve the influence of signals X_e, $X_{e'}$, X_d, issuing from other granule cell subsystems, the error signal V and mossy fiber signals U), are there any conditions for a bound output $\underline{X}$ of the GCS?

And, for the given inputs, what are the necessary conditions for a bound physiological output activity Y_i? The GCS is said to be "symmetrical" when all the X_i signals issuing from the granule cell are identical. In this case, X is the only input for the PCS, and it has been shown (Chauvet 1995) that

$$X = F_1(\underline{U}, \underline{\sigma}) - \sigma_G H_0$$
$$Y = F_2(\underline{X}, \mu_p) + H \tag{1}$$

where F_1 and F_2 are two functions depending on the anatomical structure of the network, and σ_G and $\underline{\sigma}$ are the synaptic efficacies at the level of granule cells, and μ_P the synaptic efficacy at the level of the Purkinje cell. We have proved that, in the linear case of transfer between two neurons, the following condition (**cc1**) for the Golgi cell and the granule cells must be satisfied:

$$\sum_{i=1}^{g} \sigma_{Gi}\eta_{pi} < 1 \tag{2}$$

Thus, the retrieval of patterns depends on the synaptic efficacies of the connections from the Golgi cell toward the granule cells, and vice versa. The closed loop between granule cells and Golgi cells is the cause of instabilities for the process.

Another problem concerns the possibility of learning by the Purkinje unit. As above, this problem has its origin in the existence of delays inside the unit. Learning exists if, and only if, the unit is stable, a property is defined as follows. A unit *stable for learning* is a unit connected with other identical units in the network such that: (1) the *external context* is defined by quantities H_0 and H, which involve the influence of signals X_e, $X_{e'}$, X_d, issuing from other GCSs, and the error signal V; and (2) the synaptic efficacies increase (or decrease) monotonously to a finite asymptotic value. Learning is thus characterized by a monotonous variation of synaptic efficacies. We have shown that the same condition as (**cc1**) is valid. This result has been confirmed by numerical simulation.

Function Generated by the Purkinje Unit: Input-Output Relation   The equations that describe the time course of activity in the Purkinje unit can be written in a variational form as

$$dX(t) = dG_0(t) - \sigma_G dH_0(t)$$
$$dY(t) = dG(t) + dH(t) \tag{3}$$

from which learning rules between Purkinje units can be deduced mathematically (Chauvet 1995). They are given in (table 12.1).

The meaning of these rules is condensed in figure 12.7: VLRs act on the direction of variation of the signals and not on their value. This is due to the fact that they operate at the higher level of the hierarchical structural orga-

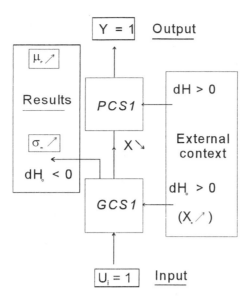

Figure 12.7 Principle of the variatim learning rules illustrated for two interactive Purkinje units. See text. (From Chauvet, 1995)

nization: the increase in complexity of the structure is compensated by an attenuation of the behavior of the function (the monotonous time course), which can be mathematically shown to be due to the hierarchically organized structure. The coordination of movement is thus explained by the relative influence of external contexts on Purkinje units which correspond to specific limbs. As in the case of a Purkinje unit, we have investigated the conditions of stability in the two cases of learning and retrieval for the network of Purkinje units submitted to VLRs. These conditions must be proved in order to establish the existence of the function.

THE NETWORK OF PURKINJE UNITS: THIRD LEVEL OF STRUCTURAL ORGANIZATION

We have considered the first and second levels of structural organization to be constituted respectively by the neuron and the Purkinje unit. As shown above, the Purkinje unit is able to learn and retrieve time-space patterns under the criteria (**cc1**). In other words, this structure provides at least the function represented by this stable process. The third level of structural organization consists of a network of Purkinje units, that is, a supernetwork of networks that are the Purkinje units (figure 12.8). Since the Purkinje units are coupled together and since each set of Purkinje units corresponds to a microzone, we may assume that the function of this supernetwork is the coordination of movements. However, we first have to define the conditions for the existence of this function.

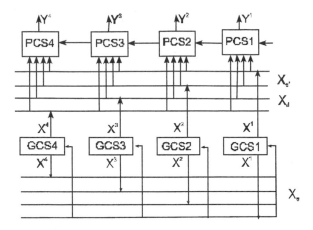

Figure 12.8   A network of four Purkinje units composed of Purkinje cell subsystem and granule cell subsystem, as in figures 12.5 and 12.6. The superscript denotes the rank of the Purkinje unit. (From Chauvet, 1995)

Existence of the Function Generated by the Network of Purkinje Units

We have to solve the same problem as the one at the level of a single Purkinje unit: given the structure of the network of Purkinje units provided by the coupling through parallel fibers, what are the conditions that allow the functioning of the network, that is, the coordination of movement? In mathematical terms, what are the conditions of stability of the dynamical process of learning and retrieving *coordinated* patterns?

The first condition that the network has to satisfy is that of stability during the retrieval phase. We have mathematically proved that a sufficient condition for stability is

$$\forall k \in \{1, \ldots, N\}, \left(\sum_{j=1}^{g} \eta_{p,j}^{(k)} + \sum_{l=1, l \neq k}^{N} \sum_{j=1}^{g} \eta_{e,j}^{(kl)} \right) \max_{1 \leq i \leq g} \sigma_{G,i}^{(k)} < 1 \tag{4}$$

The first term, which already appears in the criterion (**cc1**), is fundamental for the convergence of the dynamics of a single isolated unit, that is, a unit not included in a network:

$$C_1(k) = \left(\sum_{j=1}^{g} \eta_{p,j}^{(k)} \right) \max_{1 \leq i \leq g} \sigma_{G,i}^{(k)} \tag{5}$$

The second term represents the quality and the number of connections of the GCS in the current unit k, that is, *between units*:

$$C_2(k) = \left(\sum_{l=1, l \neq k}^{N} \sum_{j=1}^{g} \eta_{e,j}^{(kl)} \right) \max_{1 \leq i \leq g} \sigma_{G,i}^{(k)} \tag{6}$$

Therefore, the condition of stability during the retrieval phase is $C_1(k) +$

Table 12.3 Results obtained with variation learning rules for a network composed of four Purkinje units

Purkinje units			
$V^{(0)}$ constant	$X_i^{(0)} \downarrow \ (i = 1 \ldots 3)$	$Y^{(0)} \downarrow$	$\mu_{p,1}^{(0)} \downarrow$
$V^{(1)} \downarrow$	$X_i^{(1)} \uparrow \ (i = 1 \ldots 3)$	$Y^{(1)} \downarrow$	$\mu_{p,1}^{(1)} \uparrow$
$V^{(2)} \downarrow$	$X_i^{(2)} \uparrow \ (i = 1 \ldots 3)$	$Y^{(2)} \downarrow$	$\mu_{p,1}^{(2)} \uparrow$
$V^{(3)} \downarrow$	$X_i^{(3)} \uparrow \ (i = 1 \ldots 3)$	$Y^{(3)} \downarrow$	$\mu_{p,1}^{(3)} \uparrow$

$C_2(k) < 1$ for all units k between 1 and N. The condition $(C_1(k) < 1)$ is precisely the criterion (**cc1**) established above for a *linear* Purkinje unit k. However, simulations based on several delay values have shown that the networks which satisfy the two conditions, $C_1(k) < 1$ and $C_2(k) < 1$ for all unit k varying between 1 and N, converge and follow the VLRs. Moreover, this condition of stability for the retrieval phase remains valid for the learning phase. This important result can be extended to the *nonlinear* case and allows us to define the possible function of learning and retrieval in a network of Purkinje units.

Example of Learning in the Network of Purkinje Units

In order to illustrate these conditions, let us consider the above network composed of four units completely interconnected (see figure 12.8). Each unit receives eight mossy fibers ($m = 8$), and includes three granule cells ($g = 3$) and three basket cells ($b = 3$). The pattern presented to each unit is in a binary form, for example, $\underline{U} = 10001010$. The maximum of $C_1(k)$ and $C_2(k)$ equals, respectively, 0.5646 and 0.642 for all the units, that is, for k between 0 and 3. Input $V^{(0)}$ for unit 0 is constant, inputs $V^{(1)}$, $V^{(2)}$ and $V^{(3)}$ for units 1, 2, and 3, respectively, decrease.

Applying VLRs (table 12.1), it is possible to predict the time variation of activities and synaptic efficacies. The results are shown in table 12.3. Unit 0 does not receive an error signal, but it receives decreasing outputs $X_i^{(k)}$ from other units, through X_e, $X_{e'}$, and X_d. This is shown in the first row of the table, the consequence of which is the decrease in outputs $X_i^{(0)}$ and $Y^{(0)}$.

Figures 12.9 and 12.10 show the time variation of synaptic efficacies σ^{ij} and $\mu_{p,j}^{(0)}$ for completely interconnected four-unit networks. We have represented only the results for the two first Purkinje units. The observed decrease of X_1^0 is weak. However, since each unit in the cerebellar cortex is contacted by thousands of other units, outputs $\underline{X}$ of several hundreds of units may vary in the same direction and strongly influence another group of units. The direction of the time variation of synaptic efficacies also depends on the pattern presented. As shown in table 12.3, outputs $Y^{(k)}$ decrease, and the decrease in $Y^{(0)}$ is the smallest. More specifically, the coordination of movement is interpreted in terms of excitatory and inhibitory couplings

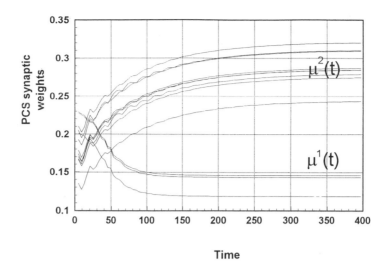

Figure 12.9 Time variation of the synaptic efficacies μp(1,2) of the Purkinje cell subsystem (PCS) for the two first Purkinje units of the network presented in figure 12.8 (four units completely interconnected). max{C1(k)} = 0.5596, max{C2(k)} = 0.6487, sum = C1(k) + C2(k) = 1.1815; g = 3; m = 8; and b = 3 for all units. Patterns: unit 0 : U = 1 0 0 0 1 0 1 0; unit 1 : U = 1 1 1 1 0 0 0 1; unit 2 : U = 1 0 1 0 1 0 1 0; unit 3 : U = 0 1 1 1 0 0 0 1.

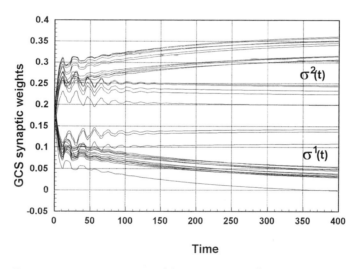

Figure 12.10 Time variation of the GCS synaptic efficacies (mij for the two first Purkinje units of the network presented in figure 12.8 (four units completely interconnected). Conditions as in figure 12.9.

between Purkinje units that operate at the higher level. This property enables us to define the Purkinje unit, or the Purkinje domain associated with cerebellar nuclei, as the functional unit of the cerebellum.

In conclusion, the conditions for the validity of VLRs are based on the structural hierarchical organization of this specific network of Purkinje units, each of which is itself composed of the network of granule cells: the condition $C_1(k) < 1$ and $C_2(k) < 1$ ensures the stability for coupled nonsymmetrical linear Purkinje units, with nonconstant inputs. This result is general and may be used for any number of Purkinje units.

DISCUSSION AND CONCLUSION: SIGNIFICANCE OF THE CONDITIONS FOR COORDINATED MOVEMENT: HIERARCHICAL ORGANIZATION

Let us discuss the significance of the above conditions. Two kinds of conditions for the validity of VLR are satisfied in the real cerebellar cortex:

1. *The validity of the emergent learning rules (VLR) is related to the functional hierarchical organization.* As recalled in table 12.1, there are two conditions for the validity of VLRs:

$$|dH_0| \gg |dG_0|, \ \text{sgn}(dH_0) = cste, \ H_0 \ \text{bounded and} \lim_{t \to \infty} dH_0 = 0$$

$$|dH| \gg |dG|, \ \text{sgn}(dH) = cste, \ H \ \text{bounded and} \lim_{t \to \infty} dH = 0 \tag{7}$$

Two quantities, representing the signals that act on the GCS, are involved in the first condition: (1) H_0, which depends on the external context X_e through a subset of parallel fibers, and on the "error signal" V; and (2) G_0, which depends on the synaptic efficacy σ_m. This first condition means that the time variation of activity is faster than the variation in time of synaptic efficacy. In real neural networks, this condition is obviously satisfied, the ratio being up to 10^{-3}.

Two quantities, representing the signals that act on the PCS, are involved in the second condition: (1) H, which depends on the external context $X_{e'}$ through another "external" set of parallel fibers, and on the "error signal" V; and (2) G, which depends on the "internal" signals X and on the synaptic efficacy μ_P. The second condition results from the difference of time scales for activity and synaptic efficacy, and from the strength of the error signal (Chauvet 1995).

Thus, the emergent VLRs depend on the functional hierarchical organization of nervous tissue, defined through different time scales for activity and synaptic efficacy. Since these very general conditions are observed in the nervous system, VLRs appear to be a new kind of learning rule emerging from the hierarchy. Classic learning rules, such as the Hebbian rules, operate at the level of individual neurons, but VLPs operate at a higher level of network organization. Learning through groups of neurons is based on the direction of variation of the inputs and the synaptic weights, while learning from neurons is based on the variations of inputs and the synaptic weights. This organizational property of the network seems to be very general.

2. *The existence of the function, that is, the coordination of movements, is based on the condition*

$$C_1(k) < 1 \quad and \quad C_2(k) < 1 \text{ for all unit } k \text{ varying between 1 and } N \qquad (8)$$

that results from Eq. (5) and Eq. (6). Thus, this condition is a consequence of the structural hierarchical organization of the cerebellar cortex network into Purkinje units, which are themselves composed of the network of granule cells: the condition $C_1(k) < 1$ and $C_2(k) < 1$ seems to be numerically sufficient. This condition insures stability for coupled nonsymmetrical linear Purkinje units, with *variable* inputs.

On the basis of anatomical and physiological data, and using a mathematical model of the cerebellum, we have proved that the cerebellum has the ability of learning and retrieving *coordinated* patterns. The operation of the cerebellum consists essentially in integrating sensory information issuing from the whole organism and, after specific transformations, in activating the efferent motor systems. Contrary to the claims of some authors, for example, Bloedel (1994), the explanation of these transformations does not call for any special hypotheses. They are due to (1) connectivity between Purkinje units, or Purkinje domains associated with specific parts of the cerebellar nuclei, which results in a coupling between them; and (2) physiological relations at the neuronal level, governed by Hebbian rules. These two mechanisms are sufficient to explain the operation of the cerebellum, the hierarchical organization of which leads to the emergence of new VLRs. The mathematical derivation of the coordination of movement is based on the proof of the stability of the system which ensures the existence of this function. These results are summed up in figure 12.11, which shows, based on figure 12.3, the coupling between the functional and structural organizations for the "coordination of movement" function of the cerebellar cortex.

Our approach also leads to consideration of the role of stability in this kind of biological system. In the case of Purkinje units with a delay of transformation inside each cell and a delay of propagation between cells, we have obtained the conditions of stability for learning and retrieval for one Purkinje unit and for a two-unit system, that is, two coupled Purkinje units. This result satisfies a paradigm introduced in our theory of functional organization of biological systems based on a hypothesis of self-association (Chauvet 1993b) which states that, from the point of view of global dynamics, the biological system appears to tend toward an increase in stability. In other words, the systems are structured such that their functional interactions increase the stability of their functioning.

The above results were obtained from a mathematical formulation established prior to the computational phase. A strictly computational approach

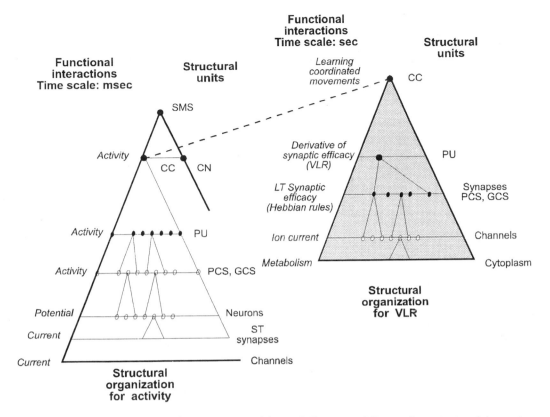

Figure 12.11 The organization of the cerebellar cortex (following figure 12.3) and the results presented in the third level of structural organization (see text). To each function (activity or co-ordination of movement, i.e., VLRs) determined by a specific time scale corresponds a structural hierarchical organization with its own structures. For each "pyramid," the functional interactions are shown on the left, with the corresponding structural units on the right. CC, cerebellar cortex; SMS, sensorimotor system; ST, short-term; LT, long-term; CN, cerebellar nuclear; PU, Purkinje unit. (From Chauvet, 1996)

would not have produced the results obtained here since these results depend strongly on the theoretical framework involving detailed anatomical and physiological mechanisms at all levels of the structure. The mathematical development proposed here applies to a realistic, well-established cerebellar circuitry (Ito 1984; Thompson 1990; Eccles 1979). New findings, such as the existence of the interneuron candelabrum (Lain and Axelrad 1994) or the possible dominant physiological influence of the granule cells associated with synapses on the ascending branch of the granule cell axon (Sultan and Bower 1996), do not affect our results which are based on very general facts, that is, the hierarchical functional organization based on time scales, and the structural organization based on space scales, corresponding to the network of Purkinje units. An important issue that arises from the present analysis concerns the degree of detail necessary for a sound interpretation of the operation of the cerebellum.

We have shown here that the coordination of movement can be explained using the hierarchical organization of the cerebellar cortex in which the Purkinje unit emerges as the functional unit of the cerebellar cortex. Two kinds of learning appear to be superimposed: supervised learning within the sensorimotor system, and unsupervised learning governed by variational learning rules. A Purkinje unit learns to associate inputs and ouputs using signals issuing from different parts of the nervous system, and then modifies the nearest Purkinje units not subjected to this supervised learning. The closer together the units, the stronger the specifications given by the VLRs. The application of VLRs in the context of a large number of Purkinje units offers considerable theoretical as well as practical advantages. This approach, based on logical relations, simplifies programming and increases the speed of calculations. As we have shown (Daya and Chauvet 1996), a learning algorithm can be used for coordinating movements in a robot.

In conclusion, the hierarchical organization of the cerebellar cortex under the form of repetitive substructures, the Purkinje units, and the existence of emergent learning rules at the higher level, lead to an algorithm for coordinating movements, that is, for coupling outputs $\psi_1(r, t)$ and $\psi_2(r, t)$, each of which corresponds to a Purkinje unit. Since each Purkinje unit may be associated with some portion of the cerebellar nuclei to form a Purkinje domain, the same results apply to this more complete architecture. We have demonstrated mathematically that the capacity of learning is then increased. In fact, the apparent functional heterogeneity associated with structural homogeneity reflects the necessary hierarchical organization which makes the system stable, that is, capable of working. From this point of view, and as already suggested for other reasons by several authors (Eccles et al. 1967; Ito 1979; Raymond et al. 1996), the cerebellum may be usefully considered as a neuronal learning machine.

REFERENCES

Albus, J. S. (1971). A theory of cerebellar function. *Math. Biosci.* 10: 25–61.

Allen, G. I., and Tsukahara, N. (1974). Cerebellar communication systems. *Physiol. Rev.* 54: 957–1006.

Bloedel, J. R. (1994). Functional heterogeneity with structural homogeneity: how does the cerebellum operate? In *Movement Control*, P. Cordo and S. Harnad, eds., pp. 64–76. Cambridge, UK, Cambridge University Press.

Braitenberg, V., Heck, D., and Sultan, F. (1997). The detection of sequences as a key to cerebellar function: experiments and theory. *Behav. Brain Sci.* 20: 2.

Chambers, W. W., and Sprague, J. M. (1951). Differential effects of cerebellar anterior lobe cortex and fastigial nuclei on postural tonus in the cat. *Science* 114: 324–325.

Chambers, W. W., and Sprague, J. M. (1955). Functional localization in the cerebellum. II. Somatotopic organization in cortex and nuclei. *Arch. Neurol. Psychiatry* 74: 653–680.

Chapeau-Blondeau, F., and Chauvet, G. A. (1991). A neural network model of the cerebellar cortex performing dynamic associations. *Biol. Cybern.* 65: 267–279.

Chauvet, G. A. (1986). Habituation rules for a theory of the cerebellar cortex. *Biol. Cybern.* 55: 201–209.

Chauvet, G. A. (1988). Correlation principle and physiological interpretation of synaptic efficacy. In *Systems with Learning and Memory Abilities*, J. Delacour and J. C. S. Levy, eds., pp. 341–364. Amsterdam, Elsevier.

Chauvet, G. A. (1993a). Hierarchical functional organization of formal biological systems: a dynamical approach. I. An increase of complexity by self-association increases the domain of stability of a biological system. *Philos. Trans. R. Soc. Lond. B. Biol. Sci.* 339: 425–444.

Chauvet, G. A. (1993b). An n-level field theory of biological neural networks. *J. Math. Biol.* 31: 771–795.

Chauvet, G. A. (1995). On associative motor learning by the cerebellar cortex: from Purkinje unit to network with variational learning rules. *Math. Biosci.,* 126: 41–79.

Chauvet, G. A. (1996). *Theoretical Systems in Biology: Hierarchical and Functional Integration*, Vol. 3: *Organisation and Regulation*. Oxford, UK, Pergamon Press.

Chauvet, P., and Chauvet, G. A. (1993). On the ability of cerebellar Purkinje units to constitute a neural network. In *WCNN'93: Proceedings of the World Congress on Neural Networks*, Vol. 2, pp. 602–605, Portland, OR, July, 11–15 1993. Hillsdale, NJ: Erlbaum.

Chauvet, P., and Chauvet, G. A. (1994). A class of functions for the adaptive control of the cerebellar cortex. In *WCNN'94: World Congress on Neural Networks*, Vol. 2, pp. 669–674, San Diego, June 5–9, 1994. Hillsdale, NJ, Erlbaum/INNS Press.

Chauvet, P., and Chauvet, G. A. (1995). Mathematical conditions for adaptive control in Marr's model of the sensorimotor system. *Neural Networks* 8: 693–706.

Chauvet, P., and Chauvet, G. A. (1996). Dynamics of delayed coupled Purkinje units in the cerebellar cortex. In *World Congress on Neural Networks*, San Diego, p. 1275. Lawrence Erlbaum Associates and INNS Press.

Daya, B., and Chauvet, G. A. (1996). Control of dynamic biped locomotion using a neural network. In *World Congress on Neural Networks*, San Diego, Sept. 15–18. Lawrence Erlbaum Associates and INNS Press.

Dickinson, P. S. (1995). Interactions among neural networks for behavior. *Curr. Opin. Neurobiol.* 5: 792–798.

Eccles, J. C. (1979). Introductory remarks. In *Cerebro-Cerebellar Interactions*, J. Massion and K. Sazaki, eds., New York, Elsevier-North Holland.

Eccles, J. C., Ito, M., and Szentagothai, J. (1967). *The Cerebellum as a Neuronal Machine*. New York, Springer-Verlag.

Fujita, M. (1982). Adaptive filter model of the cerebellum. *Biol. Cybern.* 45: 195–206.

Holmes, G. (1917). The symptoms of acute cerebellar injuries due to gunshot injuries. *Brain* 40: 461–535.

Ito, M. (1979). Is the cerebellum really a computer? *Trends Neurosci.* 5: 122–126.

Ito, M. (1984). *The Cerebellum and Neural Control*. New York, Raven Press.

Lain, C. J., Axelrad, H. (1994) The candelabrum cell: a new interneuron in the cerebellar cortex. *J. Comp. Neurol.* 339: 159–173.

Marr, D. (1969). A theory of cerebellar cortex. *J. Physiol. (Lond.)* 202: 437–470.

Melkonian, D. S., Mkrtchian, H. H., and Fanardjian, V. V. (1982). Simulation of learning processes in neuronal networks of the cerebellum. *Biol. Cybern.* 45: 79–88.

Raymond, J. L., Lisberger, S. G., and Mauk, M. D. (1996). The cerebellum: a neuronal learning machine? *Science* 272: 1126–1131.

Sultan, F., Bower, J. M. (1996). Classification of the rat cerebellar basket and stellate cells: evidence for a continuous distribution of types through principle component analysis. *Soc. Neurosc. Abstr.* 22: 502.

Thompson, R. F. (1990). Neural mechanisms of classical conditioning in mammals. *Philos. Trans. R. Soc. Lond. B. Biol. Sci.* 329: 161–170.

Tyrrell, T., and Willshaw, D. (1992). Cerebellar cortex: its simulation and the relevance of Marr's theory. *Philos. Trans. R. Soc. Lond. B. Biol. Sci.* 336: 239–257.

Uttley, A. M. (1979). *Information Transmission in the Nervous System.* New York, Academic Press.

Wu, J.-Y., Cohen, L. B., and Falk, C. X., (1994). Neuronal activity during different behaviors in *Aplysia*: a distributed organization? *Science* 263: 820–823.

13 Synaptic Plasticity: From Molecules to Behavior

Michel Baudry and Richard F. Thompson

The notion that mature organisms arise from complex interactions between a genetic program (genotype) with the environment (epigenetic regulation) to provide a unique individual (phenotype) is now well established. Such complex interactions apply to brain development as well, and it is well admitted that numerous processes referred to as "synaptic plasticity" are responsible for regulating the interactions between genotype and the environment to produce the mature phenotype not only during the developmental period but in adulthood and during aging as well (Baudry et al. 1993). Although the general principles involved in this regulation are starting to be well understood, a number of fundamental issues remain to be fully elucidated. Of particular interest in the context of learning and memory is the question of the roles of these processes in adult learning, and whether adult organisms utilize a whole new set of mechanisms to adapt to the environment. This question is of fundamental importance as it is generally admitted that the phenotype of adult organisms is relatively stable, and one has to propose and test hypotheses regarding information processing and storage that do not require epigenetic modifications (Changeux and Konishi 1987).

Of equal importance for the understanding of mature nervous system properties are questions concerning linkages between molecular and cellular processes of synaptic plasticity and adaptive processes exhibited at the network, system, and behavioral levels (Buonomano and Merzenich 1998; Marder 1998). In other words, can one predict the properties of a complex system by analyzing the properties of its components or is it the case that some properties exhibited at the system level are "emerging" from those at the lower levels? Moreover, can the understanding of the cellular mechanisms of synaptic plasticity shed any light on the behavioral properties of learning and memory? In particular, can we establish the rules used by neuronal networks to modify synaptic efficacy (if there is such a notion—see Markram et al., chapter 10), and determine how these rules define the parameters for learning? Most chapters in this book deal with these issues and our goal is to provide an overview of the field that uses particular chapters as illustrations of the various approaches used to answer the general questions raised above.

GENE TRANSCRIPTION AND SYNAPTIC PLASTICITY

The last five years have seen an explosion of work related to identifying so-called activity-dependent genes, that is, genes which are rapidly transcribed as a result of neuronal activity (Chen and Tonegawa 1997). The underlying motivation or assumption to search for such genes is indeed that synaptic plasticity requires the interaction between environment and the genotype and that neuronal activity does regulate the expression of specific genes, thus resulting in modifications of specific cellular properties. Chapters 1 and 2 illustrate one of the approaches which has been used by several laboratories to discover such genes, and underline the difficulty inherent to this type of problem, that is, the use of a stimulation paradigm that remains as close as possible to normal physiology, but at the same time activating a sufficiently large number of neurons to generate a detectable signal. As discussed in chapters 1 and 2, a number of activity-dependent genes have been identified so far, and they belong to several categories: (1) transcription factors, (2) cytoskeletal proteins, (3) growth factors, and (4) enzymes.

In some cases, the mechanisms involved in the activation of these genes have also been clearly established and so far they seem to follow the same general rules as those previously found in other tissues and cell types. A first extracellular messenger (neurotransmitter, neuromodulator, or hormone) activates a membrane-bound (or cytoplasmic) receptor which modifies the intracellular concentration of a second messenger, resulting in the activation of transcription factors, and of delayed-response genes (Morgan and Curran 1991). While it is easy to understand how such a mechanism can readily account for activity-dependent, long-lasting modifications of neuronal network properties during development or even in adulthood, it stands to reason that its activation results in cell-wide modifications, as the gene(s) whose transcription is (are) up(or down-)regulated modifies the cell phenotype, and thereby the properties of the whole cell and not of particular cellular domains. This mechanism has been well demonstrated in invertebrate preparations, where hormones, by modifying the expression of particular channels, produce dramatic alterations in network properties (Christie et al. 1995). It is conceivable that similar processes take place in vertebrate preparations, and in particular could underlie changes in network properties taking place during various biological cycles. Recent studies concerning the regulation of network properties in hippocampus during the estrous cycle of female rats appear to support the notion that this type of regulation is widespread in mammalian central nervous system (CNS) (Kawata 1995; McEwen 1988; McEwen et al. 1997). Numerous studies have also attempted to identify genes activated as a result of long-term potentiation (LTP) induction (Abraham et al. 1991, 1993; Dragunow et al. 1989; Thomas et al. 1994; see chapters 1 and 2). In most cases, several transcription factors have been shown to be induced as a result of trains of electrical activity producing LTP. However, it has been quite difficult to further establish the relationship between gene induction with mechanisms underlying LTP expression and maintenance (see below).

Examples of learning-related gene induction still remain elusive, with the exception of results from numerous studies using changes in the expression of the transcription factor, *c-fos*, to map out the circuitries activated during various phases of the learning and retrieving processes (Grimm and Tischmeyer 1997; Heurteaux et al. 1993; Zhu et al. 1996). Gall, Lynch, and colleagues have performed a number of very elegant studies to identify the networks as well as the cells engaged in initial acquisition, stable formation and retrieval of olfactory discrimination learning (Hess et al. 1995a,b, 1997). While these studies do not necessarily imply a role for *c-fos* expression in learning, they do indicate that learning is accompanied by activation of transcription factors in defined neuronal populations. In this context, it is also interesting to mention several studies indicating that the expression of several growth factors is regulated by physical activity and by learning, suggesting that the survival of neurons and the maintenance of neuronal connectivities are under constant regulation by growth factors and other trophic factors (Nawa et al. 1997; Neeper et al. 1996). Several reports describe the existence of learning-dependent gene activation. In particular, the gene encoding for the presynaptic protein syntaxin 1b has been shown to be induced in a task- and region-specific manner during learning (Davis et al. 1996). Several genes were also identified by RNA fingerprinting as being late memory-related genes after water maze acquisition. Among these genes were genes coding for the ryanodine receptor and that for glutamate dehydrogenase (Cavallaro et al. 1997).

Finally, experiments performed in one of our own laboratories indicated that acquisition of a classical conditioning response (the so-called nictitating membrane response) in rabbits is associated with the expression of a gene which belongs to a family of cyclin-dependent kinases (Gomi et al. 1997). In this case, animals receiving paired presentations of the conditioned stimulus (CS) and the unconditioned stimulus (US) showed a specific enrichment of the messenger (mRNA) coding for this kinase in the cerebellum, the structure necessary for storing the memory of the association between the CS and the US, when compared with naive animals or with animals receiving unpaired presentations of the CS and US. Again, the exact relationship between the induction of these genes and the mechanisms underlying learning of the different tasks used remains to be established. It is expected that the same type of approach, that is, subtractive hybridization protocols of the type described in chapter 1, might lead to the identification of genes involved in different types of learning in various brain structures.

Advances in molecular biology techniques, and in particular, the possibility of knocking out or knocking in specific genes (Silva et al. 1997), have produced a large number of mutant mice with various "learning and memory" impairments in addition to problems with LTP induction or maintenance (Chen et al. 1997; Huang et al. 1996; Linnarsson et al. 1997; Lu et al. 1997;

McCall et al. 1996; Oitzl et al. 1997; Silva et al. 1998, 1992). Unfortunately, the current picture emerging from these studies is far from being very clear, as technical problems of background strains as well as the existence of compensatory mechanisms have made the establishment of causal relationships between gene and function very difficult (Gerlai 1997). In addition, the mutations that have been generated often affect enzymes, receptor channels, or other cellular elements that participate in "normal" cellular functions, and are likely to modify, even in a subtle way, various aspects of brain structure and function. By analogy with work on regulation of cellular proliferation, it has recently been proposed that, in addition to positive regulatory genes involved in memory formation, there should be "memory suppressor genes," that is, genes imposing inhibitory constraints on storage of information (Abel et al. 1998). Hopefully, newer techniques, currently under development in various laboratories and aiming at producing spatially and temporally restricted modifications of gene expression, should provide a better understanding of the role gene induction plays in learning and memory and in synaptic plasticity (Mayford et al. 1997; Tsien et al. 1996).

Another approach that has been used with some success consists in preventing the translation of given genes by the administration of antisense oligonucleotides targeting specific sequences in the mRNAs for these genes (Ogawa and Pfaff 1996). Here again, a number of positive results have been reported indicating that translation of certain mRNAs encoding for transcription factors, ion channels, or growth factors is important for learning and memory and for synaptic plasticity (Guzowski and McGaugh 1997; Ma et al. 1998; Meiri et al. 1997).

The limitation on the role of gene expression in synaptic plasticity resulting from the cell-wide modifications it generally produces would be seriously eliminated if there were mechanisms coupling gene expression and local translation of the corresponding mRNAs. It has been known for quite a while that the machinery for protein synthesis is present in dendrites, and possibly in axons, and this provides for the possibility of a much more complex level of regulation of synaptic efficacy. For local protein synthesis to take place requires the dendritic targeting of mRNA and there are now a number of examples of such mRNAs, as described in chapters 1 and 2. Furthermore, there is also experimental evidence for links between synaptic transmission and regulation of local protein synthesis, as activation of glutamate metabotropic receptors in synaptoneurosomes has been shown to rapidly stimulate protein synthesis (Weiler and Greenough 1993).

There are, therefore, two types of mechanisms by which synaptic activity can produce localized modifications of synaptic properties restricted to activated synapses. In the first one, there is a small population of mRNAs constitutively present in dendrites, and in response to an appropriate signal, these mRNAs are locally translated, and the newly synthesized proteins are incorporated into the activated synapses. Note that this process is rapid and does not require gene expression, as it only depends on constitutively present mRNAs. In the second one, some locally generated signal is transmitted to the cell nucleus, triggering gene transcription, and the synthesis of mRNA. This mRNA is targeted to the dendrites and is locally translated at the appropriate site. Note that this requires the existence of a signal or signals which remain present at activated synapses for quite some time as the transcription of genes, and their targeting to the dendrites necessitates a significant period of time. This mechanism is somewhat related to the synaptic tagging described by Frey and Morris (1998). In their model, these authors propose that LTP induction is accompanied by the activation of signals they call "synaptic tags", which interact with plasticity-related newly synthesized proteins and stabilize the formation of LTP. Clearly, much more work is needed to clarify the exact mechanisms involved in this type of regulation, and to determine the types of mRNAs present in the dendrites, the mechanisms involved in targeting them to dendrites, and the signals responsible for tagging activated synapses. Finally, the types of proteins involved and their roles in regulating synaptic structure and function need to be further investigated.

REGULATION OF SYNAPTIC MORPHOLOGY AND SYNAPTIC PLASTICITY

Although it has been recognized for a long time that synapses exhibit a remarkable variety of shapes and that this property could well be responsible for regulating the strength of synaptic connections, very little is known concerning the factors responsible for determining synaptic morphology and the precise role morphology plays in controlling synaptic efficacy (Geinisman 1993; Harris et al. 1992; Harris and Stevens 1989; Wallace et al. 1991; Wilson 1988). It is quite clear that the cytoskeleton plays a major role in controlling synaptic contact morphology and the idea that the cytoskeleton is involved in learning has been recently reviewed by Dayhoff et al. (1994). On the intracellular side, a variety of cytoskeletal proteins have been shown to be present in presynaptic terminals and in dendritic spines, and evidence has been presented indicating that synaptic activity can regulate the state, distribution, and interactions of these proteins. In particular, the cytoskeletal protein spectrin has been found in postsynaptic structures, and LTP induction was shown to be associated with calpain-mediated proteolysis of spectrin (Vanderklish et al. 1995). This mechanism has been postulated to play a key role in the initiation of changes in the morphology of postsynaptic structures as a result of LTP induction (Baudry 1991; Baudry et al. 1987; Lynch et al. 1988). Another actin-binding protein, drebrin, has also been localized in dendrites where it is postulated to regulate the state of polymerization of actin filaments (Hayashi et al. 1996). Depolarization has been shown to regulate the state of phosphorylation of microtubule-associated protein 2 (MAP-2) and consequently its ability to stabilize microtubules (Quinlan and Halpain 1996). Likewise, phosphorylation reactions regulate the interactions between presynaptic proteins such as synapsin I and II and actin filaments (Nielander et al. 1997).

Recently, several families of proteins have been found to participate in the anchoring of receptors in postsynaptic structures. Thus, postsynaptic density (PSD)-95/synapse associated protein (SAP)-90 binds and clusters a number of receptors including the N-methyl-D-aspartate (NMDA) receptors (Ehlers et al. 1996; Kim et al. 1996; Kornau et al. 1995), while the glutamate reception interacting protein (GRIP) has been proposed to cluster AMPA receptors (Dong et al. 1997). In addition, other proteins such as the recently identified protein CRIPT (cysteine-Rich interceptor of PD2-3) appear to bind the PDZ domain of PSD-95 with the microtubules (Niethammer et al. 1998). It is also likely that several additional proteins play important roles in regulating the distribution of transmitter receptors in postsynaptic membranes, as well as the interaction between receptors and cytoskeleton (Kaech et al. 1997, Lin et al. 1998; Satoh et al. 1998; Wyszynski et al. 1998). Finally, it has also been demonstrated that NMDA receptor activation results in a calpain-mediated truncation of several subunits of both AMPA and NMDA receptors and this effect could be important in regulating the distribution and number of postsynaptic glutamate receptors (Bi et al. 1996, 1997, 1998; Gellerman et al. 1997; Musleh et al. 1997).

It has only recently been recognized that the extracellular matrix plays an equally important role in regulating synaptic morphology and properties. Both cell adhesion molecules (CAMs) and integrin receptors have now been shown to play critical roles in synaptic plasticity during development, as well as in adulthood (Delius et al. 1997; Lüthi et al. 1994; Xiao et al. 1991). In fact, in a number of neuronal pathways, a switch in the state of polysialication of neural CAM (NCAM) indicates the end of synaptic modifiability (see chapter 7) Furthermore, antibodies to (NCAM) and peptide inhibitors of integrin receptors have been shown to inhibit the formation of stable LTP (Bahr et al. 1997; Lüthi et al. 1994; Stäubli et al. 1998, 1990; Xiao et al. 1991). In several current models of LTP, stabilization of the modifications triggered during the induction phase of LTP is accomplished first by the disruption of the adhesive properties of synaptic contacts, possibly mediated through the proteolysis of CAM molecules, followed by the activation of integrins. In this way, synaptic contacts undergo a cycle of destabilization resulting from intracellular as well as extracellular proteolysis of proteins contributing to the morphology of synaptic contacts, followed by restabilization of a new synaptic structure implicating integrin activation and extracellular matrix components (Lynch 1998).

In this respect, it is quite interesting that the family of matrix metalloproteases (MMPs) and their endogenous inhibitors (tissue inhibitors of metalloproteinases, or TIMPs) have recently been implicated in the regulation of cell-cell interactions and more specifically in neuronal plasticity and pathological processes (see chapter 3). These proteases would be ideally suited to link synaptic activity and destabilization of the adhesive properties of synaptic contacts. It remains to be established how synaptic activity and, in particular, activation of NMDA receptors, can lead to the extracellular activation of these proteases. It is worth mentioning that plasmin and tissue plasminogen activator (t-PA) participate in the cascade leading to MMP activation, that t-PA expression has been shown to be increased following LTP induction, and that t-PA knockout mice do exhibit some impairments in LTP induction (see chapter 1). Thus, there is clearly a close relationship between synaptic plasticity mechanisms with processes regulating cellular interactions with extracellular matrix components (see chapter 3).

Although the issue is still highly debated (Sorra and Harris 1998), a large literature supports the notion that LTP is associated with modifications of synaptic structure and, in particular, that an increased number of perforated synapses might represent an intermediate stage in the establishment of LTP (see chapter 4). Here again, various models have been proposed to incorporate changes in synaptic structure with changes in synaptic function, ranging from an increase in the number of functional synaptic contacts to an increase in axodendritic synapses, with these latter types of synapses representing a more efficient type of synapse than the axospinous synapses. A popular version of these models is the notion of silent synapses, that is, synapses with functional NMDA receptors, but lacking functional AMPA receptors (Isaac et al. 1995; Liao et al. 1995; Lynch and Baudry 1991). Such synapses could become functional as a result of the coincidence of presynaptic activity with postsynaptic depolarization (conditions necessary and sufficient to activate the NMDA receptors), and the appearance of functional AMPA receptors due to their insertion in postsynaptic membranes from an intracellular pool or their redistribution from extracellular locations (Standley et al. 1996). Such hypotheses are attractive as they account for many features of the LTP debate, and satisfy the tenants of both pre- and postsynaptic modifications. What remains to be clarified are the relationships between these types of mechanisms, which imply a local regulation of synaptic structure and function quite independent of protein synthesis and gene expression, and the mechanisms discussed above. In particular, does stabilization of synaptic structures require the local synthesis of integrin molecules? Does long-lasting maintenance of synaptic structures require the expression of a selective gene(s)?

Independently of these questions, a largely ignored aspect of synaptology is the relationship between the geometrical features of synaptic contacts with synaptic function. We all reason with the simplistic view that CNS synapses are quite similar to the neuromuscular junction and that a large amount of neurotransmitter is released by the presynaptic terminal, that molecules of neurotransmitter diffuse rapidly through a narrow synaptic cleft, and readily associate with and activate postsynaptic receptors. Chapter 5 shows the results of simulation of transmitter release and receptor activation based on a model of a synapse which incorporates the geometry of synaptic contacts as well as the distribution of receptor proteins in postsynaptic densities. The results are quite astonishing as they do indeed indicate that the geometry of synaptic contacts has a much greater impact on synaptic function than one would have thought. This is true not only on the presynaptic terminals where geometry determines the probability of transmitter release but also on the postsynaptic sites where receptor location in concert with location of neurotransmitter release determines the probability that a transmitter molecule activates a postsynaptic receptor. This is quite fitting with the above discussion concerning modifications of synaptic structure as a result of LTP induction, as these simulations suggest that relatively minor modifications in synaptic structure can have profound influences on synaptic function.

A final point of discussion concerns the role of glia-neuron interactions in the regulation of synaptic structure and function. As shown in chapter 5, there is now clear evidence that glial cells respond rapidly to synaptic activity as they exhibit a variety of neurotransmitter receptors. In particular, as astrocytes express AMPA receptors lacking glutamate receptor (GluR2) subunits, they respond to synaptically released glutamate by an influx of calcium which could then induce the release of numerous molecules. In addition, glial acid fibrillary protein (GFAP) knockout mice exhibit altered neuronal physiology, including an increased LTP (McCall et al. 1996), indicating that modification of astrocyte properties affects synaptic plasticity. Considering the role of glial cells in the regulation of extracellular matrix components, it is also clear that much more remains to be discovered in regard to the role of glia-neuron interactions in the regulation of synaptic plasticity.

THE TEMPORAL STRUCTURE OF SYNAPTIC PLASTICITY

There is considerable interest at present in the possibility that information is contained in the time structure of neuronal spike trains. Recent evidence suggests that pairs of neurons may synchronize and oscillate under specific stimulus conditions (e.g., see Singer and Gray 1995). Cortical neurons in primates and other species have been observed to exhibit precise and statistically improbable sequences of neuronal activation (Abeles 1981; de Charms and Merzenick 1996). Such stimulus-induced oscillatory synchronization has also been observed in the sensorimotor system (Murthy and Fetz 1992). This synchronization was suggested by Milner (1974) as a means to bind together the neuronal elements of Hebbian cell assemblies. Von der Malsburg and Schneider (1986) proposed that synchronized oscillations could serve as a substrate for figure-ground segmentation in the visual system, whereby neurons encoding figure and ground could be segregated by their respective phase relative to a common oscillatory clock.

Perhaps the key question is whether this information is useful to the animal, that is, to the neural networks that ultimately generate behavior. In the present context, the synaptic underpinnings of stimulus-induced synchronization are particularly relevant. In chapter 9 Laurent and associates approach this problem using the locust olfactory system as a model preparation. As they note, olfactory stimuli induce complex multiple temporal response patterns in insect olfactory neurons (e.g., see Christensen and Hildebrand 1987) and in olfactory bulb neurons in vertebrates (Freeman 1992). They find that neuronal oscillatory synchronization plays a role in fine olfactory sensory discrimination tasks but not where the discrimination is between very dissimilar stimuli. Projection neurons in the antennal lobe show odor-evoked 20-Hz oscillatory local field potentials that result in synchronized action potentials in their axons. Interestingly, picrotoxin abolishes the 20-Hz oscillations, but the neurons still retain their slow and odor-specific response patterns. It would appear that local gamma aminobutyric acid (GABA) inhibition may play a key role as a synaptic mechanism for synchronized oscillatory potentials in this system. The authors conclude that spike timing and synchronization are indeed important parameters for odor sensation and perception.

A more general aspect of the temporal structure of synaptic activity concerns the overwhelming fact of the frequency dependence of synaptic transmission (Liaw and Berger 1996). In an obvious sense, alterations in monosynaptic transmission in the CA1 field of the hippocampus (Schaffer collaterals to pyramidal neurons) range from no effect at very low frequencies (0.1 Hz), to depression at low frequencies (1 Hz), to several varieties of potentiation at high frequencies. An elegantly simplified preparation is utilized by Markram and associates (see chapter 10) to explore this question. In brief they use neocortical slices and infrared microscopic methods to identify morphological neurons that are synaptically coupled. Both neurons are patched and one neuron is stimulated with a complex temporal protocol to determine the frequency-dependent properties of synaptic transmission. The overall findings are as follows:

1. Synaptic connections established via the same axon and in many cases via the same collateral from a pyramidal neuron onto a homogeneous class of pyramidal neurons differ significantly in the number and location of synapses on the dendrites.

2. Synaptic connections established via the same axon from a pyramidal neuron onto a pyramidal neuron and an interneuron can display depression onto the pyramidal neuron and facilitation onto the interneuron.

3. Synaptic connections onto two interneurons can display differential facilitation and depression.

4. Synaptic responses generated by connections established from three pyramidal neurons of the same morphological class onto a single interneuron all display facilitation of transmission, but the connections differ greatly in parameters as well as their numbers of synaptic contacts. In 65% of cases the synapses from one neuron were established on the same dendritic branch as the synapse formed by the other convergent input connection, indicating that differential synaptic properties can arise even when contacts are formed on the same dendritic branch.

These findings illustrate the potential complexities of interactions among two or three neurons. On the other hand, these complexities may result in simpler frequency dependence properties in large populations of neurons, as in long-term depression (LTD) and LTP. Indeed, when large neural networks are studied, the anatomical structures determine that a definable number of aspects of synaptic functions occur. In chapter 8, Connors and associates analyze thalamocortical relations in terms of thalamocortical, intracortical, and corticothalamic excitatory connections using thalamocortical slices. Each type of synaptic pathway has its own rules of dynamic behavior and regulation. As an example, in cortical neurons when converging thalamocortical and intracortical synapses were compared, intracortical synapses generated either weak depression or slight facilitation during stimulus trains, whereas thalamocortical synapses were always strongly depressed. In contrast, corticothalamic synapses show substantial facilitation with the same trains of stimuli. A particularly powerful resonance exists in certain thalamocortical pathways centered at about 10 Hz. Many neurons and circuits within the isolated and intact cortex have a propensity to oscillate spontaneously in this frequency range (Connors and Amitai 1997), and in vivo this activity is synchronized over large regions of neocortex.

SYNAPTIC PLASTICITY, NEURONAL NETWORKS, AND LEARNING AND MEMORY

Current views recognize several different forms or aspects of learning and memory involving different neuronal systems in the brain (figure 13.1).

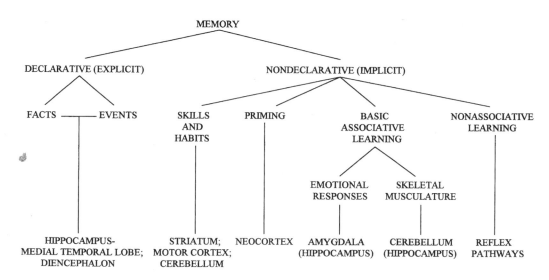

Figure 13.1

Baudry and Thompson

However, several of these systems can become engaged as a result of simple learning paradigms. Thus, in eye-blink conditioning, both hippocampal and cerebellar systems are always engaged in terms of learning-related neuronal activity, and if a strongly aversive US is used, the amygdala "fear" system also becomes engaged. We focus here on the hippocampus and cerebellum, perhaps the two most widely studied learning systems.

Interest in the critical role of the hippocampus in memory dates from the classic studies of H.M. (e.g., see Scoville and Milner 1957). In 1978, Mishkin published the first primate lesion study that appeared to mimic H.M.'s syndrome, using delayed nonmatching to sample (Mishkin 1978). In the intervening years, a large number of studies on humans, monkeys, rabbits, rats, and mice have focused on animal models of human amnesia and on the presumed role(s) of the hippocampus and related structures in memory. The memory deficit following hippocampal lesions is not global but rather much more specific for one kind of memory, termed "declarative" (or explicit or relational) (Squire 1992). Declarative memory is sometimes associated with consciousness or awareness, in contrast to many other forms of memory, including implicit (priming) memory in humans and a range of associative memory phenomena in humans and other mammals: motor and perceptual skills, classical conditioning, operant conditioning, habit formation, and so on (see figure 13.1).

The lesions in Mishkin's original study (Mishkin 1978) were designed to reproduce H.M.'s lesions and included portions of the hippocampus, amygdala, and adjacent cortical regions bilaterally. It now seems relatively clear that the amygdala per se is not critical, at least for declarative memory, but the hippocampus and related cortical structures are, for example, perirhinal, parahippocampal, and entorhinal cortex (Squire and Zola-Morgan 1991). Lesions including all these structures produce the most profound amnesia and lesions including subsets produce substantial but less profound amnesia.

Learning of a number of tasks in infraprimate mammals is sensitive to hippocampal damage, for example, water maze (Morris et al. 1986); odor discriminations (Eichenbaum et al. 1986; Lynch 1986); event timing (Olton et al. 1987); cue relationships (Sutherland et al. 1989); spatial memory (O'Keefe and Nadel 1978); spatial alternation (Aggleton et al. 1989); radial arm maze (Becker et al. 1980); conditional learning (Ross et al. 1984); discrimination reversal (Berger and Orr 1983); trace classical conditioning (Moyer et al. 1990; Solomon et al. 1986); contextual conditioning (Kim and Fanselow 1992; Phillips and LeDoux 1992). Although it is difficult to generalize, common threads in many of these tasks include relational memories, that is, memories for relations among stimuli and events, and memories that utilize spatial-contextual information, both of which would seem reasonable analogs of primate declarative memory in lower mammals (see also Eichenbaum et al. 1996). For neurobiological analysis, one would ideally wish to utilize preparations where much of the essential neuronal circuitry generating the behavior is known. Only a few of the animal models meet this modest requirement to some degree.

Perhaps the most widely proposed mechanism of memory storage in the hippocampus and neocortex is the process of LTP. In general, evidence does support this hypothesis but as yet there have been no clear and detailed demonstrations of causal chains from hippocampal (or cortical) LTP to learned behaviors, as we noted in our earlier volume (Baudry et al. 1993). But evidence grows.

In chapter 11, Roman and associates explore learning-induced alterations in field potentials in piriform cortex and the hippocampal dentate gyrus evoked by stimulation of the lateral olfactory tract and the lateral perforant path (dentate recordings only) (see also Roman et al. 1987). Animals (rats) were trained in two different discriminations, one between two odors and the other between a natural odor and a patterned electrical stimulus to the lateral olfactory tract. Results for monosynaptic field potentials in piriform cortex were striking—a marked enhancement of the potential evoked by the training electrode. Interestingly, in pseudoconditioned animals there was a pronounced depression in the response over trials. Polysynaptic responses in the dentate gyrus to lateral olfactory tract stimulation over trials also showed enhancement as a result of training, but monosynaptic responses of the same tissue to perforant path stimulation showed no changes as a result of training.

This study (see chapter 11) is illustrative of many experiments showing enhancement of field potentials in the hippocampus and other structures as a result of training (see Baudry et al. 1993). The evidence is correlational and suggestive but not yet causal. The recent spate of studies using gene knock-out mice is certainly supportive of LTP as a memory mechanism (see Chen and Tonegawa 1997; Silva et al. 1998 for reviews). Thus knockout mice that show impaired hippocampal LTP also show impaired spatial learning, although this is not invariable (Hölscher 1997).

There is an extensive literature documenting the critical role of the cerebellum in certain aspects of learning and memory. Examples include plasticity of the vestibulo-ocular reflex (Ito 1984, 1889), learning of multijoint movements (Thach et al. 1992), and basic sensorimotor associative learning and memory (Thompson and Krupa 1994; see also Thompson et al. 1997). Classical conditioning of discrete behavioral responses learned with aversive unconditioned stimuli provides a particularly clear case where the cerebellum and its associated brainstem circuitry forms the essential (necessary and sufficient) circuitry for learning and memory. The conditioned eye-blink response has been the most widely used paradigm, but others have also been used, for example, limb flexion, head-turning, and so forth. Further, evidence strongly supports the hypothesis that the memory traces are formed and stored in the cerebellum (see Thompson et al. 1997).

Lesion, neuronal recording, electrical microstimulation, and anatomical procedures have been used to identify the essential CS circuit as including the pontine mossy fiber projections to the cerebellum; the essential US reinforcing or teaching circuit as including neurons in the inferior olive (dorsal accessory olive) projecting to the cerebellum as climbing fibers; and the essential conditioned response (CR) circuit as including the interpositus nucleus, its projection via the superior cerebellar peduncle to the magnocellular red nucleus, and rubral projections to premotor and motor nuclei. Each major component of the eye-blink CR circuit was reversibly inactivated both in trained animals and over the course of training. In all cases in trained animals, inactivation abolished the CR (and the unconditioned response as well when motor nuclei were inactivated). When animals were trained during inactivation (and not exhibiting CRs) and then tested without inactivation, animals with inactivation of the motor nuclei, red nucleus, and superior peduncle had fully learned, whereas animals with inactivation of a very localized region of the cerebellum (anterior interpositus and overlying cortex) had not learned at all. Consequently, the memory traces would seem to be formed and stored in the cerebellum. Evidence suggests that a process like LTD may be a mechanism of memory storage in cerebellar cortex (Ito 1989; Linden and Connor 1995; Thompson et al. 1997).

In chapter 12, Chauvet and Chauvet present a comprehensive model of the circuitry in the cerebellar cortex. They define a functional unit as the Purkinje neuron and associated neural network: A granule cell, denoted gc, belongs to the unit containing the nearest Purkinje cell it contacts. Then gc is considered to belong to a specific unit numbered k if the following conditions apply: gc has synapses with at least one Purkinje cell of the unit k, the distance between gc and the Purkinje cells corresponds to the smallest distance between gc and any Purkinje cell it contacts outside the unit, and gc has synapses with at least one Golgi cell of the unit k. The basket and stellar cells included in unit k are those which are contacted by the granule cells of the unit k and which are connected to the Purkinje cell of the unit k. This unit may be separated into two subsystems, that is, the granule cell neural network and the Purkinje cell subsystem.

They propose that the Purkinje neuron itself exhibits synaptic plasticity (e.g., LTD), and the functional unit serves to code the learning and memory of patterns, that sets of Purkinje neurons corresponding to microzones code learning of coordinated patterns, and that together with the deep nucleus neurons learn much more extensive coordinated patterns, for example, associative learning. Their model is comprehensive, quantitative, and elegant. The unique geometry of the cerebellum (200,000 parallel fiber synapses and one climbing fiber synapse) has inspired many models of the cerebellum as a learning machine (see, e.g., Bartha and Thompson 1996), beginning with the classic models of Marr (1969) and Albus (1971). In our view, the approach developed by Chauvet and Chauvet is extremely promising as it illustrates the possibility of describing the properties of complex neuronal networks with a formal mathematical analysis.

CONCLUSIONS

One of the purposes of this book was to evaluate progress in the field of synaptic plasticity over the last five years. It is clear (at least to us) that there has been tremendous progress at all levels of analysis. At the molecular level, technologies that did not exist five years ago (or at best were in their infancy) are now available to delineate with an exquisite degree of precision the involvement of any gene in synaptic plasticity and to delineate the possible role(s) of the corresponding gene product. At the cellular level, although some details remain to be clarified, the mechanisms underlying different forms of LTP and LTD are starting to be well understood. No doubt that the considerable progress in modeling and simulation techniques will allow a much more rapid testing and evaluation of different hypotheses regarding the intimate details which have resisted traditional investigation. At the network level, the rules determining alterations in synaptic efficacy at various types of synapses are being unraveled and the computational properties of various networks are starting to be well understood. At the behavior level, although there still remains a lot to learn concerning how even relatively simple behavior can be described in terms of functioning of neuronal assemblies, initial steps in this direction are being taken in a number of laboratories. As shown in the chapter 12, it is not too far before simple behaviors will be described by a set of mathematical equations. Let us hope we will still discover new phenomena worth investigating and return to Angers to discuss them.

REFERENCES

Abel, T., Martin, K. C., Bartsch, D., and Kandel, E., R. (1998). Memory suppressor genes: inhibitory constraints on the storage of long-term memory. *Science* 279: 338–341.

Abeles, M. (1981). *Corticonics. Neural Circuits of the Cerebral Cortex*. Cambridge, UK, Cambridge University Press.

Abraham, W. C., Dragunow, M., and Tate, W. P. (1991). The role of immediate early genes in the stabilization of long-term potentiation. *Mol. Neurobiol.* 5: 297–314.

Abraham, W. C., Mason, S. E., Demmer, J., Williams, J. M., Richardson, C. L., Tate, W. P., Lawlor, P. A., and Dragunow, M. (1993). Correlations between immediate early gene induction and the persistence of long-term potentiation. *Neuroscience* 56: 717–727.

Aggleton, J. P., Blindt, H. S., and Rawlins, J. N. P. (1989). Effects of amygdaloid and amygdaloid-hippocampal lesions on object recognition and spatial working memory in rats. *Behav. Neurosci.* 103: 962–974.

Albus, J. S. (1971). A theory of cerebellar function, *Math. Biosci.* 10: 25–61.

Bahr, B. A., Staubli, U., Xiao, P., Chun, D., Ji, Z. X., Esteban, E. T., and Lynch, G. (1997). Arg-Gly-Asp-Ser-selective adhesion and the stabilization of long-term potentiation—pharmacological studies and the characterization of a candidate matrix receptor. *J. Neurosci.* 17: 1320–1329.

Bartha, G. T., and Thompson, R. F. (1996). Cerebellum and conditioning. In *The Handbook of Brain Theory and Neural Networks*, M. A. Arbib, ed., pp. 169–172. Cambridge, MA, MIT Press.

Baudry, M. (1991). An integrated biochemical model for long-term potentiation. In *Long-Term Potentiation: A Debate of Current Issues*, M. Baudry and J. L. Davis, eds., pp. 169–182. Cambridge, MA, MIT Press.

Baudry, M., Seubert, P., and Lynch, G. (1987). A possible second messenger system for the production of long-term changes in synapses. *Adv. Exp. Med. Biol.* 221: 291–311.

Baudry, M., Davis, J. L., and Thompson, R. F. eds. (1993). *Synaptic Plasticity: Molecular and Functional Aspects*. Cambridge, MA, MIT Press.

Becker, J. T., Walker, J. A., and Olton, D. S. (1980). Neuroanatomical bases of spatial memory. *Brain Res.* 200: 307–320.

Berger, T. W., and Orr, W. B. (1983). Hippocampectomy selectively disrupts discrimination reversal conditioning of the rabbit nictitating membrane response. *Behav. Brain Res.* 8: 49–68.

Bi, X., Chang, V., Molnar, E., McIlhinney, J., and Baudry, M. (1996). The C-terminal domain of GluR1 subunits is a target for calpain-mediated proteolysis. *Neuroscience* 73: 903–906.

Bi, X., Chen, J., and Baudry, M. (1998). Calpain-mediated proteolysis of GluR, subunits in organotypic hippocampal cultures following kainic and treatment. *Brain Res.* 781: 355–357.

Bi, X., Chen, J., Dang, S., Wenthold, R. J., Tocco, G., and Baudry, M. (1997). Characterization of calpain-mediated proteolysis of GluR1 subunits of alpha-amino-3-hydroxy-5-methylisoxazole-4-propionate receptors in rat brain. *J. Neurochem.* 68: 1484–1493.

Buonomano, D. V., and Merzenich, M. M. (1998). Cortical plasticity—from synapses to maps. *Annu. Rev. Neurosci.* 21: 149–186.

Cavallaro, S., Meiri, N., Yi, C. L., Musco, S., Ma, W., Goldberg, J., and Alkon, D. L. (1997). Late memory-related genes in the hippocampus revealed by RNA fingerprinting. *Proc. Natl. Acad. Sci. USA* 94: 9669–9673.

Changeux, J. P., and Konishi, M., eds. (1987). *The Neural and Molecular Bases of Learning. Dahlem Konferenzen*. New York, John Wiley & Sons d.

Chen, C., and Tonegawa, S. (1997). Molecular-genetic analysis of synaptic plasticity, activity-dependent neural development, learning, and memory in the mammalian brain. *Annu. Rev. Neurosci.* 20: 157–184.

Chen, K. S., Nishimura, M. C., Armanini, M. P., Crowley, C., Spencer, S. D., and Phillips, H. S. (1997). Disruption of a single allele of the nerve growth factor gene results in atrophy of basal forebrain cholinergic neurons and memory deficits. *J. Neurosci.* 17: 7288–7296.

Christensen, T. A., and Hildebrand, J. G. (1987). Male-specific, sex pheromone—selective projection neurons in the antennal lobes of the moth *Manduca sexta*. *J. Comp. Physiol.* [A] 160: 553–569.

Christie, A. E., Skiebe, P., and Marder, E. (1995). Matrix of neuromodulators in neurosecretory structures of the crab *Cancer borealis*. *J. Exp. Biol.* 198: 2431–2439.

Connors, C. W., and Amitai, Y. (1997). Making waves in the neo cortex. *Neuron* 18: 1–20.

Davis, S., Rodger, J., Hicks, A., Mallet, J., and Laroche, S. (1996). Brain structure and task-specific increase in expression of the gene encoding syntaxin 1b during learning in the rat—a potential molecular marker for learning-induced synaptic plasticity in neural networks. *Eur. J. Neurosci.* 8: 2068–2074.

Dayhoff, J., Hameroff, S., Lahozbeltra, R., and Swenberg, C. E. (1994). Cytoskeletal involvement in neuronal learning—a review. *Eur. Biophys. J.* 23: 79–93.

DeCharms, R. C., and Merzenich, M. M. (1996). Primary cortical representation of sounds by the coordination of action potential timing. *Nature* 381: 610–613.

Delius, J. A. M., Kramer, I., Schachner, M., and Singer, W. (1997). NCAM-180 in the postnatal development of cat visual cortex—an immunohistochemical study. *J. Neurosci. Res.* 49: 255–267.

Dong, H., O'Brien, R. J., Fung, E. T., Lanahan, A. A., Worley, P. F., and Huganir, R. L. (1997). GRIP: a synaptic PDZ domain-containing protein that interacts with AMPA receptors. *Nature* 386: 279–288.

Dragunow, M., Abraham, W. C., Goulding, M., Mason, S. E., Robertson, H. A., and Faull, R. L. (1989). Long-term potentiation and the induction of *c-fos* mRNA and proteins in the dentate gyrus of unanesthetized rats. *Neurosci. Lett.* 101: 274–280.

Ehlers, M. D., Mammen, A. L., Lau, L. F., and Huganir, R. L. (1996). Synaptic targeting of glutamate receptors. *Curr. Opin. Cell Biol.* 8: 484–489.

Eichenbaum, H., Fagan, A., and Cohen, N. J. (1986). Normal olfactory discrimination learning set and facilitation of reversal learning after medial-temporal damage in rats: implications for an account of preserved learning abilities in amnesia. *J. Neurosci.* 6: 1876–1884.

Eichenbaum, H., Schoenbaum G., Young, B., and Baudry M. (1996). Functional organization of the hippocampal memory system. *Proc. Natl. Acad. Sci. USA* 93: 13500–13507.

Freeman, W. J. (1992). Nonlinear dynamics in olfactory information processing. In: *Olfaction, a Model System for Computational Neuroscience*, J. L. Davis and H. Eichenbaum, eds., pp. 225–249. Cambridge, MA, MIT Press.

Frey, U., and Morris, G. M. (1998). Synaptic tagging: implications for late maintenance of hippocampal long-term potentiation. *Trends Neurosci.* 21: 181–188.

Geinisman, Y. (1993). Perforated axospinous synapses with multiple, completely partitioned transmission zones—probable structural intermediates in synaptic plasticity. *Hippocampus* 3: 417–434.

Gellerman, D., Bi, X., and Baudry, M. (1997). NMDA receptor–mediated regulation of AMPA receptor properties in organotypic culture. *J. Neurochem.* 69: 131–136.

Gerlai, R. (1997). A causal relationship between LTP and learning—has the question been answered by genetic approaches? *Behav. Brain Sci.* 20: 617.

Gomi, H., Sun, W., Chun, J. T., Finch, C. E., and Thompson, R. F. (1997). Learning induces RNA encoding a *cdc2*-related kinase. *Soc. Neurosci. Abstr.* 23: 780.

Grimm, R., and Tischmeyer, W. (1997). Complex patterns of immediate-early gene induction in rat brain following brightness-discrimination training and pseudotraining. *Behav. Brain Res.* 84: 1–2.

Guzowski, J. F., and McGaugh, J. L. (1997). Antisense oligodeoxynucleotide-mediated disruption of hippocampal cAMP response element–binding protein levels impairs consolidation of memory for water maze training. *Proc. Natl. Acad. Sci. USA* 94: 2693–2698.

Harris, K. M., and Stevens, J. K. (1989). Dendritic spines of CA1 pyramidal cells in the rat hippocampus: serial electron microscopy with reference to their biophysical characteristics. *J. Neurosci.* 9: 2982–2997.

Harris, K. M., Jensen, F. E., and Tsao, B. (1992). 3-Dimensional structure of dendritic spines and synapses in rat hippocampus CA1 at postnatal day 15 and adult ages—implications for the maturation of synaptic physiology and long-term potentiation. *J. Neurosci.* 12: 2685–2705.

Hayashi, K., Ishikawa, R., Ye, L. H., He, X. L., Takata, K., Kohama, K., and Shirao, T. (1996). Modulatory role of drebrin on the cytoskeleton within dendritic spines in the rat cerebral cortex. *J. Neurosci.* 16: 7161–7170.

Hess, U. S., Lynch, G., and Gall, C. M. (1995a). Changes in *c-fos* messenger RNA expression in rat brain during odor discrimination learning—differential involvement of hippocampal subfields Ca1 and Ca3. *J. Neurosci.* 15: 4786–4795.

Hess, U. S., Lynch, G., and Gall, C. M. (1995b). Regional patterns of *c-fos* messenger RNA expression in rat hippocampus following exploration of a novel environment versus performance of a well-learned discrimination. *J. Neurosci.* 15: 7796–7809.

Hess, U. S., Gall, C. M., Granger, R., and Lynch, G. (1997). Differential patterns of *c-fos* messenger RNA expression in amygdala during successive stages of odor discrimination-learning. *Learn. Mem.* 4: 262–283.

Heurteaux, C., Messier, C., Destrade, C., and Lazdunski, M. (1993). Memory processing and apamin induce immediate early gene expression in mouse brain. *Mol. Brain Res.* 18: 1–2.

Hölscher[?], C. (1997). Long-term potentiation: a good model for learning and memory. *Prog. Neuropsychopharmacol. Biol. Psychiatry* 21: 47–68.

Huang, Y. Y., Bach, M. E., Lipp, H. P., Zhuo, M., Wolfer, D. P., Hawkins, R. D., Schoonjans, L., Kandel, E. R., Godfraind, J. M., Mulligan, R., Collen, D., and Carmelieb, P. (1996). Mice lacking the gene encoding tissue-type plasminogen-activator show a selective interference with late-phase long-term potentiation in both schaffer collateral and mossy fiber pathways. *Proc. Natl. Acad. Sci. USA* 93: 8699–8704.

Isaac, J. T. R., Nicoll, R. A., and Malenka, R. C. (1995). Evidence for silent synapses: implications for the expression of LTP. *Neuron* 15: 427–434.

Ito, M. (1984). *The Cerebellum and Neural Control*. New York, Appleton Century-Crofts.

Ito, M. (1989). Long-term depression. *Annu. Rev. Neurosci.* 12: 85–102.

Kaech, S., Fischer, M., Doll, T., and Matus, A. (1997). Isoform specificity in the relationship of actin to dendritic spines. *J. Neurosci.* 17: 9565–9572.

Kawata, M. (1995). Roles of steroid-hormones and their receptors in structural organization In the nervous system. *Neurosci. Res.* 24: 1–46.

Kim, E., Cho, K. O., Rothschild, A., and Sheng, M. (1996). Heteromultimerzation and NMDA receptor–clustering activity of Chapsyn-110, a member of the PSD-95 family of protein. *Neuron* 17: 103–113.

Kim, J. J., and Fanselow, M. S. (1992). Modality-specific retrograde amnesia of fear. *Science* 256: 675–677.

Kornau, H. C., Schenker, L. T., Kennedy, M. B., and Seeburg, P. H. (1995). Domain interaction beween NMDA receptor subunits and the postsynaptic density protein PSD-95. *Science* 269: 1737–1740.

Liao, D. Z., Hessler, N. A., and Malinow, R. (1995). Activation of postsynaptically silent synapses during pairing-induced LTP in CA1 region of hippocampal slice. *Nature* 375: 400–404.

Liaw, J. S., and Berger, T. (1996). Dynamic synapse: a new concept of neural representation and computation. *Hippocampus* 6: 591–600.

Lin, J. W., Wyszynski, M., Madhavan, R., Sealock, R., Kim, J. U., and Sheng, M. (1998). Yotiao, a novel protein of neuromuscular junction and brain that interacts with specific splice variants of NMDA receptor subunit Nr1. *J. Neurosci.* 18: 2017–2027.

Linden, D. J., and Connor, J. A. (1995). Long-term synaptic depression. *Annu. Rev. Neurosci.* 18: 319–357.

Linnarsson, S., Bjorklund, A., and Ernfors, P. (1997). Learning deficit in BDNF mutant mice. *Eur. J. Neurosci.* 9: 2581–2587.

Lu, Y. M., Jia, Z. P., Janus, C., Henderson, J. T., Gerlai, R., Wojtowicz, J. M., and Roder, J. C. (1997). Mice lacking metabotropic glutamate receptor-5 show impaired learning and reduced Ca1 long-term potentiation (LTP) but normal Ca3 LTP. *J. Neurosci.* 17: 5196–5205.

Lüthi, A., Laurent, J. P., Figurov, A., Muller, D., and Schachner, M. (1994). Hippocampal long-term potentiation and neural cell-adhesion molecules L1 and NCAM. *Nature* 372: 777–779.

Lynch, G. (1986). *Synapses, Circuits, and the Beginnings of Memory.* Cambridge, MA, MIT Press.

Lynch, G. (1998). Memory and the brain: unexpected chemistries and a new pharmacology. *Neurobiol. Learn. Mem.* 70: 82–100.

Lynch, G., and Baudry, M. (1991). Re-evaluating the constraints on hypothesis regarding LTP expression. *Hippocampus* 1: 9–14.

Lynch, G., Bodsch, W., and Baudry, M. (1988). Cytoskeletal proteins and the regulation of synaptic structure. In *Intrinsic Determinants of Neuronal Form and Function*, R. J. Lasek and M. M. Black, eds., pp. 217–243. New York, Alan R. Liss, Inc.

Ma, Y. L., Wang, H. L., Wu, H. C., Wei, C. L., and Lee, E. H. Y. (1998). Brain-derived neurotrophic factor antisense oligonucleotide impairs memory retention and inhibits long-term potentiation in rats. *Neuroscience* 82: 957–967.

Marder, E. (1998). From biophysics to models of network function. *Annu. Rev. Neurosci.* 21: 25–45.

Marr, D. (1969). A theory of cerebellar cortex. *J. Physiol.* 202: 437–470.

Mayford, M., Mansuy, I. M., Muller, R. U., and Kandel, E. R. (1997). Memory and behavior—a 2nd generation of genetically-modified mice. *Curr. Biol.* 7: R580–R589.

McCall, M. A., Gregg, R. G., Behringer, R. R., Brenner, M., Delaney, C. L., Galbreath, E. J., Zhang, C. L., Pearce, R. A., Chiu, S. Y., and Ressing A. (1996). Targeted deletion in astrocyte intermediate filament (Gfap) alters neuronal physiology. *Proc. Natl. Acad. Sci. USA* 93: 6361–6366.

McEwen, B. S. (1988). Steroid hormones and the brain: linking "nature" and "nurture." *Neurochem. Res.* 13: 663–669.

McEwen, B. S., Alves, S. E., Bulloch, K., and Weiland, N. G. (1997). Ovarian steroids and the brain—implications for cognition and aging. *Neurology* 48: S8–S15.

Meiri, N., Ghelardini, C., Tesco, G., Galeotti, N., Dahl, D., Tomsic, D., Cavallaro, S., Quattrone, A., Capaccioli, S., Bartolini, A., and Allzan, D. L. (1997). Reversible antisense inhibition of shaker-like Kv1.1 potassium channel expression impairs associative memory in mouse and rat. *Proc. Natl. Acad. Sci. USA* 94: 4430–4434.

Milner, P. (1974). A model for visual shape recognition. *Psychol. Rev.* 81: 521–535.

Mishkin, M. (1978). Memory in monkeys severely impaired by combined but not separate removal of amygdala and hippocampus. *Nature* 273: 297–298.

Morgan, J. I., and Curran, T. (1991). Stimulus-transcription coupling in the nervous system: involvement of the inducible proto-oncogenes *fos* and *jun*. *Annu. Rev. Neurosci.* 14: 421–451.

Morris, R. G. M., Anderson, E., Lynch, G. S., and Baudry, M. (1986). Selective impairment of learning and blockade of long-term potentiation by an N-methyl-D-asparate receptor antagonist, AP5. *Nature* 319: 774–775.

Moyer, J., Jr., Deyo, R. A., and Disterhoft, J. F. (1990). Hippocampectomy disrupts trace eyeblink conditioning in rabbits. *Behav. Neurosci.* 104: 243–252.

Murthy, V. N., and Fetz, E. E. (1992). Coherent 25–35 Hz oscillations in the sensorimotor cortex of the awake behaving monkey. *Proc. Natl. Acad. Sci. USA* 89: 5670–5674.

Musleh, W., Bi, X., Tocco, G., Yaghoubi, S., and Baudry, M. (1997). Glycine-induced long-term potentiation is associated with structural and functional modifications of AMPA receptors. *Proc. Natl. Acad. Sci. USA* 94: 9451–9456.

Nawa, H., Saito, M., and Nagano, T. (1997). Neurotrophic factors in brain synaptic plasticity. *Crit. Rev. Neurobiol.* 11: 91–100.

Neeper, S. A., Gomez-Pinilla, F., Choi, J., and Cotman, C. W. (1996). Physical activity increases messenger RNA for brain-derived neurotrophic factor and nerve growth factor in rat brain. *Brain Res.* 726: 1–2.

Nielander, H. B., Onofri, F., Schaeffer, E., Menegon, A., Fesce, R., Valtorta, F., Greengard, P., and Benfenati, F. (1997). Phosphorylation-dependent effects of synapsin IIa on actin polymerization and network formation. *Eur. J. Neurosci.* 9: 2712–2722.

Niethammer, M., Valtschanoff, J. G., Kapoor, T. M., Allison, D. W., Weinberg, R. J., Craig, A. M., and Sheng, M. (1998). Cript, a novel postsynaptic protein that binds to the 3rd PDZ domain of PSD-95/SAP90. *Neuron* 20: 693–707.

Ogawa, S., and Pfaff, D. W. (1996). Application of antisense DNA method for the study of molecular bases of brain function and behavior. *Behav. Genet.* 26: 279–292.

Oitzl, M. S., Dekloet, E. R., Joels, M., Schmid, W., and Cole, T. J. (1997). Spatial learning deficits in mice with a targeted glucocorticoid receptor gene disruption. *Eur. J. Neurosci.* 9: 2284–2296.

O'Keefe, J., and Nadel, L. (1978). *The Hippocampus as a Cognitive Map.* London, Oxford University Press.

Olton, D. S., Meck, W. H., and Church, R. M. (1987). Separation of hippocampal and amygdaloid involvement in temporal memory dysfunction. *Brain Res.* 404: 180–188.

Phillips, R. G., and LeDoux, J. E. (1992). Differential contribution of amygdala and hippocampus to cued and contextual fear conditioning. *Behav. Neurol.* 106: 274–285.

Quinlan, E. M., and Halpain, S. (1996). Emergence of activity-dependent, bidirectional control of microtubule-associated protein (MAP-2) phosphorylation during postnatal development. *J. Neurosci.* 16: 7627–7637.

Roman, F. S., Staubli, U., and Lynch G. (1987). Evidence for synaptic potentiation in a cortical network during learning. *Brain Res.* 418: 221–226.

Ross, R. T., Orr, W. B., Holland, P. C., and Berger, T. W. (1984). Hippocampectomy disrupts acquisition and retention of learned conditional responding. *Behav. Neurosci.* 98: 211–225.

Satoh, A., Nakanishi, H., Obaishi, H., Wada, M., Takahashi, K., Satoh, K., Hirao, K., Nishioka, H., Hata, Y., Mizoguchi, A., and Takai Y. (1998). Neurabin-Ii/spinophilin—an actin filament–binding protein with one PDZ domain localized at cadherin-based cell-cell adhesion sites. *J. Biol. Chem.* 273: 3470–3475.

Scoville, W. B., and Milner, B. (1957). Loss of recent memory after bilateral hippocampal lesions. *J. Neurol. Neurosurg. Psychiatry* 20: 11–21.

Silva, A. J., Kogan, J. H., Frankland, P. W., and Kida, S. (1998). CREB and Memory. *Annu. Rev. Neurosci.* 21: 127–148.

Silva, A. J., Smith, A. M., and Giese, K. P. (1997). Gene targeting and the biology of learning and memory. *Annu. Rev. Genet.* 31: 527–546.

Silva, A. J., Stevens, C. F., Tonegawa, S., and Wang, Y. (1992). Deficient hippocampal long-term potentiation in calcium-calmodulin kinase II mutant mice. *Science* 257: 201–206.

Singer, W., and Gray, C. M. (1995). Visual feature integration and the temporal correlation hypothesis. *Annu. Rev. Neurosci.* 18: 555–586.

Solomon, P. R., Vander Schaaf, E. R., Thompson, R. F., and Weisz, D. J. (1986). Hippocampus and trace conditioning of the rabbit's classically conditioned nictitating membrane response. *Behav. Neurosci.* 100: 729–744.

Sorra, K., E., and Harris, K., M. (1998). Stability in synapse number of size at 2hr after long-term potentiation in hippocampal area CA1. *J. Neurosci.* 18: 658–671.

Squire, L. R. (1992). Memory and the hippocampus: a synthesis from findings with rats, monkeys, and humans. *Psychol. Rev.* 99: 195–231.

Squire, L. R., and Zola Morgan, S. (1991). The medial temporal lobe memory system. *Science* 253: 1380–1386.

Standley, S., Bi, X., and Baudry, M. (1996). Glutamate receptor regulation and synaptic plasticity. In *Long-Term Potentiation*, Vol. 3, M. Baudry and J. L. Davis, eds., pp. 17–40. Cambridge, MA, MIT Press.

Staubli, U., Vanderklish, P., and Lynch, G. (1990). An inhibitor of integrin receptors blocks long-term potentiation. *Neurobiol. Learn. Mem.* 53: 1–5.

Staubli, U., Chun, D., and Lynch, G. (1998). Time-dependent reversal of long-term potentiation by an integrin antagonist. *J. Neurosci.* 18: 3460–3469.

Sutherland, R. W., McDonald, R. J., Hill, C. R., and Rudy, J. W. (1989). Damage to the hippocampal formation in rats selectively impairs the ability to learn cue relationships. *Behav. Brain Res.* 52: 321.

Thach, W. T., Goodkin, H. G., and Keating, J. G. (1992). The cerebellum and the adaptive coordination of movement. *Annu. Rev. Neurosci.* 15: 403–442.

Thompson, R. F., and Krupa, D. J. (1994). Organization of memory traces in the mammalian brain. *Annu. Rev. Neurosci.* 17: 519–549.

Thompson, R. F., Bao, S., Chen, L., Cipriano, B. D., Grethe, J. S., Kim, J. J., Thompson, J. K., Tracy, J., Weninger, M. S., and Krupa, D. J. (1997). *Int. Rev. Neurobiol.* 41: 151–189.

Thomas, K. L., Laroche S., Errington, M. L., Bliss, T. V. P., and Hunt, S. P. (1994). Spatial and temporal changes in signal transduction pathways during LTP. *Neuron* 13: 737–745.

Tsien, J. Z., Chen, D. F., Gerber, D., Tom, C., Mercer, E. H., Anderson, D. J., Mayford, M., Kandel, E. R., and Tonegawa, S. (1996). Subregion-restricted and cell type—restricted gene knockout in mouse brain. *Cell* 87: 1317–1326.

Vanderklish, P., Saido, T. C., Gall, C., and Lynch, G. (1995). Proteolysis of spectrin by calpain accompanies theta-burst stimulation in cultured hippocampal slices. *Mol. Brain Res.* 32: 25–35.

Von der Malsburg, C., and Schneider, W. (1986). A neural cocktail-party processor. *Biol. Cybern.* 54: 29–40.

Wallace, C. S., Hawrylak, N., and Greenough, W. T. (1991). Studies of synaptic structural modifications after long-term potentiation and kindling: context for a molecular morphology. In *Long-Term Potentiation: A Debate of Current Issues*, M. Baudry and J. L. Davis, eds., pp. 189–232. Cambridge, MA, MIT Press.

Weiler, I. J., and Greenough, W. T. (1993). Metabotropic glutamate receptors trigger post-synaptic protein synthesis. *Proc. Natl. Acad. Sci. USA* 90: 7168–7171.

Wilson, C. J. (1988). Cellular mechanisms controlling the strength of synapses. *J. Electron Microsc. Tech.* 10: 293–313.

Wyszynski, M., Kharazia, V., Shanghvi, R., Rao, A., Beggs, A. H., Craig, A. M., Weinberg, R., and Sheng, M. (1998). Differential regional expression and ultrastructural localization of alpha-actinin-2, a putative NMDA receptor–anchoring protein in rat brain. *J. Neurosci.* 18: 1383–1392.

Xiao, P., Bahr, B. A., Staubli, U., Vanderklish, P. W., and Lynch, G. (1991). Evidence that matrix recognition contributes to stabilization but not induction of LTP. *Neuroreport* 2: 461–464.

Zhu, X. O., McCabe, B. J., Aggleton, J. P., and Brown, M. W. (1996). Mapping visual recognition memory through expression of the immediate-early gene *c-fos*. *Neuroreport* 7: 1871–1875.

Contributors

Yael Amitai
Department of Physiology
Ben-Gurion University of the Negev
Beersheba, Israel

Michel Baudry
Department of Biological Sciences
University of Southern California
Los Angeles, CA

Theodore W. Berger
Department of Biomedical
Engineering
University of Southern California
Los Angeles, CA

Pierre-Alain Buchs
Division of Neuropharmacology
Centre Médical Universitaire
Geneva, Switzerland

A. K. Butler
Department of Neurology
UCLA School of Medicine
Los Angeles, CA

Franck A. Chaillan
Laboratoire de Neurobiologie des
Comportements
Université de Provence
Marseille, France

Gilbert A. Chauvet
Institute of Theoretical Biology
University of Angers
Angers, France

Pierre Chauvet
Institute of Theoretical Biology
University of Angers
Angers, France

Marie-Françoise Chesselet
Department of Neurology
UCLA Department of Medicine
Los Angeles, CA

Barry W. Connors
Department of Neuroscience
Brown University
Providence, RI

Taraneh Ghaffari
Department of Biomedical
Engineering
University of Southern California
Los Angeles, CA

Jay R. Gibson
Department of Neuroscience
Brown University
Providence, RI

Ziv Gil
Department of Physiology
Ben-Gurion University of the Negev
Beersheba, Israel

Michel Khrestchatisky
INSERM U29
Hospital de Port Royal
Paris, France

Dietmar Kuhl
Center for Molecular Neurobiology
University of Hamburg
Hamburg, Germany

Carole E. Landisman
Department of Neuroscience
Brown University
Providence, RI

Gilles Laurent
Division of Biology
California Institute of Technology
Pasadena, CA

Jim-Shih Liaw
Department of Biomedical
Engineering
University of Southern California
Los Angeles, CA

David J. Linden
Department of Neuroscience
Johns Hopkins School of Medicine
Baltimore, MD

Katrina MacLeod
Division of Biology
California Institute of Technology
Pasadena, CA

Henry Markram
Department of Neurobiology
Weizmann Institute for Science
Rehovot, Israel

W. V. Morehouse
Department of Neurology
UCLA School of Medicine
Los Angeles, CA

Dominique Muller
Centre Médical Universitaire
Geneva, Switzerland

J. A. Napieralski
Department of Neurology
UCLA School of Medicine
Los Angeles, CA

Santiago Rivera
INSERM U29
Paris, France

François S. Roman
Laboratoire de Neurobiologie des
Comportements
Université de Provence
Marseille, France

Bernard Soumireu-Meurat
Laboratoire de Neurobiologie des
Comportements
Université de Provence
Marseille, France

Oswald Steward
Department of Neurosciences
University of Virginia Medical
School
Charlottesville, VA

Mark Stopfer
Division of Biology
California Institute of Technology
Pasadena, CA

F. G. Szele
Department of Neurology
UCLA School of Medicine
Los Angeles, CA

Richard F. Thompson
Department of Biological Sciences
University of Southern California
Los Angeles, CA

Bruno Truchet
Laboratoire de Neurobiologie des
Comportements
Université de Provence
Marseille, France

Nicolas Toni
Division of Neuropharmacology
Centre Médical Universitaire
Geneva, Switzerland

Misha Tsodyks
Department of Neurobiology
Weizmann Institute of Science
Rehovot, Israel

K. Uryu
Department of Neurology
UCLA School of Medicine
Los Angeles, CA

Ascher Uziel
Department of Neurobiology
Weizmann Institute of Science
Rehovot, Israel

Christopher S. Wallace
Center for Research on Occupational
and Environmental Toxicology
Oregon Health Sciences University
Portland, OR

Yun Wang
Department of Neurobiology
Weizmann Institute for Science
Rehovot, Israel

Michael Wehr
Division of Biology
California Institute of Technology
Pasadena, CA

Paul F. Worley
Department of Neuroscience
Johns Hopkins University School of
Medicine
Baltimore, MD

Xiaping Xie
Department of Biomedical
Engineering
University of Southern California
Los Angeles, CA

Index

Perforated synapses (cont.)
  dentate gyrus, 91
  electron microscopy, 116
  mathematical model, 114–122
  morphology, 93, 113
  release probability, 117
  spatial effects, 121, 124
  symmetrical terminal, 118
Pericellular proteolysis, 66
Peripheral nervous system (PNS), 63, 239
Phagemid subtraction, 5
Phenotypes, 299
Pheochromocytoma, 67
Pheromones, odorant receptors, 225
Phosphocans, 59
Pial blood vessels, thermocoagulation, 174
Picrotoxin, 11, 13
Piriform cortex
  associative memory, 265
  field potentials, 269, 310
  odor discrimination, 266–274
  synaptic plasticity, 266–274
  unusual synaptoids, 145
Plasmids, trihybrid system, 21
Plasmin, 13
Plasticity. *See also* Synaptic plasticity
  anatomical, 168–174
  animal models, 167
  axonal, 167, 174
  corticostriatal, 180–187
  development, 167
  frequency-dependent synapses, 253–256
  molecular basis, 3
  neuronal, 67–73
  short-term, 201
  single synapses, 253
  tissue-plasminogen activator, 9–14
Plexins, 60
Polypeptides, *arg3.1* interaction, 23
Polysialic acid (PSA), 60, 96
Postnatal cortical lesions, 174–176
Postsynaptic density, 90
Postsynaptic realignment, 135–137
Post-tetanus potentiation, 134
Posture equilibrium, 277
Potassium release, glial cells, 143
Presynaptic terminal, model structure, 107
Projection neurons
  coding hypothesis, 229
  intercoupling, 229
  mechanisms, 229–231
  odorant receptors, 225

oscillations, 227
phase-locking, 228
spatiotemporal features, 226–229
synchronization, 228
temporal patterns, 228
Proteases, brain function, 11
Proteinases. *See* Metalloproteinases
Protein kinase C (PKC), 62, 87
Proteins
  autoradiography, 39
  biochemical assays, 18
  functions, 37
  identifying, 18
  phosphorylation, 87–90
  RNA interactions, 18–22
  selective targeting, 48
  synaptic activity, 33
  types, 37
Proteoglycans, 57–59
Proteolysis, pericellular, 66
Protooncogenes, 3
Purkinje cells
  cerebellar, 150, 152
  function and property, 284
  learning and memory, 311
  subsystem activity, 287
  synaptic currents, 145
Purkinje networks, 289–293
  function generation, 290
  learning example, 291–293
  subsystem diagram, 290
  synaptic efficacy, 291
  variational learning rules, 291
Purkinje units
  cerebellar cortex, 283
  coordinated movement, 293–296
  external contexts, 287
  functions, 284, 287
  hierarchical organization, 293–296
  input-output relation, 287–289
  learning and retrieving, 287
  motor functions, 277
  nervous system, 277–280
  neural networks, 278
  resting state, 287
  stability, 294
  structural organization, 287–289

Quantal properties, synapses, 199

Realignment, postsynaptic, 135–137
Rearing, environmental, 103